Non-invasive Medical Devices for Detection and Monitoring within Healthcare

Non-invasive Medical Devices for Detection and Monitoring within Healthcare

Editor

Ronny Priefer

MDPI • Basel • Beijing • Wuhan • Barcelona • Belgrade • Manchester • Tokyo • Cluj • Tianjin

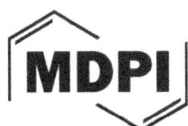

Editor
Ronny Priefer
MCPHS University
Boston
USA

Editorial Office
MDPI
St. Alban-Anlage 66
4052 Basel, Switzerland

This is a reprint of articles from the Special Issue published online in the open access journal *Biosensors* (ISSN 2079-6374) (available at: https://www.mdpi.com/journal/biosensors/special_issues/non_invasive_medical).

For citation purposes, cite each article independently as indicated on the article page online and as indicated below:

LastName, A.A.; LastName, B.B.; LastName, C.C. Article Title. *Journal Name* **Year**, *Volume Number*, Page Range.

ISBN 978-3-0365-6984-0 (Hbk)
ISBN 978-3-0365-6985-7 (PDF)

© 2023 by the authors. Articles in this book are Open Access and distributed under the Creative Commons Attribution (CC BY) license, which allows users to download, copy and build upon published articles, as long as the author and publisher are properly credited, which ensures maximum dissemination and a wider impact of our publications.

The book as a whole is distributed by MDPI under the terms and conditions of the Creative Commons license CC BY-NC-ND.

Contents

About the Editor vii

Hyun Jin Jung and Ronny Priefer
Non-Invasive Breath Analysis for Disease Screening and Diagnoses
Reprinted from: *Biosensors* **2022**, *12*, 235, doi:10.3390/bios12040235 1

Meysam Rezaei, Sajad Razavi Bazaz, Dorsa Morshedi Rad, Olga Shimoni, Dayong Jin, William Rawlinson and Majid Ebrahimi Warkiani
A Portable RT-LAMP/CRISPR Machine for Rapid COVID-19 Screening
Reprinted from: *Biosensors* **2021**, *11*, 369, doi:10.3390/bios11100369 3

Soumyasanta Laha, Aditi Rajput, Suvra S. Laha and Rohan Jadhav
A Concise and Systematic Review on Non-Invasive Glucose Monitoring for Potential Diabetes Management
Reprinted from: *Biosensors* **2022**, *12*, 965, doi:10.3390/bios12110965 9

Murad Althobaiti
In Silico Investigation of SNR and Dermis Sensitivity for Optimum Dual-Channel Near-Infrared Glucose Sensor Designs for Different Skin Colors
Reprinted from: *Biosensors* **2022**, *12*, 805, doi:10.3390/bios12100805 29

Fabiane Fantinelli Franco, Richard A. Hogg and Libu Manjakkal
Cu_2O-Based Electrochemical Biosensor for Non-Invasive and Portable Glucose Detection
Reprinted from: *Biosensors* **2022**, *12*, 174, doi:10.3390/bios12030174 39

Omar Alkedeh and Ronny Priefer
The Ketogenic Diet: Breath Acetone Sensing Technology
Reprinted from: *Biosensors* **2021**, *11*, 26, doi:10.3390/bios11010026 51

Tasbiraha Athaya and Sunwoong Choi
Real-Time Cuffless Continuous Blood Pressure Estimation Using 1D Squeeze U-Net Model: A Progress toward mHealth
Reprinted from: *Biosensors* **2022**, *12*, 655, doi:10.3390/bios12080655 67

Silvano Dragonieri, Vitaliano Nicola Quaranta, Enrico Buonamico, Claudia Battisti, Teresa Ranieri, Pierluigi Caratu and Giovanna Elisiana Carpagnano
Short-Term Effect of Cigarette Smoke on Exhaled Volatile Organic Compounds Profile Analyzed by an Electronic Nose
Reprinted from: *Biosensors* **2022**, *12*, 520, doi:10.3390/bios12070520 83

Chen-Wei Lin, Yuan-Hsiung Tsai, Yen-Pei Lu, Jen-Tsung Yang, Mei-Yen Chen, Tung-Jung Huang, et al.
Application of a Novel Biosensor for Salivary Conductivity in Detecting Chronic Kidney Disease
Reprinted from: *Biosensors* **2022**, *12*, 178, doi:10.3390/bios12030178 91

Jiancheng Mo and Ronny Priefer
Medical Devices for Tremor Suppression: Current Status and Future Directions
Reprinted from: *Biosensors* **2021**, *11*, 99, doi:10.3390/bios11040099 109

Cheng-Hsu Chen, Teh-Ho Tao, Yi-Hua Chou, Ya-Wen Chuang and Tai-Been Chen
Arteriovenous Fistula Flow Dysfunction Surveillance: Early Detection Using Pulse Radar Sensor and Machine Learning Classification
Reprinted from: *Biosensors* **2021**, *11*, 297, doi:10.3390/bios11090297 131

Yuri Kang, Hyeok Jung Kim, Sung Hoon Lee and Hyeran Noh
Paper-Based Substrate for a Surface-Enhanced Raman Spectroscopy Biosensing Platform—A Silver/Chitosan Nanocomposite Approach
Reprinted from: *Biosensors* **2022**, *12*, 266, doi:10.3390/bios12050266 . . . . **145**

Posen Lee, Tai-Been Chen, Chin-Hsuan Liu, Chi-Yuan Wang, Guan-Hua Huang and Nan-Han Lu
Identifying the Posture of Young Adults in Walking Videos by Using a Fusion Artificial Intelligent Method
Reprinted from: *Biosensors* **2022**, *12*, 295, doi:10.3390/ bios12050295 . . . . **157**

Felipe Acácio de Paiva, Kariny Realino Ferreira, Michelle Almeida Barbosa and Alexandre Carvalho Barbosa
Masticatory Myoelectric Side Modular Ratio Asymmetry during Maximal Biting in Women with and without Temporomandibular Disorders
Reprinted from: *Biosensors* **2022**, *12*, 654, doi:10.3390/bios12080654 . . . . **169**

Hayeon Min, Sophie Zhu, Lydia Safi, Munzer Alkourdi, Bich Hong Nguyen, Akshaya Upadhyay and Simon D. Tran
Salivary Diagnostics in Pediatrics and the Status of Saliva-Based Biosensors
Reprinted from: *Biosensors* **2023**, *13*, 206, doi:10.3390/bios13020206 . . . . **179**

About the Editor

Ronny Priefer

Dr. Priefer is the Associate Dean of Graduate Studies at MCPHS University in Boston, MA. He completed his doctoral work at McGill University in Montreal, Canada, focusing on organic and polymer chemistry. After working in two industrial settings, Starks Associate and Neurochem Inc., he entered academia. Prior to joining MCPHS, he spent seven years working in the chemistry department of Niagara University and another seven years working at Western New England University. He has almost 100 journal publications ranging from organic synthesis, physical organic, analytical, medicinal, educational, and material chemistry. He is also the pioneering investigator of the recently introduced new class of polyelectrolytes in the realm of multilayer polyelectrolytes (i.e., pseudo-polyelectrolytes) which has made inroads in detection technology for diabetes and Alzheimer's disease as well as proton exchange membranes.

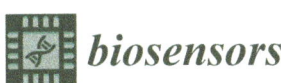

Editorial

Non-Invasive Breath Analysis for Disease Screening and Diagnoses

Hyun Jin Jung and Ronny Priefer *

Department of Pharmaceutical Sciences, Massachusetts College of Pharmacy and Health Sciences University, Boston, MA 02115, USA; hjung1@stu.mcphs.edu
* Correspondence: ronny.priefer@mcphs.edu

Lower respiratory infections are a deadly communicable disease ranked as the fourth leading cause of death globally, with nearly 2.6 million succumbing annually [1]. Acute lower respiratory tract infections in children have sadly been shown to increase the risk of developing a chronic respiratory disease later in life. Additionally, respiratory tract infections caused by influenza kill between 250,000 and 500,000 people globally and costs between USD 71 and 167 billion annually [2]. Early detection and accurate diagnosis of infectious disease are important to ultimately improve the effectiveness of treatments, determine the correct use of antibiotics, avoid long-term complications, and help prevent or stop an outbreak.

Many different laboratory tests are currently used to identify infectious microorganisms. These include tests on blood, urine, tissue, cerebrospinal fluid, stool, sputum, and mucus from the nose or throat, as well as fluid from the genital area [3]. These existing methods can also be divided into either invasive or non-invasive. Invasive methods include esophagogastroduodenoscopy (EGD), with collection for gastric biopsies and subsequent histological staining. It is often used to detect Helicobacter pylori infection in the gut. This is expensive, causes patient discomfort, and sometimes yields false negative results due to sampling errors. However, there are a growing number of non-invasive methods for detecting H. pylori infection, such as serological, fecal antigen, and ^{13}C-urea breath testing (^{13}C-UBT) [4,5].

Utilizing the breath to screen or diagnose diseases has become increasingly popular. Human-exhaled breath contains over 3000 volatile organic compounds (VOCs). Breath VOCs are produced by our own biologic processes, as well as by microorganisms as part of their metabolism. These can be detected and quantified utilizing various instrumentations, such as gas chromatography/mass spectrometry or eNose detection [6]. These and other advanced technologies specifically examine the volatile metabolic fingerprints generated by our body and its microorganism flora in order to discriminate between different aliments. Thus, VOCs are being evaluated extensively as potential biomarkers and as a non-invasive approach to analyze a multitude of diseases, such as diabetes, lactose intolerance, cancer, infections, [7–9] and/or lifestyle choices, such as keto-diet [10] or cannabis use [11]. For example, Gastric Emptying Breath Test (GEBT), H_2 breath monitoring, and NIOX® are FDA-approved tests [7,12,13]. GEBT is used to diagnose gastroparesis, H_2 breath analysis is used for the diagnosis of lactose intolerance [9], and NIOX measures markers for airway inflammation. By identifying disease-specific biomarkers, early detection could prevent serious complications, lowering mortality rates and reducing the unnecessary use of medicines.

With the fantastic advances in technology, especially nanotechnology, the opportunity to use these in the realm of healthcare, specifically to detect small quantities of biomarkers, is an obvious next step. This Special Issue, "Non-invasive Medical Devices for Detection and Monitoring within Healthcare", is designed not only to showcase what has already been

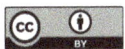

accomplished to improve detection efficacy, but also the translation of these advancements into improving patient experiences and outcomes.

Funding: This research received no external funding.

Institutional Review Board Statement: Not applicable.

Informed Consent Statement: Not applicable.

Data Availability Statement: Data sharing not applicable.

Acknowledgments: The authors wish to thank the School of Pharmacy at the Massachusetts College of Pharmacy and Health Sciences University for their financial support of this project.

Conflicts of Interest: The authors declare no conflict of interest.

References

1. World Health Organization. *The Top 10 Causes of Death Fact Sheet*; World Health Organization: Geneva, Switzerland, 2020.
2. Forum of International Respiratory Societies. *The Global Impact of Respiratory Disease*, 2nd ed.; European Respiratory Society: Sheffield, UK, 2017.
3. Ratiu, I.A.; Ligor, T.; Bocos-Bintintan, V.; Szeliga, J.; Machała, K.; Jackowski, M.; Buszewski, B. GC-MS application in determination of volatile profiles emitted by infected and uninfected human tissue. *J. Breath Res.* **2019**, *13*, 026003. [CrossRef] [PubMed]
4. BreathTek UBT [Package Insert]. U.S. Food and Drug Administration Website. Available online: https://www.accessdata.fda.gov/drugsatfda_docs/label/2001/20586s4lbl.pdf (accessed on 9 May 2021).
5. Maity, A.; Som, S.; Ghosh, C.; Banik, G.D.; Daschakraborty, S.B.; Ghosh, S.; Chaudhuri, S.; Pradhan, M. Oxygen-18 stable isotope of exhaled breath CO_2 as a non-invasive marker of helicobacter pylori infection. *J. Anal. At. Spectrom.* **2014**, *29*, 2251–2255. [CrossRef]
6. Licht, J.-C.; Grasemann, H. Potential of the electronic nose for the detection of respiratory diseases with and without infection. *Int. J. Mol. Sci.* **2020**, *21*, 9416. [CrossRef] [PubMed]
7. Argnani, F.; Di Camillo, M.; Marinaro, V.; Foglietta, T.; Avallone, V.; Cannella, C.; Vernia, P. Hydrogen breath test for the diagnosis of lactose intolerance, is the routine sugar load the best one? *World J. Gastroenterol.* **2008**, *14*, 6204–6207. [CrossRef] [PubMed]
8. Mazzatenta, A.; Pokorski, M.; Di Giulio, C. Real-time breath analysis in type 2 diabetes patients during cognitive effort. *Adv. Exp. Med. Biol.* **2013**, *788*, 247–253. [PubMed]
9. Robles, L.; Priefer, R. Lactose Intolerance: What Your Breath Can Tell You. *Diagnostics.* **2020**, *10*, 412. [CrossRef] [PubMed]
10. Alkedeh, O.; Priefer, R. The Ketogenic Diet: Breath Acetone Sensing Technology. *Biosensors* **2021**, *11*, 26. [CrossRef] [PubMed]
11. Ramzy, V.; Priefer, R. THC detection in the breath. *Talanta* **2021**, *222*, 121528. [CrossRef] [PubMed]
12. Bharucha, A.E.; Camilleri, M.; Veil, E.; Burton, D.; Zinsmeister, A.R. Comprehensive assessment of gastric emptying with a stable isotope breath test. *Neurogastroenterol. Motil.* **2013**, *25*, e60–e69. [CrossRef] [PubMed]
13. Silkoff, P.E.; Carlson, M.; Bourke, T.; Katial, R.; Ogren, E.; Szefler, S.J. The Aerocrine exhaled nitric oxide monitoring system NIOX is cleared by the US Food and Drug Administration for monitoring therapy in asthma. *J. Allergy Clin. Immunol.* **2004**, *114*, 1241–1256. [CrossRef] [PubMed]

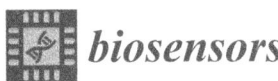

Communication

A Portable RT-LAMP/CRISPR Machine for Rapid COVID-19 Screening

Meysam Rezaei [1,2,3], Sajad Razavi Bazaz [1,2], Dorsa Morshedi Rad [1], Olga Shimoni [2], Dayong Jin [2,4], William Rawlinson [5,6] and Majid Ebrahimi Warkiani [1,2,3,*]

1. School of Biomedical Engineering, University of Technology Sydney, Sydney, NSW 2007, Australia; meysam.rezaei@genea.com.au (M.R.); Sajad.RazaviBazaz@student.uts.edu.au (S.R.B.); Dorsa.MorshediRad@student.uts.edu.au (D.M.R.)
2. Institute for Biomedical Materials & Devices (IBMD), Faculty of Science, University of Technology Sydney, Sydney, NSW 2007, Australia; Olga.Shimoni@uts.edu.au (O.S.); Dayong.Jin@uts.edu.au (D.J.)
3. Genea, Sydney, NSW 2000, Australia
4. SUStech-UTS Joint Research Centre for Biomedical Materials & Devices, Southern University of Science and Technology, Shenzhen 518055, China
5. Serology and Virology Division, NSW Health Pathology, Prince of Wales Hospital, Sydney, NSW 2031, Australia; w.rawlinson@unsw.edu.au
6. School of Women's and Children's Health, University of New South Wales, Sydney, NSW 2052, Australia
* Correspondence: majid.warkiani@uts.edu.au

Abstract: The COVID-19 pandemic has changed people's lives and has brought society to a sudden standstill, with lockdowns and social distancing as the preferred preventative measures. To lift these measurements and reduce society's burden, developing an easy-to-use, rapid, and portable system to detect SARS-CoV-2 is mandatory. To this end, we developed a portable and semi-automated device for SARS-CoV-2 detection based on reverse transcription loop-mediated isothermal amplification followed by a CRISPR/Cas12a reaction. The device contains a heater element mounted on a printed circuit board, a cooler fan, a proportional integral derivative controller to control the temperature, and designated areas for 0.2 mL Eppendorf® PCR tubes. Our system has a limit of detection of 35 copies of the virus per microliter, which is significant and has the capability of being used in crisis centers, mobile laboratories, remote locations, or airports to diagnose individuals infected with SARS-CoV-2. We believe the current methodology that we have implemented in this article is beneficial for the early screening of infectious diseases, in which fast screening with high accuracy is necessary.

Keywords: SARS-CoV-2; COVID-19; point of care testing; rapid diagnostics

Citation: Rezaei, M.; Razavi Bazaz, S.; Morshedi Rad, D.; Shimoni, O.; Jin, D.; Rawlinson, W.; Ebrahimi Warkiani, M. A Portable RT-LAMP/CRISPR Machine for Rapid COVID-19 Screening. *Biosensors* **2021**, *11*, 369. https://doi.org/10.3390/bios11100369

Received: 26 August 2021
Accepted: 28 September 2021
Published: 2 October 2021

Publisher's Note: MDPI stays neutral with regard to jurisdictional claims in published maps and institutional affiliations.

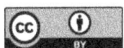

Copyright: © 2021 by the authors. Licensee MDPI, Basel, Switzerland. This article is an open access article distributed under the terms and conditions of the Creative Commons Attribution (CC BY) license (https://creativecommons.org/licenses/by/4.0/).

1. Introduction

The SARS-CoV-2 virus causes COVID-19, a serious and life-threatening disease with a wide spectrum of symptoms, ranging from fever and cough to dyspnea, and in severe cases, resulting in intensive care unit (ICU) admission of patients, organ failure, and death [1,2]. The continuing spread of COVID-19 and its high transmissibility have become a major concern and prompted the rapid development of diagnostic methods. Conventional diagnostic methods such as quantitative reverse transcription polymerase chain reaction (RT-qPCR) have been developed and are used routinely for SARS-CoV-2 detection [3]. Although RT-qPCR is the gold standard technique to diagnose SARS-CoV-2, laboratories with RT-qPCR capabilities are often centralized, making this method less suitable in settings such as aged care facilities and ports of entry where on-site screening is required [4]. In addition, other diagnostic methods have been developed based on the detection of antibodies and antigens, which are simple, quick, and cheap and do not necessitate the use of specific instrumentation or trained users [5]. Since antibodies against SARS-CoV-2 take days to weeks to be produced in the patient's body, antigen-based methods are not recommended to diagnose acute COVID-19 cases. Moreover, these diagnostic tests targeting the viral proteins are usually less sensitive than RT-qPCR tests detecting the viral nucleic acids. Therefore, these tests may not be considered highly sensitive methods for early detection of COVID-19 [6].

Recent studies have focused on the development of integrated molecular diagnostic devices based on microfabrication technologies to provide rapid and reliable methods for SARS-CoV-2 detection, enabling faster clinical decisions [7]. In this study, we report the development and validation of a portable, integrated, and semi-automated device for in vitro COVID-19 molecular diagnosis. This device involves nucleic acid reverse transcription and isothermal amplification using loop-mediated amplification (RT-LAMP) of viral ribonucleic acid (RNA) extracted from nasopharyngeal or oropharyngeal swabs followed by Cas12a detection and readout with lateral flow assay (LFA) strips. Given the low reagent consumption, the compact size, and integration capability with a power bank, this wireless device can be conveniently used in crisis centers, mobile laboratories, remote locations, or airports to diagnose individuals infected with SARS-CoV-2. Our device consists of a small thermocycler machine integrated into a portable box containing sample tubes that can be potentially used for simultaneous testing of five tests in just 35 min with minimal hands-on processing.

A total of 10 samples were collected from Serology and Virology laboratories at the Prince of Wales Adult Hospital (Sydney, NSW, Australia) under the Biosafety (ETH-5127) protocol. Each patient, who had symptoms of respiratory disease and a positive RT-qPCR result for COVID-19, participated in this study voluntarily after signing an informed consent form. Next, the patient's nasopharyngeal or oropharyngeal swab sample was collected in the Copan universal transport medium for viruses and vortexed at maximum speed for 1–2 min followed by passing through the 0.45 μm Minisart® filter (Sartorius Stedim Biotech, Goettingen, Germany). Then viral RNA was extracted from 200 μL of samples using the MagNA Pure LC Total Nucleic Acid Isolation Kit (Roche Diagnostics, Sydney, Australia) according to the manufacturer's instructions. Then, the purity and quantity of extracted RNA samples were evaluated using NanoDrop (One UV-Vis Spectrophotometer, Thermofisher Scientific, Waltham, MA, USA) and stored at -80 °C for further analysis. First, we set the RT-LAMP primers to target the E (envelope) and N (nucleoprotein) genes of SARS-CoV-2, covering the regions followed by protocols validated by the World Health Organization (WHO) and US Centers for Disease Control and Prevention (CDC) assays, as well as the RNase P gene as a control [8]. To this aim, the RT-Lamp reaction for the preamplification of viral RNA has been performed by preparing 25 μL of a reaction mix containing the WarmStart LAMP master mix ($2\times$), fluorescent dye ($50\times$), and 4 μM LAMP primer mix followed by incubation at 65 °C for 30 min [9]. Then, we set the Cas12a gRNAs to detect the control gene, E gene, and specifically the N gene in SARS-CoV-2 [8]. We conducted a series of experiments using a higher concentration of SARS-CoV-2 RNA (1×10^5 copies/μL) to assess the functionality of the RT-LAMP reactions in a q-PCR machine (CFX Connect™ Real-Time PCR System. Bio-Rad, Hercules, CA, USA). Using this q-PCR apparatus and fluorescent intercalating dye in the first place enabled us to track the RT-LAMP reaction in real-time and optimize the optimal temperature and time for SARS-CoV-2 RNA gene target amplification. The amplification was performed at a temperature gradient of 58 to 70 °C for 30 min. The optimal amplification proceeded at 65 °C for 25 min (Figure 1A), and no amplification was observed in negative samples (containing all the reaction materials except viral RNA). We then evaluated the performance of the detection step by combining pre-amplified viral and control RNA targets with the Cas12a-gRNA ribonucleoprotein (RNP) assays followed by the LFA strips readout (Figure 1B). Each pre-amplified target was added to a separate tube containing a specific Cas12a-gRNA and a FAM-biotin reporter molecule, prepared as suggested by the assay manufacturer (New England Biolabs, Ipswich, MA, USA) [9]. After incubation for 10 min at 37 °C, the completed reaction was read out using LFA strips placed into the tubes, showing the results after 2 min.

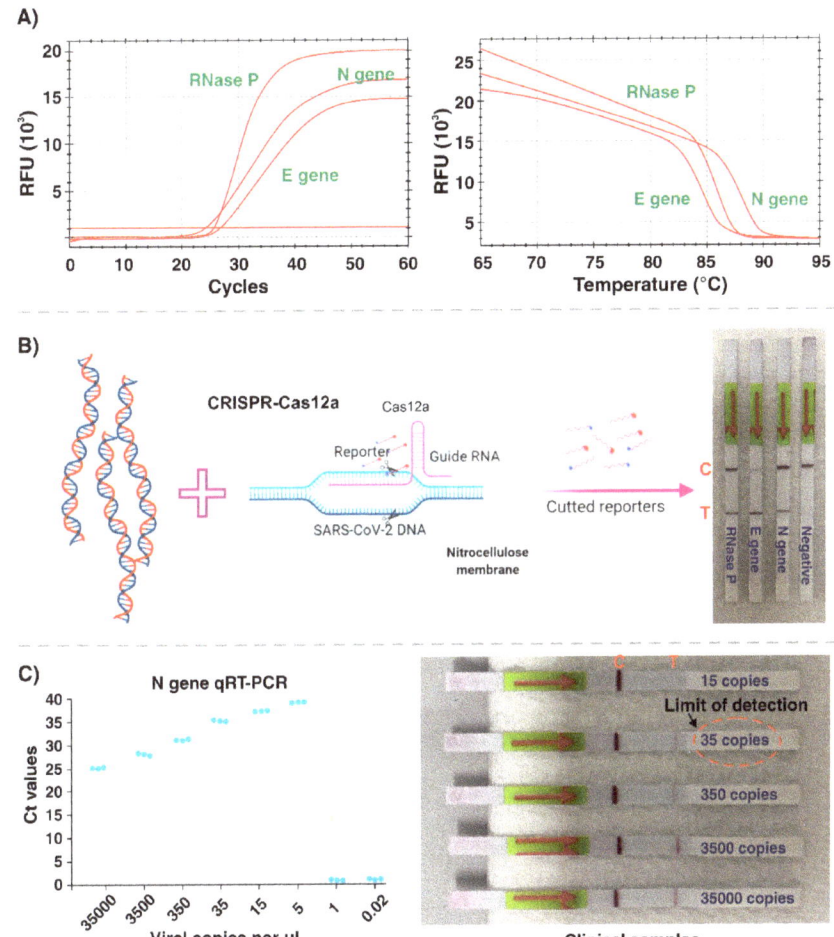

Figure 1. (**A**) RT-LAMP reaction performed in an RT-qPCR machine using N, E, and RNase P primers at an optimal temperature and time. (**B**) Schematic illustration of CRISPR-Cas12a reaction on pre-amplified SARS-CoV-2 target genes, followed by visualization with lateral flow strips. (**C**) The detection limit of the RT-qPCR assay (left) using PCR machine and RT-LAMP/Cas12a assay (right) using clinical samples.

We observed concordance between our results from fluorescence-based readouts for positive/negative RT-LAMP samples in q-PCR and those from lateral flow strips by the appearance of one (negative sample) or two (positive sample) lines. With the presence of N, E, and Rnase P target genes amplified during the RT-LAMP step, Cas12a can specifically bind to targets using its gRNAs, resulting in the activation of indiscriminate Cas12a cleavage and cutting of the FAM-biotin reporter molecules. Visualization of the Cas12a cleavage activity was achieved by applying LFA strips designed to capture FAM- and Biotin-tagged nucleic acids (Milenia HybriDetect 1, TwistDx, Cambridge, UK). For the positive samples, two lines were observed on the lateral flow strips: Uncut reporters captured at the first line (control) and cut reporters captured at the second line (test); while in negative samples, only one line (control) of captured uncut reporters was detected.

After validating the feasibility of our approach for detecting the SARS-CoV-2 virus, we determined the limit of detection (LoD) in a controlled situation using lab-based instruments before the final design and production of our portable RT-LAMP/CRISPR machine for rapid COVID-19 screening. First, we quantified the number of viral copies in one sample using q-PCR (N = 3) after preparing a standard curve using a GenScript RT-qPCR detection assay. The standard curve was prepared using six dilutions of N-positive control plasmids (3×10^5 copies/μL) with three replicates at each dilution. After determining the RNA copy numbers in our selected sample, we prepared a series of diluted samples with concentrations of 35,000, 3500, 350, 35, 15, 5, 1, and 0.02 copies per μL. The copy number of each sample was confirmed and the LoD of commercial RT-qPCR assay for SARS-CoV-2 detection was determined using the cycle threshold (Ct) values (Figure 1C). Finally, we determined the LoD of the RT-LAMP/Cas12a assay by assessing the ability to generate visible test and control lines on lateral flow strips after testing three replicates of all eight diluted samples. The minimum copy numbers that could be detected using the RT-qPCR assay was 5 copies per μL (consistent in all 3 replicates), compared with 35 copies per μL of targets with the RT-LAMP/CRISPR-Cas12a approach (Figure 1C).

Having shown the proof of concept of our approach in the laboratory setting, modifications were made to build a portable device to be utilized for SARS-CoV-2 point-of-care testing. The RT-LAMP step requires a heater that should have accurate thermal stability, i.e., the temperature at each step should be accurate and consistent without variation. Although laboratory instruments for thermal control of various tubes and vessels exist, these facilities are often bulky and expensive. Moreover, in some of these facilities, condensation occurs on the tube walls and lid, resulting in performance loss and reduced efficiency [10]. As a result, they are not favorable for point-of-care devices, especially in resource-poor settings. Although there are ongoing efforts to improve lab-scale heaters' temperature uniformity, this feature is yet to be optimized and is not fully functional [11]. To address this issue and make the process semi-automated, we designed a portable machine for accurate control of the heating process during the experiment. In our design, a heater element is mounted on a printed circuit board (PCB). A small fan that is directly connected to the board was used to reduce the temperature. The device is able to reach any temperatures within the range of 20 to 95 °C. The system's temperature is controlled and regulated using a proportional integral derivative (PID) controller, which is among the most stable, reliable, and accurate controllers and uses a loop feedback approach to control the system [12]. These components were mounted on a PCB board, programmed using Python and layout software packages. Tubes with reagents were placed on the heater with a closed lid for better temperature control and enhanced efficiency. The device operates on power obtained from a USB Type-C connection, meaning that it can be connected to a USB port of any computer, Power Bank, or battery with a minimum rating of 2A. The device can fit in a single hand or a pocket, with approximate dimensions of 3.5 cm × 3 cm × 13 cm, and can handle up to 10 samples in the sample position and reaction zone (Figure 2). Python programing of the system enabled us to turn on the device at a specific time and increase or decrease the temperature of the system at a specific point. This means that amplification and detection in our system are essentially automated (except for tube handling). Because the PID controller adjusts the temperature, and the reaction zone (Figure 2) is relatively small, there is no heat loss or temperature variation in the system, with minimum condensation on tube lids and walls. To decrease the temperature for the CRISPR/Cas12a reaction, the fan reduces the temperature of the RT-LAMP step to 37 °C directly via the PID controller.

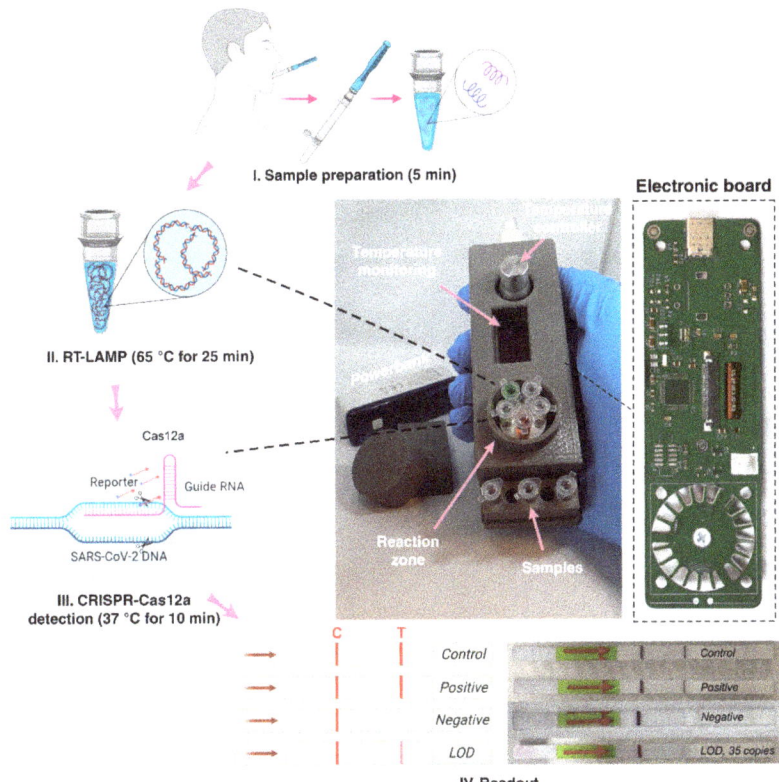

Figure 2. Schematic representation of the experimental procedure for the detection of SARS-CoV-2 with a portable device using an RT-LAMP/CRISPR-Cas12a approach. The workflow includes SARS-CoV-2 virus sampling from confirmed patients, virus deactivation and RNA extraction, RNA transcription and amplification by RT-LAMP, Cas12a reaction, and lateral flow strips visualization. Our portable device, along with its integrated electronic board, is demonstrated at the center of the figure. Samples in red and green are food dye for better illustration.

We have repeated SARS-CoV-2 detection for all 10 patient samples using the modified portable device. The device was connected to a 2600 mAh Cellularline Power Bank, which has an estimated battery life of up to 10 h without the need of recharging, representing a significant step forward for a point-of-care diagnostic device. For the RT-LAMP stage, the temperature was set at 65 °C for 25 min. After completing this stage, the temperature was set at 37 °C for 10 min for the CRISPR/Cas12a reaction. To minimize the risk of cross-contamination between the test samples, microtubes are moved and opened in the sample position once the RT-LAMP reaction has been completed. Finally, the LFA strips were placed in the tubes and the results were analyzed. As shown in Figure 2, all the results were replicable, and an LOD of 35 copies was achieved, similar to that obtained using a lab-based PCR machine.

In conclusion, we were able to successfully design and develop a low-cost, portable, and semi-automated device leveraging RT-LAMP/CRISPR technologies that can be used for early SARS-CoV-2 detection with an LOD of 35 copies per microliter. Through multiplexing our portable machine and increasing the number of wells in the reaction zone, up to 500 samples can be processed simultaneously in just 35 min. Moreover, with multiplexing the CRISPR/Cas technology, our device can offer co-detection of SARS-CoV-2 and the flu in a single reaction with minimal sample requirements. After further screening of different SARS-CoV-2 variants in several patient populations, our portable machine holds significant potential for being rapidly used as a point-of-care testing device in crisis centers and mobile laboratories.

Author Contributions: Conceptualization, M.E.W.; methodology, M.R.; validation, M.R.; investigation, M.R.; resources, M.E.W., O.S. and D.J.; writing—original draft preparation, M.R., S.R.B. and D.M.R.; writing—review and editing, M.R., S.R.B., D.M.R., O.S., D.J., W.R. and M.E.W.; visualization, S.R.B.; supervision, M.E.W. and D.J.; funding acquisition, M.E.W., O.S. and D.J. All authors have read and agreed to the published version of the manuscript.

Funding: This research was funded by the Australian Research Council through Discovery Project Grants (DP170103704 and DP180103003), the National Health and Medical Research Council through the Career Development Fellowship (APP1143377), IH150100028, and the Australia-China Joint Research Center.

Institutional Review Board Statement: The study was conducted according to the guideline of the Declaration of Helsinki, and approved by the Ethics Committee of University of Technology Sydney (Application ID: ETH20 4890, date of approval: 13/07/2020).

Informed Consent Statement: Informed consent was obtained from all subjects involved in the study.

Data Availability Statement: The data presented in this study are available on request from the corresponding author.

Acknowledgments: M.E.W. would like to acknowledge the support of the Australian Research Council through Discovery Project Grants (DP170103704 and DP180103003) and the National Health and Medical Research Council through the Career Development Fellowship (APP1143377). O.S. and D.J. acknowledge the support of IH150100028 and the Australia-China Joint Research Center.

Conflicts of Interest: The authors declare no conflict of interest.

References

1. Zhou, F.; Yu, T.; Du, R.; Fan, G.; Liu, Y.; Liu, Z.; Xiang, J.; Wang, Y.; Song, B.; Gu, X. Clinical course and risk factors for mortality of adult inpatients with COVID-19 in Wuhan, China: A retrospective cohort study. *Lancet* **2020**, *395*, 1054–1062. [CrossRef]
2. Rezaei, M.; Razavi Bazaz, S.; Zhand, S.; Sayyadi, N.; Jin, D.; Stewart, M.P.; Ebrahimi Warkiani, M. Point of Care Diagnostics in the Age of COVID-19. *Diagnostics* **2021**, *11*, 9. [CrossRef] [PubMed]
3. Wu, F.; Zhao, S.; Yu, B.; Chen, Y.-M.; Wang, W.; Song, Z.-G.; Hu, Y.; Tao, Z.-W.; Tian, J.-H.; Pei, Y.-Y. A new coronavirus associated with human respiratory disease in China. *Nature* **2020**, *579*, 265–269. [CrossRef] [PubMed]
4. Zu, Z.Y.; Jiang, M.D.; Xu, P.P.; Chen, W.; Ni, Q.Q.; Lu, G.M.; Zhang, L.J. Coronavirus disease 2019 (COVID-19): A perspective from China. *Radiology* **2020**, *296*, E15–E25. [CrossRef] [PubMed]
5. Udugama, B.; Kadhiresan, P.; Kozlowski, H.N.; Malekjahani, A.; Osborne, M.; Li, V.Y.; Chen, H.; Mubareka, S.; Gubbay, J.B.; Chan, W.C. Diagnosing COVID-19: The disease and tools for detection. *ACS Nano* **2020**, *14*, 3822–3835. [CrossRef]
6. Muhi, S.; Tayler, N.; Hoang, T.; Ballard, S.A.; Graham, M.; Rojek, A.; Kwong, J.C.; Trubiano, J.A.; Smibert, O.; Drewett, G.; et al. Multi-site assessment of rapid, point-of-care antigen testing for the diagnosis of SARS-CoV-2 infection in a low-prevalence setting: A validation and implementation study. *Lancet Reg. Health West. Pac.* **2021**, *9*, 100115. [CrossRef] [PubMed]
7. Wang, C.; Liu, M.; Wang, Z.; Li, S.; Deng, Y.; He, N. Point-of-care diagnostics for infectious diseases: From methods to devices. *Nano Today* **2021**, *37*, 101092. [CrossRef]
8. Broughton, J.P.; Deng, X.; Yu, G.; Fasching, C.L.; Servellita, V.; Singh, J.; Miao, X.; Streithorst, J.A.; Granados, A.; Sotomayor-Gonzalez, A. CRISPR–Cas12-based detection of SARS-CoV-2. *Nat. Biotechnol.* **2020**, *38*, 870–874. [CrossRef] [PubMed]
9. Biolabs, N.E. *In Vitro Digestion of DNA with EnGen®Lba Cas12a (Cpf1) (M0653)*; New England Biolabs: Ipswich, MA, USA, 2015.
10. Sapcariu, S.C.; Kanashova, T.; Weindl, D.; Ghelfi, J.; Dittmar, G.; Hiller, K. Simultaneous extraction of proteins and metabolites from cells in culture. *MethodsX* **2014**, *1*, 74–80. [CrossRef] [PubMed]
11. Jin, W.; Xing, C.; Lu, Y.; Baoshou, S.; Li, D. A novel method improving the temperature uniformity of hot-plate under induction heating. *Proc. Inst. Mech. Eng. Part C J. Mech. Eng. Sci.* **2020**, *235*, 190–201. [CrossRef]
12. Kiam Heong, A.; Chong, G.; Yun, L. PID control system analysis, design, and technology. *IEEE Tran. Control Syst. Technol.* **2005**, *13*, 559–576. [CrossRef]

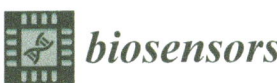

Review

A Concise and Systematic Review on Non-Invasive Glucose Monitoring for Potential Diabetes Management

Soumyasanta Laha [1,*], Aditi Rajput [1], Suvra S. Laha [2,*] and Rohan Jadhav [3,*]

1. Department of Electrical and Computer Engineering, California State University, Fresno, Fresno, CA 93740, USA
2. Centre for Nano Science and Engineering (CeNSE), Indian Institute of Science, Bangalore 560012, India
3. Department of Public Health, California State University, Fresno, Fresno, CA 93740, USA
* Correspondence: laha@csufresno.edu (S.L.); suvralaha@iisc.ac.in (S.S.L.); rjadhav@csufresno.edu (R.J.)

Abstract: The current standard of diabetes management depends upon the invasive blood pricking techniques. In recent times, the availability of minimally invasive continuous glucose monitoring devices have made some improvements in the life of diabetic patients however it has its own limitations which include painful insertion, excessive cost, discomfort and an active risk due to the presence of a foreign body under the skin. Due to all these factors, the non-invasive glucose monitoring has remain a subject of research for the last two decades and multiple techniques of non-invasive glucose monitoring have been proposed. These proposed techniques have the potential to be evolved into a wearable device for non-invasive diabetes management. This paper reviews research advances and major challenges of such techniques or methods in recent years and broadly classifies them into four types based on their detection principles. These four methods are: optical spectroscopy, photoacoustic spectroscopy, electromagnetic sensing and nanomaterial based sensing. The paper primarily focuses on the evolution of non-invasive technology from bench-top equipment to smart wearable devices for personalized non-invasive continuous glucose monitoring in these four methods. With the rapid evolve of wearable technology, all these four methods of non-invasive blood glucose monitoring independently or in combination of two or more have the potential to become a reality in the near future for efficient, affordable, accurate and pain-free diabetes management.

Keywords: optical spectroscopy; photoacoustic spectroscopy; electromagnetic sensing; nanomaterials; diabetes management

1. Introduction

Diabetes mellitus ranks among the top ten lethal disease globally as approximately 451 million people suffer from diabetes across the world according to WHO estimates [1]. As of 2020, in the US alone, the prevalence of diabetes is officially estimated to be around 37.3 million [2], approximately 11% of the total US population. The actual number could be much higher because of unavailability of adequate/efficient infrastructure and/or lack of willingness to preventive check-ups among the population.

The non invasive blood glucose monitoring has the potential to become wearable and continuous in the near future is particularly important for patients with hypoglycemia which is known to cause death during sleep due to unexpected changes in blood glucose levels and is a common occurrence among insulin-dependent diabetics [3]. Hypoglycemia unawareness results from reduced sympathetic adrenal response and patients have difficulty to recognize hypoglycemia events which puts them at high risk of adverse health events [3].These adverse health events include cardiovascular ischemia [4], dementia [5], falls [6], and even deaths [7]. Hypoglycemia-related events resulted in 100,000 visits to emergency rooms and 30,000 hospital admissions between 2007 and 2011 in the US [8]. On the other hand, poorly managed hyperglycemia can also lead to adverse health events such as

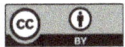

cerebrovascular accidents, cardiovascular events, and peripheral vascular disease [9]. Diabetic ketoacidosis (DK) and Hyperglycemic hyperosmolar state (HHS) are life-threatening emergencies among diabetic patients. Patients with oliguria, unconsciousness for a period tend to have poor prognosis. Complications like cerebral edema, hypokalemia, rhabdomyolysis (more common during HHS) and respiratory failure due to secondary infection can occur [10]. Blood sugar reaches more than 250 mg/dL in DK and 600 plus in HHS [11]. Thus, prompt and real time identification of rapid fluctuations in the blood sugar is the key to successful management of diabetes-related emergencies and increases the likelihood of better prognosis. Thus, noninvasive blood glucose monitoring which has the potential for real time diagnosis can be used to identify the development of DK and HHS early and avoid all the aforementioned complications without any pain.

As a result of these, there have been multiple research articles published on various types and techniques of noninvasive glucose monitoring in the last two decades. Multiple review articles have also been published highlighting and discussing the progresses and challenges of these original research. The current review paper *distinguishes* from the previously published review articles by discussing recent papers in a concise manner using four detection methods widely investigated for noninvasive glucose monitoring. In this paper, the classification of these four methods are based on the detection principles as explained in Section 3. Furthermore, the *uniqueness* of the paper comes from the systematic progress in reporting original research papers on noninvasive glucose monitoring starting with tabletop *in-vitro* sensing to *in-vivo* wearable/compact/portable continuous blood glucose monitoring with advanced technology (such as Machine learning/Internet of Things (IoT)/advanced nanomaterials etc.) or its high possibility in near future. To exemplify, the classification of sensing in the current paper is based on the principles of excitation and detection of glucose unlike [12] that is based on the location where the sensor is placed or on the types of human excretion (saliva, tears, urine etc.). In [13], developments of seven optical noninvasive glucose monitoring techniques are reviewed without reporting on the electromagnetic and nanomaterial based sensing, whereas in [14], the use of microwave planar resonant sensors to track changes in glucose concentration has been only assessed. In [13,15], photoacoustic spectroscopy has been classified under optical methods unlike the current paper where it has been differentiated from the optical approach based on its detection principle of acoustics. Recent developments on non-invasive machine learning and neural network methods are discussed in [16]. None of these papers focus on the technology evolution from bench-top to a wearable device.

2. Background

This section describes the two currently used modes of blood glucose monitoring for diabetes management. They are the conventional invasive blood extraction and pricking technique and the recently popular minimally invasive continuous glucose monitoring.

2.1. Diabetes Management via Conventional Blood Pricking Invasive Device

The gold standard for the determination of blood glucose concentration is the Hexokinase Method [17]. This procedure involves the extraction of a 1.5 mL blood sample using a specialised laboratory equipment. The method is not portable, real time and cannot be operated in home environment. Due to this, a method that relies on using an invasive finger pricking approach has become the most widely used standard of successful management and effective treatment of diabetes. This makes use of capillary glucometers, where a test strip interacts with with a drop of blood, extracted by the pricking in the finger [18]. However, the finger prick technique is not necessarily accurate [19].

Some techniques have evolved to make the these sensors to be more accurate. To make insulin prediction with less amount of invasive procedure and some degree of accuracy, a local fuzzy reconstruction method based on chaos theory for predicting fasting blood glucose at peak time was reported in [20]. The prediction achieves a 70–90% success rate.

In recent times, techniques based on machine learning has been introduced for insulin prediction [21] for similar reasons.

However, these techniques do not eliminate the greatest agony of the invasive procedure: pain and discomfort. In addition, there is always a high probability for the finger pricking procedure to cause infection. The daily usage of lancets and testing strips causes potentially unsafe bio-hazards. Furthermore, a pre-emptive action on the part of the patient or caretaker is always necessary for the drawing and testing of blood. As earlier explained, for patients with complex medical conditions and aggressive forms of type-2 diabetes, continuous monitoring is highly desired so that unexpected changes in blood glucose levels, known to cause death due to sudden hypoglycemia during sleep, can be detected.

2.2. Diabetes Management via Minimally Invasive Continuous Glucose Monitoring

The extreme fluctuations in the blood sugar level can cause cardiovascular events [4,22] and even deaths. Therefore, there is a need to monitor blood glucose levels continuously [23]. Continuous glucose monitoring (CGM) devices can be helpful to identify these extreme fluctuations in the blood sugar and can alert the patient thereby enhancing self or parental management which can lead to avoidance of severe outcomes related to hypo or hyperglycemia. Very recently, multiple such commercial (CGM) devices (Dexcom [24], Adobe FreeStyleLibre [25], Eversense [26] etc.) have come up but none of them is completely non-invasive and wearable as it needs some part to be periodically implanted subcutaneously. Current versions of CGM uses a metal inserted into the skin and remains in contact with blood. It monitors blood sugar level by measuring the charge on the electrical current which emerges from the oxidation of glucose from the enzymes that the device releases. Besides the painful insertion, discomfort and the risk due to the presence of a foreign body under the skin always remains active. Moreover, the adhesives used in CGM systems can cause skin irritation and contact dermatitis in some cases [27]. These skin problems can cause emotional distress among diabetics and can inversely affect adherence to CGM [28]. Current versions of CGM are semi-invasive where a metal is inserted into the skin and serves as a sensor. It emits blood sugar oxidizing enzyme. The interaction of this enzyme with blood sugar molecules results in the formation of hydrogen peroxides amongst other compounds. The reaction also results in the generation of a current. The charge on this current is measured and it corresponds to the appropriate amount of blood sugar in the interstitial cells. The lag time currently is 1 to 5 min [23]. Although the CGM systems have been quite accurate and efficient in monitoring blood glucose levels among insulin-dependent diabetics [29], high costs particularly among those who are uninsured or underinsured and difficulty in placement of these devices on the body and the dislike of skin attachment of the subcutaneous implant were among the major barriers, particularly among adolescents [30,31]. Therefore, there is a need of a strategy that is non-invasive, affordable but accurate at the same time at par with CGM and traditional invasive methods. To this end, numerous research findings thus far suggest that a workable complete non-invasive blood glucose monitoring solution is feasible and multiple techniques are being pursued to build a glucose monitor that is non-invasive, accurate, wearable, low-cost and continuous.

3. Principles of Non Invasive Glucose Monitoring

Multitude principles and techniques of non-invasive glucose monitoring have been pursued in academic research as well as in industry in recent times. Among them, broadly four particular non-invasing glucose monitoring principles are widely investigated and reported. These four principles are differentiated based on the their principles of detection of glucose. They are as follows:

- Optical Spectroscopy (Optical Detection)
- Photoacoustic Spectroscopy (Acoustic Detection)
- Electromagnetic Sensing (Electromagnetic Detection)
- Nanomaterial Based Sensing (Electrochemical Detection)

These four techniques are illustrated in Figure 1 and are reviewed in Sections 4–7. The principles of these four techniques are explained in the following subsections.

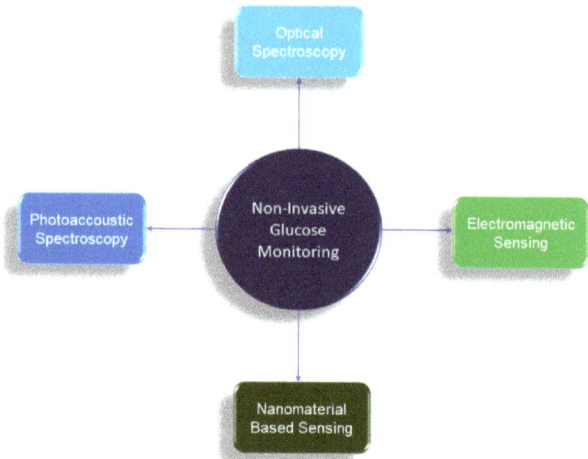

Figure 1. The four different types of noninvasive glucose monitoring technique are illustrated based on their principle of detection.

3.1. Optical Spectroscopy

The detection principle of the Optical Spectroscopy is based on the fact that glucose influences the optical signal passing through it by absorption of light at some particular overtones and combination band wavelengths in the mid infrared (mid-IR) and near infrared (NIR) spectrum regions. Among the mid-IR spectrum of glucose light interactions, a first OH overtone band is designated at 1408 nm. The 1536 nm band can be designated as an OH and CH combination band whereas, the 1688 nm band is designated as a CH overtone band [32]. In the NIR spectrum, the combination bands are a second OH overtone band at 939 nm and a second harmonic CH overtone band at 1126 nm [32]. Due to this absorbance at these particular wavelengths, the intensity of light transmitted through the glucose either *in-vitro* or *in-vivo* decreases as concentration of the glucose increases and vice versa. Using optical sensors like photodiodes, this phenomenon is utilized in the measurement of the blood glucose concentration from the transmitted or reflected intensity of light [32]. Another way to measure glucose concentration using optical detection is Surface Plasmon Resonance (SPR), where a beam of light is passed through the prism on the back of the SPR metal surface which then bends on to the detector. Unlike the intensity of the light, the method exploits information on angular shift to identify the glucose concentration. At a certain resonance angle (refractive index), the light excites the electrons on the metal part of the chip. When an analyte is introduced to the SPR surface, the shift of the reflection intensity curve is observed. The direct measurement of blood sugar is based on the change in angle of the SPR reflection intensity curve [33].

3.2. Photoacoustic Spectroscopy

The photoacoustic glucose monitoring is a hybrid approach, which combines optical excitation and acoustic detection in determining the glucose concentration. Here, the optical energy from the excitation is converted into an acoustic energy by a multistage energy conversion process [34]. The optical excitation of the glucose molecules in blood leads to the localized heating of the solution, which produces a small temperature rise, resulting in the volumetric thermal expansion of the optical interaction region. The associated ultrasonic pressure pulse is then measured by an ultrasonic piezoelectric transducer, which is then converted into electrical signals for determining the glucose concentration.

3.3. Electromagnetic Sensing

The frequency dependency of body tissue has been investigated since early 20th century. The propagation of electromagnetic waves through any media depends on the permittivity of that media. The permittivity is a frequency-dependent parameter unique for each material. These investigations have found that the complex permittivity of tissue is strongly frequency dependent. The underlying mathematical principle is derived from the Debye's relaxation theory. The mathematical equations can be written as [35,36]:

$$\epsilon_r(\omega, \chi) = \epsilon_\infty(\chi) + \frac{\epsilon_{stat}(\chi) - \epsilon_\infty(\chi)}{1 + j\omega\tau(\chi)} \quad (1)$$

where, $\epsilon_r(\omega)$ is the complex and frequency-dependent relative permittivity of a dispersive material, ϵ_{stat} is the static permittivity at lower frequencies, ϵ_∞ is the permittivity at high frequencies and τ is the characteristic relaxation time of the medium. ω and χ are the angular frequency and the concentration, respectively.

Human blood consists of 55% of plasma. The blood plasma consists of around 90% of water. Water being a dipolar compound, the polarization is high. This makes the relative permittivity to be high as well. In contrast, glucose has a smaller relative permittivity, being less polarized. Thus, the overall increase or decrease in glucose concentration in the same volume of blood sample reduces or elevates the relative permittivity of blood plasma, respectively. The measure of the relative permittivity by multiple techniques of electromagnetic sensing at a particular microwave/mm-wave frequency gives the value of the glucose concentration in blood in the form of measured electrical power in a very effective manner which helps in the measurement of blood glucose. In other words, the common measurement principle of these sensors is the electromagnetic interaction between the sensor and the material under test (MUT) (either blood or glucose solutions in cuvette) where the amplitude and/or phase variations in the scattering parameters are measured, when the dielectric properties of the MUT change. It is important to note that the dielectric properties of blood are modified because the change in blood glucose levels is of much greater extent than due to changes of other compounds present in the blood [37,38].

3.4. Nanomaterial Based Sensing

The emergence of nanomaterials, starting from metallic gold, silver, copper oxide, iron oxide to polymer composites, carbon nanotubes and graphene, as primary components in sensing technologies, has significantly upgraded the modern-day biosensors, extracting valuable physiological data and useful information from essential body fluids like urine, saliva, sweat and tears. The impact of nanomaterials in sensing applications is remarkable as they exhibit large surface area, enhanced sensitivity and selectivity, improved catalytic activities which are essential prerequisites for an accurate and precise estimation of glucose levels in humans [39,40].

4. Optical Spectroscopy

The optical spectroscopy is perhaps the most popular among all the four methods for non-invasive blood glucose monitoring. As explained earlier, glucose responses to light at specific wavelengths in the near infra red (NIR) and mid-infra red (mid-IR) regions. The Light Emitting Diode (LED) is mostly used for the excitation in the NIR region with some exceptions [41], however, the use of laser is seen in all cases of mid-IR regions. The signal from either the LED or the laser is pulsed at a certain frequency and is allowed to fall and pass through the glucose. One of the wavelengths at the NIR region is at 940 nm and multiple experiments have been reported at this wavelength using the transmittance principle of glucose light from using a simple operational amplifier [42] to digital detection and processing [41,43]. In the method transmittance spectroscopy, the excited optical light is allowed to transmit through the layers of epidermis, dermis and subcutaneous tissue of the finger tip, before it is detected by a photodetector.

In addition to the transmittance another method was proposed using the dermis tissue spectra [44]. Here the glucose content in dermis tissue traces the variations in blood glucose and the epidermis acts as an interference in skin tissue. This method is termed diffused reflectance. Multiple other works that have used this technique to determine the blood glucose solution are reported in [45–48]. In [49], a phase sensitive front end based compact design has been reported for continuous wearable applications. The protocols of Oral Glucose Tolerant Test (OGTT) was used to compare with the invasive blood pricking technique. This work uses both the transmittance and the diffused reflectance approach. This work has been depicted in Figure 2 as an example of optical spectroscopy with both transmittance and diffused reflectance techniques.

Cardoso et al. [50] implemented an architecture composed of two light emitters, with a wavelength of 940 nm and 805 nm. Another work [51] used 950 nm in addition to 940 nm and have shown that the output voltages are nearly linear with the increment of glucose concentration. In [52], average value of three different wavelengths was used to determine the blood glucose concentration. Besides the popular 940 nm, two other wavelengths at 850 nm and 880 nm were used. Comparative analysis with an invasive technique following either OGTT protocol or Clarke Error Grid gives a good accuracy for the non-invasive device.

Analysis with classification based machine learning models was carried out in [53]. In this work, in addition to 940 nm, transmission measurements show a high correlation value of 0.98 between glucose concentration and transmission intensity for three other wavelengths: 485 nm, 645 nm and 860 nm. The feasibility of a cellular automata based tracking method of blood glucose through skin impedance measurement was introduced in [54]. Recently, Yan et al. [55] using a portable NIR Spectrometer and advanced machine learning models have shown the model based on the combination of synergy interval, genetic algorithm and extreme learning machine as the most accurate for blood glucose detection. A partial least squares method was used in [56] to obtain a correlation coefficient of 93.2% and a prediction error of 0.23 mmol/L.

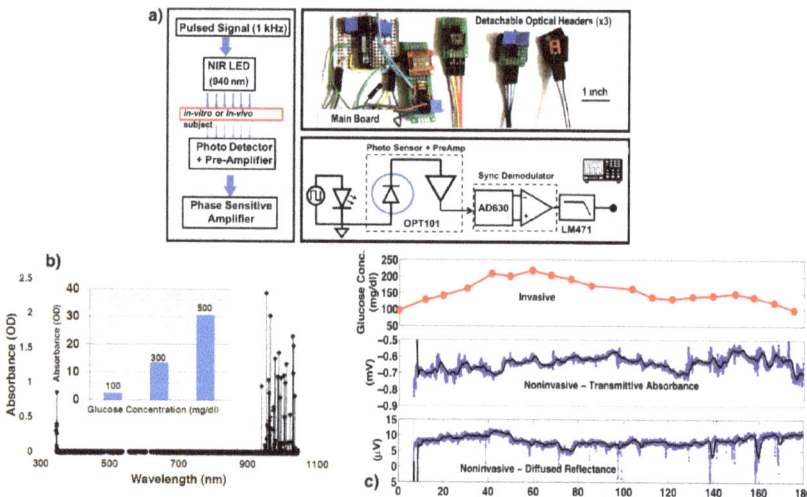

Figure 2. (**a**) Experimental set up of NIR spectroscopy with LED (**b**) *In-vitro* NIR spectra of glucose in water solution. Light absorption is proportional to glucose concentration (Inset). (**c**) *In-vivo* results from experiments on a human subject. Comparison of the transmittance and diffused reflectance techniques with the blood-pricking invasive technique following OGTT protocol. Reproduced with permission from [49]. Copyright 2018, IEEE.

Mid-infra red spectroscopy is another mode within the optical spectroscopy used to determine glucose concentration. The glucose has a better response in some selected mid infrared bands than the NIR bands as reported in [32]. Using a laser diode, the prospect of mid-infrared spectroscopy was reported in [57] for concentrations between 75 and 160 mg/dL. Partial least squares regression was employed to predict the glucose concentration. An average error of 2% in comparison to a commercial electrochemical sensor was observed. In another study [58], the mid-infrared spectroscopy is used in the range of 3333~2857 nm and a strong correlation between the transmittance approach and blood glucose concentration was presented. Using Fourier transform infrared spectroscopy (FT-IR) of attenuated total reflection, the spectra of a human finger was measured. Further, in [59–61], the techniques of Fourier transform infrared spectroscopy (FT-IR) of attenuated total reflection (ATR) were used to accurately determine the glucose concentration.

A customised multi-modal spectroscopy combining impedance spectroscopy and multi-wavelength infrared spectroscopy is proposed in [62] as an application specific integrated circuit (ASIC) in 0.18 µm 1P6M CMOS technology. It occupies an area of 12.5 mm^2 and dissipates a peak power of 38 mW. The three wavelengths used are 850 nm, 950 nm and 1300 nm. The work further uses an artificial neural network (ANN) algorithm to achieve high accuracy in glucose estimation value. The use of ASIC together with ANN enabled the sensor to be area and power efficient for practical wearable applications of blood glucose monitoring with high accuracy. Together with the application of Healthcare IoT [63], the potential of this approach for diabetes management seems to be very bright.

In the technique of SPR, the researchers used attached glucose/galactase binding protein to SPR surface and detected blood glucose and determined the binding equilibrium of glucose molecules to the SPR surface [64]. The analysis of this equilibrium can be a key in continuous glucose monitoring. The SPR method can yield a high sensitivity in the detection of blood glucose at 1050 nm/refractive index unit [33] The sensitivity was reported to be highest at the refractive index of 0.982 nm [65]. Another study reported similar result with greatest sensitivity with refractive index in the range of 1.0000 to 1.0007 [66]. In [67], imprinted hybrid microgels achieved root-mean-squared error of predication (RMSEC) as low as ~0.2 mg/dL over a clinically relevant glucose concentration range of 1.8–360 mg/dL. In case of SPR techniques and other similar techniques that resort to large bench-top equipment for measurement and analysis, the prospect of down-scaling the technique in form-factor to that of a wearable device is minimal. Those techniques such as Optical Polarimetry, Raman Spectroscopy, Optical Coherence Tomography are not discussed in this review and can be referred in [13,15].

The accuracy of optical spectroscopy is affected by several factors which include, skin color and temperature and therefore an algorithmic correction is required [15]. According to some studies, skin can cause birefringence of light due to scattering of contents in the skin leading to lesser degree of polarization of light than expected [15,68]. The detection requires person specific calibration to mitigate the skin color and advanced machine learning algorithm to separate signals coming out of proteins and lipids [69].

5. Photoacoustic Spectroscopy

A large amount of work on glucose monitoring with photoacoustic spectroscopy have been also reported. As earlier explained, although this technique shares the same excitation principle with the optical spectroscopy however the detection mechanism is entirely different and is based on the principles of acoustics. The feasibility of photoacoustic spectroscopy with the depth profiling of a skin model for non-invasive glucose measurement was reported in [70]. The measurable depth of 2–3 mm with a modulation frequency of 1000–2000 Hz provided the necessary confidence to work with this technique. This led to an early work that investigated the feasibility of photoacoustic spectroscopy as an independent technique for blood glucose monitoring and reported in [71]. This work implemented a laser diode to excite the glucose medium and the signal was detected using a piezoelectric transducer followed by a low noise amplifier. The validation was implemented using the established OGTT method. It is important to note that the laser excitation in the cases described above, were pulsed at a certain frequency and is allowed to fall and pass through the glucose.

Optical excitation, where laser was not pulsed but continuous were also reported. Such continuous laser excitation with desktop based lock-in-amplifiers were reported for accurate phase-sensitive detections in [72] and later differential continuous-wave photoacoustic spectroscopy (DCW-PAS) in [73]. The DCW-PAS technique utilizes amplitude modulation of dual wavelengths of light to determine changes in glucose concentration. Both of these works also use the laser diode for the optical excitation. Very recently, Faheem et al., has implemented a laser based photoacoustic glucose monitoring system using a phase sensitive amplifier in wearable form factor as reported in [74]. This work replaces the desktop based lock-in amplifier with an integrated modulator/demodulator microchip working as a lock-in-amplifier for practical wearable applications in diabetes management. The work further analyzes the results using classification based machine learning algorithms and achieve a correlation coefficient of 97% and p-value 5.6e-6. This work has been depicted in Figure 3 as an example of photoacoustic spectroscopy with compact instruments for potential wearable applications. In [75], a portable photoacoustic embedded system is implemented using field programmable gate array (FPGA). The glucose measurement technique is verified both *in-vitro* and *in-vivo*. This work further advances to include a kernel-based regression algorithm using multiple features of the photoacoustic signal to estimate glucose concentration [76]. The work also uses cloud service using a mobile device in as an example of Healthcare IoT for glucose monitoring. Some other works that were reported and used laser diodes are [77–80].

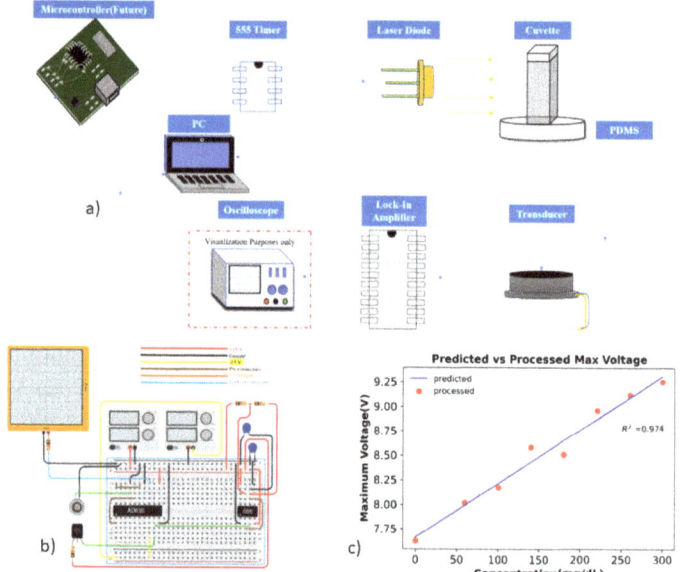

Figure 3. (**a**) Compact instrumentation for in vitro glucose measurement with phase sensitive detection using PAS. All the instruments are portable and can be replicated for wearable in vivo glucose monitoring (**b**) The electronics circuit for the optical stimulation and the phase sensitive detection of the proposed compact instrumentation system using the micrchip AD630 (**c**) Linear regression calculations of the Amplitude of the signal. Reproduced with permission [74]. Copyright 2022 IEEE under CC BY

In comparison to the optical spectroscopy, this technique is yet to gain similar popularity. This is because the optical excitation in this technique depends mostly on laser, unlike an LED as in the case of the NIR Optical Spectroscopy. The laser has multiple safety concerns and health issues and is therefore not recommended for continuous blood glucose monitoring. A major challenge to replace it with NIR/mid-IR LED that has the potential to be a continuous wearable system will be to compromise on the signal to noise ratio (SNR) of the detected signal. In this method, the SNR is comparatively less than the optical approach because the acoustic signal coming as an electric signal out of a transducer is relatively weak in comparison to a direct optical detection with a photodetector as in the case of an optical approach. A few works have attempted to mitigate this issue. In [81], an NIR LED based photoacoustic glucose monitoring system is reported. They make use of a box that has a good sound shielding characteristic to attenuate noise from outside without compromising on the SNR. The challenge to improve the SNR quality can be further resolved by implementing different signal processing techniques such as signal averaging reported in [82,83] in the context of photoacoustic imaging.

The measurement of blood glucose using this method is also challenged by skin thickness, roughness and moisture and other skin conditions [69]. These factors interfere the absorption of light in the skin and the glucose signal will not be as strong. The presence of other contents in the blood such as lipids and proteins. Similar to the optical approach, person specific calibration, signal averaging and advanced machine learning techniques will be able to mitigate these effects.

6. Electromagnetic Sensing

The electromagnetic sensing can be further categorized broadly into Planar Microwave Resonant Sensors and Antenna Sensing, based on the instrument used and principles of microwave theory. They are described as follows:

6.1. Planar Microwave Resonant Sensors

Planar microwave sensors are considered an attractive choice to non-invasively probe the dielectric attributes of biological tissues due to their low cost, simple fabrication, miniature scale, and minimum risk to human health. This method relies on the change in the permittivity of blood due to the variation in glucose content resulting out of small shifts in the sensor's frequency response. However, there are certain challenges that should be taken into consideration. In [84], Volkan et al., has investigated the external factors those play a major role in the resonant sensor's response, making it challenging to achieve the accuracy needed for blood glucose measurements in these small shifts in frequency.

A split-ring resonator has been used in [85], to measure the glucose concentration at 1.4 GHz. The sensor has two spatially separated rings, one of which interacts with the change in glucose level of the device under test while the second ring is used as a reference. The observed OGTT trend showed nice correlation of frequency shift and the glucose concentration comparable to a commercial sensor, including a CGM device and a blood pricking device. This work has been depicted in Figure 4 as an example of planar microwave sensors. In [86], the sensor has a microfluidic container on top and works at a frequency of 2 GHz in-vitro. The sensor responds to permittivity change with glucose solutions at varying concentrations. The range of glucose concentrations used are from 50 mg/dL to 300 mg/dL. A multi-layer is approach is proposed in [87]. The paper analyses three different microwave resonator structure and finds the ground plane coplanar waveguide to be the most suitable amongst them. In [88], a microwave resonator comparable to the size of a coin has been fabricated. The device was sensitive enough to detect as low as 10 mg/dL change in glucose concentration.

In [89], a metamaterial structure monitors the variation of blood glucose concentration on human body and increases the sensitivity by the addition of a diode. The change in frequency and magnitude (reflection loss) of 1.4 MHz and 0.7 dB, respectively, increases to 5.2 MHz and 1.2 dB, respectively. The improvements exploit the nonlinear effects of the diode. Another microwave sensor is suggested with a sensitivity performance of about 6.2 dB/(mg/mL) that operates in the range of 1–6 GHz [90]. The sensor gets excited by a coupled microstrip transmission-line that is etched on the bottom side of the substrate and monitor the glucose concentration changes by recording the frequency response of the maximum reflection and transmission loss. An interdigital capacitor sensor was reported in [91] at 4.080 GHz. The measurement principle here is based on the fringing electric field produced on top of the interdigital capacitor sensor of the MUT. In [92], an ultrawideband microwave technique has been proposed for non-invasive blood glucose monitoring in the frequency range of 3–10 GHz. In this frequency range, there is a regularity of the energy of the received signal in the blood glucose concentration of varied from 70 to 400 mg/dL. The technique uses a single pair of antennas to achieve this. The gain ranges from 0 to 2 dB for blood glucose level from 50 to 400 mg/dL.

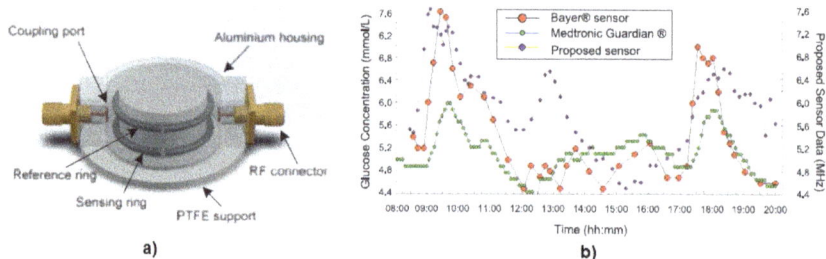

Figure 4. (a) A 3D structure of a double split-ring resonator sensor. (b) Noninvasive sensor data against the commercially available continuous invasive sensor (Medtronic) and blood strip glucometer (Bayer). Reproduced with permission [85]. Copyright 2014 IEEE.

The transmission properties of glucose solutions with different concentrations, including the amplitude and phase responses, are reported in [93]. With modeling and experiment, two glucose solutions utilizing saline and distilled water are studied at 17 GHz Ku-band. At 40 GHz, a sensitivity of 0.2° phase shift per 10 mg/dL was achieved in [94]. The transmission phase of glucose solutions is shown to have a linear response to glucose concentration from hypoglycemia to hyperglycemia, indicating that microwave technology in the Ku-band has a lot of promise for developing non-invasive glucose monitoring systems [95]. In [96], two spatially separated split-ring resonators are reported, with one interacts with the change in glucose level of a sample under test while the other ring is used as a reference. The comparative analysis of the two split rings following the OGTT protocol is used for validation purposes.

6.2. Antenna as Sensors

The change in permittivity with varying glucose concentration can effect both an antenna in near field coupling and electromagnetic transmission. This enables an antenna to work as a sensor following the principles of electromagnetic sensing. To this end, several research work has been reported. In [97], two different antennas: a patch and integrated slot antenna have been designed. The two-port analysis shows the measured gain responds to the glucose concentration change at a frequency of 5.5 GHz using the patch antenna. The slot antenna on the other hand did not produce any glucose sensitive measurements. In [98], the sensor is modeled as a microstrip antenna made of flat sheet of metal separated by a dielectric substrate at a frequency of 2.4 GHz. The return loss for an antenna with microstrip feed is determined to be 36 dB at that frequency. However, the paper does not give any information on the return loss change with varying glucose concentrations. In [99], the sensitivity of the antenna is determined by swarm optimization with a frequency shift of 85.5 MHz corresponding to change in aqueous glucose of 50% and 10%.

In [100], the sensor output is an amplitude-only measurement of the standing wave with frequency on a microstrip line that is spiral shaped with an open-terminated end. A comparative analysis similar to Clarke Error Grid with a commercial device shows promising results. The response of a single-spiral microstrip sensor has been demonstrated to alter significantly in response to changes in recorded blood glucose levels in numerous test participants [101]. A monopole antenna is placed in a cuff and wrapped around the wrist in [102]. Using a realistic tissue model of a human hand, simulations have been performed to obtain the antenna input impedance. The shift in resonant frequency was used to determine the blood glucose level. The frequency targeted for this study is in the range of 1.5–2 GHz. The maximum reflection loss shifts to 1.45 GHz, 1.48 GHz, 1.43 GHz for normoglycemia, hypoglycemia and hyperglycemia, respectively, from 1.78 GHz that is observed in the absence of tissue.

At an operating frequency of 19 GHz, a two-port microstrip line sensor was designed in [103]. A water solution which mimics the permittivity of blood glucose is kept at a tank under the model to fill a slot between the two parts of the substrate. The slot is used for electromagnetic waves to interact with the water glucose solution underneath. The sensor achieves a sensitivity of 2° phase change per 10 mg/dL glucose concentration variation. A truncated microstrip patch antenna was designed in [104]. The sensitivity of the antenna could detect minor changes (10%) in blood's dielectric characteristics from the transmission coefficient in the range of 21 GHz to 29.6 GHz. In [105], two facing microstrip patch antennas operating at 60 GHz that are placed across the glucose solution are designed. The measured transmission coefficient which depends on the permittivity change along the signal path, was correlated with determine the change in glucose concentration. The work was extended in [106], by utilizing an Intravenous Glucose Tolerance Test for in vivo applications.

Chaithanya et al., has implemented the power level of the Received Signal Strength Indicator (RSSI) of a Blutooth Low Energy (BLE) signal at 2.4 GHz to identify the blood glucose level in [107] in a wearable form-factor. Concurrent measurements with the commercial invasive finger pricking approach using the OGTT protocol have shown promising results. This work has been depicted in Figure 5 as an example of sensing with antenna.

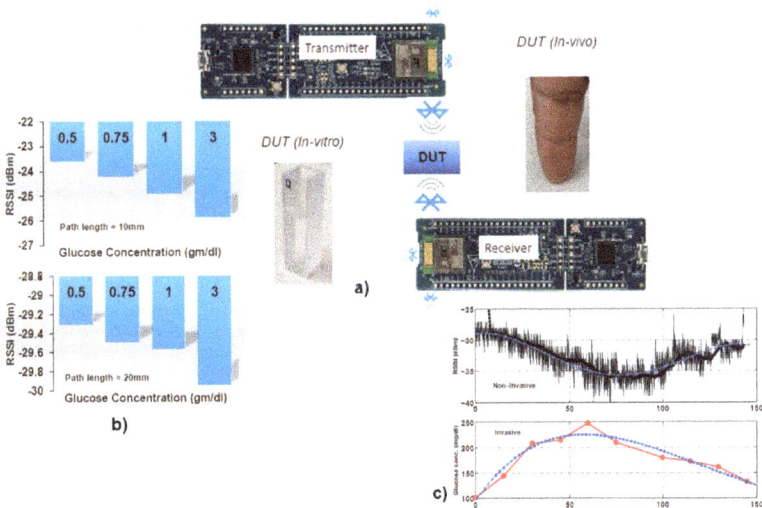

Figure 5. (a) Experimental set-up for both the *in-vitro* and *in-vivo* measurements with a bluetooth enabled MCU (Antenna as Sensors) (b) The RSSI power level dependence on glucose concentration with *in-vitro* experiment (c) Comparison with *in-vivo* experimental results of the noninvasive device with the blood-pricking invasive technique following OGTT protocol on a human subject. Reproduced with permission [107]. Copyright 2019 IEEE.

The challenges in the detection of blood glucose using electromagnetic method is limited by uncertainty of change in dielectric properties of blood glucose. The sensitivity and selectivity need improvement using advanced machine learning and signal averaging techniques that can mitigate background noise in the data from the contents in the blood to separate high and low amplitude signaling effectively improving the accuracy. Unlike to the previous two optical excitation approaches, this method does not require person specific calibration for skin color differentiation. With the custom development of smart minuscule transceiver system in advanced CMOS technology, the future of this method seems very promising for continuous detection of blood glucose as a non-invasive wearable device (see Figure 5).

7. Nanomaterial Based Sensing

Nanomaterial-based precise glucose monitoring strategies for early-stage detection of diabetes in patients have largely been explored and investigated. Here, we will primarily be discussing nanomaterial-based biosensors which have witnessed extensive applications for precise detection of glucose levels in human urine, saliva, sweat and tears. These techniques are depicted in Figure 6.

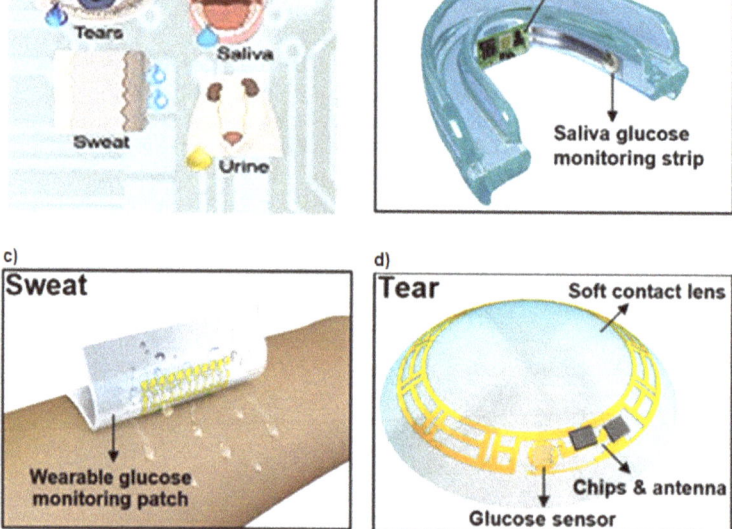

Figure 6. (a)The important bio-fluids like tears, saliva, sweat, and urine used to build non-invasive glucose monitoring devices. Typical biosensors based on (**b**) saliva, (**c**) sweat and (**d**) tear. Reproduced with permission [108] Copyright 2022, Ivyspring International Publisher under CC BY. Reproduced with permission [109] Copyright 2018, John Wiley & Sons.

Metallic, metal alloy, metal oxide and magnetic nanostructures, carbon-based nanomaterials and even their hybrid/composite structures have been significantly used for non-invasive glucose sensing technologies [110–113]. Most of these nanomaterials, in particular, metal oxides and ferrite nanoparticles exhibit intrinsic peroxidase-like activity which plays a catalytic role in glucose detection [111,114–117].

When sugar levels in human blood is on the higher side, excess glucose gets excreted out through urine. The ready availability of urine and its easy collection makes urine-based glucose sensing a non-invasive approach for the diagnosis of diabetes [110]. Su et al. have successfully demonstrated the application of $ZnFe_2O_4$ nanoparticles for the detection of glucose levels in urine [111]. The method is based on colorimetric sensing using glucose oxidase (GOx). Recently, colorimetric based sensor using plasmonic gold nanoparticles on graphitic carbon nitride nanosheets (Au nanoparticles @g-C_3N_4) was used to determine the urine glucose levels [118]. Furthermore, hybrid nanostructures like Co_3O_4/graphene nanocomposites have been employed as electrode material to detect sugar concentration in urine samples. This is a non-enzymatic electrochemical-based sensor having a detection limit of 0.5 mM [119].

The glucose content in human saliva can also carry useful information regarding the diabetic condition in humans. An early glucose analyzing sensor was developed in [120]. The transducer used here is an enzyme amperometric glucose sensor and has three electrodes. The working electrode made with platinum is covered with an albumin membrane, over which H_2O_2 based immobilized enzyme membrane is placed. The concentration of H_2O_2 determines the output current from sensor and which is detected by the amperometry circuit of the saliva analyzing system. A similar study was carried out in [121]. Chakraborty et al. reported fabrication of a non-enzymatic porous CuO nanostructures based electrochemical sensor for salivary glucose monitoring [122]. Similarly, in a recent study, porous NiO nanostructures have been utilized as electrode materials for estimating salivary glucose levels with a detection limit as low as 84 nM [123].

Sometimes morphological changes in nanomaterials have been introduced to offer an enhanced diagnosis approach. Very recently, non-enzymatic and highly sensitive glucose sensors based on composite nanosystems like cuprous oxide nanocubes embedded on graphene have been adopted for a systematic probing of salivary glucose levels [124]. Several other enzyme-free electrochemical-based salivary glucose sensors developed in the recent past based on composite structures include Au nanoparticles on CuO nanorods (~2009 $\mu A\ mM^{-1}$), IrO_2@NiO core–shell nanowires (1439.4 $\mu A\ mM^{-1}cm^{-2}$), CuBr@CuO nanoparticles (3096 $\mu A\ mM^{-1}cm^{-2}$), Cu-Pt nanoparticles on glassy carbon electrode (2209 $\mu A\ mM^{-1}cm^{-2}$), and many more [112,125–127].

The physiological data obtained from human sweat or perspiration also possess valuable imprints regarding the glucose concentration in humans. In an attempt to modernize non-invasive glucose detection approaches, several sweat sensors have been developed using nanomaterials of zinc oxide, gold, silver, graphene oxide, carbon nanotubes and their composite systems [128–134].

Tear based sensing approach using nanomaterials have also gathered significant attention in the development of this kind of non-invasive biosensors [135–138]. Nanostructures embedded in highly sophisticated and biocompatible contact lenses are capable of detecting glucose levels accurately, sometimes having a detection limit as low as 211 nM [139]. In the commercial arena, a small and flexible spring like device was introduced and termed Noviosense [140].

In the last decade, the nanomaterials have been hugely exploited for advanced biomedical applications [141–145]. As already stated, mostly nano-ferrites and metal oxide nanomaterials as well as graphene oxides and carbon nanotubes show intrinsic peroxidase-like activities [111,116,117,146,147]. Consequently, it is advisable to employ more of these nanostructures, particularly in the form of composites to design and fabricate sophisticated glucose monitoring devices having a much higher degree of sensitivity. Ferrite-based nanostructures are already established candidates in gas sensing applications [148,149]. There lies a good possibility of further exploring these iron oxide-based ferrites for non-invasive glucose sensing applications. Tailoring the physicochemical properties of ferrites and some prominent metal oxide nanostructures, primarily by incorporating suitable dopants (transition metals, rare-earths etc.) and also by introducing shape and surface anisotropies in the system, creating structures like nanowires, nanorods, nano-octopods etc. can possibly have a significant impact in better quantification of glucose levels in humans.

Therefore, these nanomaterial-based sensors have a tremendous future ahead particularly in the design and development of highly sensitive, cost-effective non-invasive glucose monitoring devices. This non-invasive mode of quantifying glucose levels in pre-diabetic and diabetic patients carry immense possibility which could register a giant leap in the healthcare industry as opposed to the traditional blood glucose sensing invasive strategies. These nanomaterial-based biosensors could be the next generation non-invasive technology for efficient and precise quantification of sugar levels in diabetic patients.

8. Hybrid, Integrated and Other Methods

Besides these four techniques, some other approaches have also been investigated such as Nuclear Magnetic Resonance [150] at 400 MHz. In [151], a feasibility study of a non-invasive sensor integrating three different types of techniques: electromagnetic, acoustic speed and near infra-red spectroscopy with compensation techniques results. Another study [152] involved an integrated approach combining Near Infra Red (NIR) absorption and bio-impedance measurements using artificial neural network and stochastic methods. An attempt was made to measure the blood glucose level using a capacitance measurement technique in [153] using a parallel plate capacitor, with the forearm in between acting as a dielectric medium. Two metal plates of equal dimensions were placed near left wrist as electrodes. A semi-cylindrical capacitive sensor was similarly proposed in [154]. In [155], the change in dielectric permittivity of saliva estimates the glucose concentration. A correlation between blood glucose levels with saliva glucose was investigated. A microwave biosensor was used at the microwave frequency to measure the shift in resonant frequency of the resonator. However, these techniques or approaches are not widely pursued and investigated so far.

9. Conclusions

The aim of this concise and systematic review is to highlight the clinical significance of non-invasive methods in glucose monitoring and bring out the progression of these methods for potential diabetes management in the near future. There are four methods of non-invasive glucose monitoring that were reviewed here and classified primarily based on their principles of detection of the signal from the MUT, which is either a glucose solution (*in-vitro*) or blood glucose (*in-vivo/ex-vivo*). These four methods are optical spectroscopy, photoacoustic spectroscopy, electromagnetic sensing and nanomaterial based sensing. Furthermore, integration of these different approaches to bring out a cohesive and hybrid blood monitoring device were also reviewed. The developments observed from all of these investigations suggest that the non-invasive glucose monitoring has a huge potential to replace the current standard of invasive and minimally invasive approaches with a *pain-free*, efficient and accurate diabetes management in the near future.

Author Contributions: Conceptualization, S.L.; Methodology, S.L.; Formal Analysis, S.L., A.R., S.S.L., R.J.; Investigation, S.L., A.R., S.S.L., R.J.; Writing—Original Draft Preparation, S.L., A.R., S.S.L., R.J.; Writing—Review and Editing, S.L., S.S.L., R.J. All authors have read and agreed to the published version of the manuscript.

Funding: This research was partially supported by the California Department of Food & Agriculture under the Fresno-Merced Future of Food (F3) Innovation Program.

Institutional Review Board Statement: Not applicable.

Informed Consent Statement: Not applicable.

Data Availability Statement: Not applicable.

Conflicts of Interest: The authors declare no conflict of interest.

References

1. Diabetes Overview, World Health Organization. Available online: https://www.who.int/health-topics/diabetes#tab=tab_1 (accessed on 19 March 2022).
2. National Diabetes Statistics Report. Available online: https://www.cdc.gov/diabetes/data/statistics-report/index.html (accessed on 19 August 2022).
3. Jameson, J.L.; Fauci, A.S.; Kasper, D.L.; Hauser, S.L.; Longo, D.L.; Loscalzo, J. *Harrison's Principles of Internal Medicine*; Mc-Graw Hill Education: New York City, NY, USA, 2011.

4. Desouza, C.V.; Bolli, G.B.; Fonseca, V. Hypoglycemia, Diabetes, and Cardiovascular Events. *Diabetes Care* **2010**, *33*, 1389–1394. [CrossRef] [PubMed]
5. Whitmer, R.A. Type 2 diabetes and risk of cognitive impairment and dementia. *Curr. Neurol. Neurosci.* **2007**, *7*, 373–380. [CrossRef] [PubMed]
6. Schwartz, A.V.; Vittinghoff, E.; Sellmeyer, D.E.; Feingold, K.R.; de Rekeneire, N.; Strotmeyer, E.S.; Shorr, R.I.; Vinik, A.I.; Odden, M.C.; Park, S.W.; et al. Diabetes-related complications, glycemic control, and falls in older adults. *Diabetes Care* **2008**, *33*, 391–396. [CrossRef]
7. McCoy, R.G.; Houten, H.K.V.; Ziegenfuss, J.Y.; Shah, N.D.; Wermers, R.A.; Smith, S.A. Increased mortality of patients with diabetes reporting severe hypoglycemia. *Diabetes Care* **2012**, *35*, 1897–1901. [CrossRef] [PubMed]
8. Geller, A.I.; Shehab, N.; Lovegrove, M.C.; Kegler, S.R.; Weidenbach, K.N.; Ryan, G.J.; Budnitz, D.S. National estimates of insulin-related hypoglycemia and errors leading to emergency department visits and hospitalizations. *JAMA Intern. Med.* **2010**, *174*, 678–686. [CrossRef]
9. Mouri, M.; Badireddy, M. *Hyperglycemia*; StatPearls Publishing LLC: Treasure Island, FL, USA, 2022.
10. Lizzo, J.M.; Goyal, A.; Gupta, V. *Adult Diabetic Ketoacidosis*; StatPearls Publishing LLC: Treasure Island, FL, USA, 2021.
11. Gosmanov, A.R.; Gosmanova, E.O.; Kitabchi, A.E. Hyperglycemic Crises: Diabetic Ketoacidosis and Hyperglycemic hyperosmolar State. Endotext. 2021. Available online: https://www.ncbi.nlm.nih.gov/sites/books/NBK279052/ (accessed on 15 October 2022).
12. Bolla, A.; Priefer, R. Blood glucose monitoring- an overview of current and future non-invasive devices. *Diabetes Metab. Syndr.* **2017**, *14*, 739–751. [CrossRef]
13. Alsunaidi, B.; Althobaiti, M.; Tamal, M.; Albaker, W.; Al-Naib, I. A Review of Non-Invasive Optical Systems for Continuous Blood Glucose Monitoring. *Sensors* **2021**, *21*, 6820. [CrossRef]
14. Juan, C.G.; Potelon, B.; Quendo, C.; Bronchalo, E. Microwave Planar Resonant Solutions for Glucose Concentration Sensing: A Systematic Review. *Appl. Sci.* **2021**, *11*, 7018. [CrossRef]
15. Tang, L.; Chang, S.J.; Chen, C.J.; Liu, J.T. Non-Invasive Blood Glucose Monitoring Technology: A Review. *Sensors* **2020**, *20*, 6925. [CrossRef]
16. Gusev, M.; Poposka, L.; Spasevski, G.; Kostoska, M.; Koteska, B.; Simjanoska, M.; Ackovska, N.; Stojmenski, A.; Tasic, J.; Trontelj, J.; et al. Noninvasive Glucose Measurement Using Machine Learning and Neural Network Methods and Correlation with Heart Rate Variability. *J. Sens.* **2020**, *2020*, 9628281. [CrossRef]
17. Bondar, J.L.; Mead, D.C. Evaluation of glucose-6-phosphate dehydrogenase from Leuconostoc mesenteroides in the hexokinase method for determining glucose in serum. *Clin. Chem.* **1974**, *20*, 586–590. [CrossRef] [PubMed]
18. Finger Prick. Available online: https://dtc.ucsf.edu/types-of-diabetes/type1/treatment-of-type-1-diabetes/monitoring-diabetes/monitoring-your-blood/ (accessed on 19 March 2022).
19. Bond, M.M.; Richards-Kortum, R.R. Drop-to-Drop Variation in the Cellular Components of Fingerprick Blood: Implications for Point-of-Care Diagnostic Development. *Am. J. Clin. Pathol.* **2015**, *144*, 885–894. [CrossRef] [PubMed]
20. do Amaral, C.E.F.; Wolf, B. Current Development in Non-Invasive Glucose Monitoring. *Med. Eng. Phys.* **2008**, *30*, 541–549. [CrossRef] [PubMed]
21. Obeidat, Y.; Ammar, A. A System for Blood Glucose Monitoring and Smart Insulin Prediction. *IEEE Sens. J.* **2021**, *21*, 13895–13909. [CrossRef]
22. Laakso, M. Hyperglycemia and cardiovascular disease in type 2 diabetes. *Diabetes* **1999**, *48*, 937–942. [CrossRef]
23. Cappon, G.; Vettoretti, M.; Sparacino, G.; Facchinetti, A. Continuous glucose monitoring sensors for diabetes management: A review of technologies and applications. *Diabetes Metab. J.* **2019**, *43*, 383–397. [CrossRef]
24. Dexom CGM. Available online: https://www.dexcom.com/g6/how-it-works (accessed on 19 March 2022).
25. Libre CGM. Available online: https://www.freestylelibre.us/cgm-difference/benefits-of-cgm.html (accessed on 19 March 2022).
26. Eversense CGM. Available online: https://www.eversensediabetes.com/why-eversense-cgm (accessed on 12 August 2022).
27. Messer, L.H.; Berget, C.; Beatson, C.; Polsky, S.; Forlenza, G.P. Preserving skin integrity with chronic device use in diabetes. *Diabetes Technol. Ther.* **2018**, *20*, S2-54–S2-64. [CrossRef]
28. Christensen, M.O.; Berg, A.K.; Rytter, K.; Hommel, E.; Thyssen, J.P.; Svensson, J.; Nørgaard, K. Skin problems due to treatment with technology are associated with increased disease burden among adults with type 1 diabetes. *Diabetes Technol. Ther.* **2019**, *21*, 215–221. [CrossRef]
29. Mastrototaro, J.; Shin, J.; Marcus, A.; Sulur, G. STAR 1 Clinical Trial Investigators The accuracy and efficacy of real-time continuous glucose monitoring sensor in patients with type 1 diabetes. *Diabetes Technol. Ther.* **2008**, *10*, 385–390. [CrossRef]
30. Engler, R.; Routh, T.L.; Lucisano, J.Y. Adoption barriers for continuous glucose monitoring and their potential reduction with a fully implanted system: Results from patient preference surveys. *Clin. Diabetes* **2018**, *36*, 50–58. [CrossRef]
31. Messer, L.H.; Tanenbaum, M.L.; Cook, P.F.; Wong, J.J.; Hanes, S.J.; Driscoll, K.A.; Hood, K.K. Cost, hassle, and on-body experience: Barriers to diabetes device use in adolescents and potential intervention targets. *Diabetes Technol. Ther.* **2020**, *22*, 760–767. [CrossRef] [PubMed]
32. Khalil, O.S. Spectroscopic and Clinical Aspects of Noninvasive Glucose Measurements. *Clin. Chem.* **1999**, *45*, 165–177. [CrossRef]
33. Omidniaee, A.; Karimi, S.; Farmani, A. Surface Plasmon Resonance-Based SiO_2 Kretschmann Configuration Biosensor for the Detection of Blood Glucose. *Silicon* **2021**, *14*, 3081–3090. [CrossRef]

34. MacKenzie, H.A.; Ashton, H.S.; Spiers, S.; Shen, Y.; Freeborn, S.S.; Hannigan, J.; Lindberg, J.; Rae, P. Advances in Photoacoustic Noninvasive Glucose Testing. *Clin. Chem.* **1999**, *45*, 1587–1595. [CrossRef]
35. Debye, P.J.W. *Polar Molecules*; Dover Publications: Mineola, NY, USA, 1960.
36. Cole, K.S.; Cole, R.H. Dispersion and Absorption in Dielectrics I. Alternating Current Characteristics. *J. Chem. Phys.* **1941**, *9*, 341–351. [CrossRef]
37. Kim, N.-Y.; Adhikari, K.K.; Dhakal, R.; Chuluunbaatar, Z.; Wang, C.; Kim, E.-S. Rapid, sensitive and reusable detection of glucose by a robust radiofrequency passive device biosensor chip. *Nat. Sci. Rep.* **2015**, *5*, 7807. [CrossRef] [PubMed]
38. Adhikary, K.; Kim, N.Y. Ultrahigh sensitive mediator free biosensor based on a microfabricated microwave sensor for the detection of micromolar glucose concentrations. *IEEE Trans. Microw. Theory Tech.* **2016**, *64*, 319–327. [CrossRef]
39. Makaram, P.; Owens, D.; Aceros, J. Trends in Nanomaterial-Based Non-Invasive Diabetes Sensing Technologies. *Diagnostics* **2014**, *4*, 27–46. [CrossRef]
40. Rahman, M.M.; Ahammad, A.J.; Jin, J.H.; Ahn, S.J.; Lee, J.J. A comprehensive review of glucose biosensors based on nanostructured metal-oxides. *Sensors* **2010**, *10*, 4855–4886. [CrossRef]
41. Haxha, S.; Jhoja, J. Optical Based Noninvasive Glucose Monitoring Sensor Prototype. *IEEE Photonics J.* **2016**, *8*, 1–11. [CrossRef]
42. Asekar, M.S. Development of Portable Non-Invasive Blood Glucose Measuring Device Using NIR Spectroscopy. In Proceedings of the 2018 Second International Conference on Intelligent Computing and Control Systems (ICICCS), Madurai, India, 14–15 June 2018; pp. 572–575.
43. Zheng, T.; Li, W.; Liu, Y.; Ling, B.W.-K. A noninvasive blood glucose measurement system by Arduino and near-infrared. In Proceedings of the 2016 IEEE International Conference on Consumer Electronics-China (ICCE-China), Guangzhou, China, 19–21 December 2016; pp. 1–3.
44. Maruo, K.; Tsurugi, M.; Chin, J.; Ota, T.; Arimoto, H.; Yamada, Y.; Tamura, M.; Ishii, M.; Ozaki, Y. Noninvasive Blood Glucose Assay Using a Newly Developed Near-Infrared System. *IEEE J. Sel. Top. Quantum Electron.* **2003**, *9*, 322–330. [CrossRef]
45. Arefin, M.S.; Khan, A.H.; Islam, R. Non-invasive Blood Glucose Determination using Near Infrared LED in Diffused Reflectance Method. In Proceedings of the 2018 10th International Conference on Electrical and Computer Engineering (ICECE), Dhaka, Bangladesh, 20–22 December 2018; pp. 93–96.
46. Udara, S.S.W.I.; Alwis, A.K.D.; Silva, K.M.W.K.; Ananda, U.V.D.M.A.; Kahandawaarachchi, K.A.D.C.P. DiabiTech- Non-Invasive Blood Glucose Monitoring System. In Proceedings of the 2019 International Conference on Advancements in Computing (ICAC), Malabe, Sri Lanka, 5–7 December 2019; pp. 145–150.
47. Lawand, K.; Parihar, M.; Patil, S.N. Design and development of infrared LED based non invasive blood glucometer. In Proceedings of the 2015 Annual IEEE India Conference (INDICON), New Delhi, India, 17–20 December 2015; pp. 1–6.
48. Noor, Y.; Mohd, N.; Mohd, Z.Z.; Zuli, J.M.; Md, Y.Z.; Rehman, L.A.; Hafiz, L.M.; Hafizulfika, H.M. Noninvasive glucose level determination using diffuse reflectance near infrared spectroscopy and chemometrics analysis based on in vitro sample and human skin. In Proceedings of the 2014 IEEE Conference on Systems, Process and Control (ICSPC 2014), Kuala Lumpur, Malaysia, 12–14 December 2014; pp. 30–35.
49. Laha, S.; Kaya, S.; Dhinagar, N.; Kelestemur, Y.; Puri, V. A Compact Continuous non-Invasive Glucose Monitoring System with Phase-Sensitive Front End. In Proceedings of the 2018 IEEE Biomedical Circuits and Systems Conference (BioCAS), Cleveland, OH, USA, 17–19 October 2018; pp. 1–4.
50. Cardoso, S.D.S.; Machado, M.B.; Ruzicki, J.C.M. A Non-Invasive Infrared Glucose Monitor Double Wavelength Based. *IEEE Lat. Am. Trans.* **2020**, *18*, 1572–1580. [CrossRef]
51. Abidin, M.T.B.Z.; Rosli, M.K.R.; Shamsuddin, S.A.B.; Madzhi, N.K. Initial quantitative comparison of 940nm and 950nm infrared sensor performance for measuring glucose non-invasively. In Proceedings of the 2013 IEEE International Conference on Smart Instrumentation, Measurement and Applications (ICSIMA), Kuala Lumpur, Malaysia, 25–27 November 2013; pp. 1–6.
52. Kassem, A.; Hamad, M.; Harbieh, G.G.; Moucary, C.E. A Non-Invasive Blood Glucose Monitoring Device. In Proceedings of the 2020 IEEE 5th Middle East and Africa Conference on Biomedical Engineering (MECBME), Amman, Jordan, 27–29 October 2020; pp. 1–4.
53. Shokrekhodaei, M.; Cistola, D.P.; Roberts, R.C.; Quinones, S. Non-Invasive Glucose Monitoring Using Optical Sensor and Machine Learning Techniques for Diabetes Applications. *IEEE Access* **2021**, *9*, 73029–73045. [CrossRef] [PubMed]
54. Li, C.K.; Tsai, C.W. Skin Impedance Measurement in Wearable Non-invasive Optical Blood Glucose Monitors. In Proceedings of the 2020 IEEE 2nd International Workshop on System Biology and Biomedical Systems (SBBS), Taichung, Taiwan, 3–4 December 2020; pp. 1–4.
55. Yu, Y.; Huang, J.; Zhu, J.; Liang, S. An Accurate Noninvasive Blood Glucose Measurement System Using Portable Near-Infrared Spectrometer and Transfer Learning Framework. *IEEE Sens. J.* **2021**, *21*, 3506–3519. [CrossRef]
56. Wang, S.; Yuan, X.; Zhang, Y. Non-invasive blood glucose measurement scheme based on near-infrared spectroscopy. In Proceedings of the 2017 Conference on Lasers and Electro-Optics Pacific Rim (CLEO-PR), Singapore, 31 July–4 August 2017; pp. 1–4.
57. Liakat, S.; Bors, K.A.; Xu, L.; Woods, C.M.; Doyle, J.; Gmachl, C.F. Noninvasive in vivo glucose sensing on human subjects using mid-infrared light. *Biomed. Opt. Express* **2014**, *5*, 2397–2404. [CrossRef]

58. Chen, Y.; Liu, J.; Pan, Z.; Shimamoto, S. Non-invasive Blood Glucose Measurement Based on mid-Infrared Spectroscopy. In Proceedings of the 2020 IEEE 17th Annual Consumer Communications & Networking Conference (CCNC), Las Vegas, NV, USA, 10–13 January 2020; pp. 1–5.
59. Koyama, S.; Miyauchi, Y.; Horiguchi, T.; Ishizawa, H. Non-invasive blood glucose measurement based on ATR infrared spectroscopy. In Proceedings of the 2008 SICE Annual Conference, Chofu, Japan, 20–22 August 2008; pp. 321–324.
60. Koyama, S.; Miyauchi, Y.; Horiguchi, T.; Ishizawa, H. Non-invasive measurement of blood glucose of diabetic based on IR spectroscopy. In Proceedings of the SICE Annual Conference, Taipei, Taiwan, 18–21 August 2010; pp. 3425–3426.
61. Morikawa, T.; Saiki, F.; Ishizawa, H.; Toba, E. Noninvasive Measurement of Blood Glucose Based on Optical Sensing and Internal Standard Method. In Proceedings of the IEEE Instrumentation and Measurement Technology Conference Proceedings, Ottawa, ON, Canada, 16–19 May 2005; pp. 1433–1437.
62. Song, K.; Ha, U.; Park, S.; Yoo, H.-J. An impedance and multi-wavelength near-infrared spectroscopy IC for non-invasive blood glucose estimation. *IEEE J.-Solid-State Circuits* **2015**, *50*, 1025–1037. [CrossRef]
63. Dantu, V.; Vempati, J.; Srivilliputhur, S. Non-invasive blood glucose monitor based on spectroscopy using a smartphone. In Proceedings of the 36th Annual International Conference of the IEEE Engineering in Medicine and Biology Society, Chicago, IL, USA, 26–30 August 2014; pp. 3695–3698.
64. Hsieh, H.V.; Pfeiffer, Z.A.; Amiss, T.J.; Sherman, D.B.; Pitner, J.B. Direct detection of glucose by surface plasmon resonance with bacterial glucose/galactose-binding protein. *Biosens. Bioelectron.* **2004**, *19*, 653–660. [CrossRef]
65. Srivastava, S.K.; Arora, V.; Sapra, S.; Gupta, B.D. Localized Surface Plasmon Resonance-Based Fiber Optic U-Shaped Biosensor for the Detection of Blood Glucose. *Plasmonics* **2012**, *7*, 261–268. [CrossRef]
66. Panda, A.; Pukhrambam, P.D.; Keiser, G. Performance analysis of graphene-based surface plasmon resonance biosensor for blood glucose and gas detection. *Appl. Phys.* **2020**, *126*, 153 [CrossRef]
67. Wu, W.; Shen, J.; Li, Y.; Zhu, H.; Banerjee, P.; Zhou, S. Specific glucose-to-SPR signal transduction at physiological pH by molecularly imprinted responsive hybrid microgels. *Biomaterials* **2012**, *33*, 7115–7125. [CrossRef]
68. Pravdin, A.B.; Spivak, V.A.; Yakovlev, D.A. On the possibility of noninvasive polarimetric determination of glucose content in skin. *Opt. Spectrosc.* **2016**, *120*, 45–49. [CrossRef]
69. Jin, Y.; Yin, Y.; Li, C.; Liu, H.; Shi, J. Non-Invasive Monitoring of Human Health by Photoacoustic Spectroscopy. *Sensors* **2022**, *22*, 1155. [CrossRef] [PubMed]
70. Wadamori, N.; Shinohara, R.; Ishihara, Y. Photoacoustic depth profiling of a skin model for non-invasive glucose measurement. In Proceedings of the 30th Annual International Conference of the IEEE Engineering in Medicine and Biology Society, Vancouver, BC, Canada, 20–25 August 2008; pp. 5644–5647.
71. Kulkarni, O.C.; Mandal, P.; Das, S.S.; Banerjee, S. A Feasibility Study on Noninvasive Blood Glucose Measurement Using Photoacoustic Method. In Proceedings of the 4th International Conference on Bioinformatics and Biomedical Engineering, Chengdu, China, 18–20 June 2010; pp. 1–4.
72. Camou, S.; Ueno, Y.; Tamechika, E. Towards non-invasive and continuous monitoring of blood glucose level based on CW photoacoustics: New concept for selective and sensitive measurements of aqueous glucose. In Proceedings of the Fifth International Conference on Sensing Technology, Palmerston North, New Zealand, 28 November–1 December 2011; pp. 193–197.
73. Tanaka, Y.; Tajima, T.; Seyama, M.; Waki, K. Differential Continuous Wave Photoacoustic Spectroscopy for Non-Invasive Glucose Monitoring. *IEEE Sens. J.* **2020**, *20*, 4453–4458. [CrossRef]
74. Shaikh, F.; Haworth, N.; Wells, R.; Bishop, J.; Chatterjee, S.K.; Banerjee, S.; Laha, S. Compact Instrumentation for Accurate Detection and Measurement of Glucose Concentration Using Photoacoustic Spectroscopy. *IEEE Access* **2022**, *10*, 31885–31895. [CrossRef]
75. Pai, P.P.; Sanki, P.K.; Banerjee, S. A photoacoustics based continuous non-invasive blood glucose monitoring system. In Proceedings of the IEEE International Symposium on Medical Measurements and Applications (MeMeA), Turin, Italy, 7–9 May 2015; pp. 106–111.
76. Pai, P.P.; Sanki, P.K.; Sahoo, S.K.; De, A.; Bhattacharya, S.; Banerjee, S. Cloud Computing-Based Non-Invasive Glucose Monitoring for Diabetic Care. *IEEE Trans. Circuits Syst. I Regul. Pap.* **2018**, *65*, 663–676. [CrossRef]
77. Zhao, S.; Tao, W.; He, Q.; Zhao, H. A new approach to non-invasive blood glucose measurement based on 2 dimension photoacoustic spectrum. In Proceedings of the International Conference on Electronics Instrumentation & Information Systems (EIIS), Harbin, China, 3–5 June 2017; pp. 1–5.
78. Priya, B.L.; Jayalakshmy, S.; Bhuvaneshwar, R.; Kumar, J.K. Non—Invasive Blood Glucose Monitoring based on Visible LASER Light. In Proceedings of the 2018 3rd International Conference on Communication and Electronics Systems (ICCES), Coimbatore, India, 15–16 October 2018; pp. 938–941.
79. Ali, H.; Bensaali, F.; Jaber, F. Novel Approach to Non-Invasive Blood Glucose Monitoring based on Transmittance and Refraction of Visible Laser Light. *IEEE Access* **2017**, *5*, 9163–9177. [CrossRef]
80. Naam, H.A.A.; Idrees, M.O.; Awad, A.; Abdalsalam, O.S.; Moham, F. Non invasive blood glucose measurement based on Photo-Acoustic Spectroscopy. In Proceedings of the 2015 International Conference on Computing, Control, Networking, Electronics and Embedded Systems Engineering (ICCNEEE), Khartoum, Sudan, 7–9 September 2015; pp. 1–4.

81. Jahana, T.; Higa, H. Non-Invasive Blood Glucose Monitoring Device Using Photoacoustic Spectroscopy. In Proceedings of the 5th International Conference on Intelligent Informatics and Biomedical Sciences (ICIIBMS), Okinawa, Japan, 18–20 November 2020; pp. 85–88.
82. Allen, T.J.; Beard, P.C. High power visible light emitting diodes as pulsed excitation sources for biomedical photoacoustics. *Biomed. Opt. Express* **2016**, *7*, 1260–1270. [CrossRef]
83. Zhu, Y.; Xu, G.; Yuan, J.; Jo, J.; Gandikota, G.; Demirci, H.; Agano, T.; Sato, N.; Shigeta, Y.; Wang, X. Light Emitting Diodes based Photoacoustic Imaging and Potential Clinical Applications. *Nat. Sci. Rep.* **2018**, *8*, 1–12 [CrossRef]
84. Turgul, V.; Kale, I. Simulating the Effects of Skin Thickness and Fingerprints to Highlight Problems With Non-Invasive RF Blood Glucose Sensing From Fingertips. *IEEE Sens. J.* **2017**, *17*, 7553–7560. [CrossRef]
85. Choi, H.; Nylon, J.; Luzio, S.; Beutler, J.; Porch, A. Design of continuous non-invasive blood glucose monitoring sensor based on a microwave split ring resonator. In Proceedings of the IEEE MTT-S International Microwave Workshop Series on RF and Wireless Technologies for Biomedical and Healthcare Applications, London, UK, 8–10 December 2014; pp. 1–3.
86. Schwerthoeffer, U.; Weigel, R.; Kissinger, D. Highly sensitive microwave resonant near-field sensor for precise aqueous glucose detection in microfluidic medical applications. In Proceedings of the IEEE International Instrumentation and Measurement Technology Conference Proceedings, Montevideo, Uruguay, 12–15 May 2014; pp. 919–922.
87. Cebedio, M.C.; Rabioglio, L.A.; Gelosi, I.E.; Ribas, R.A.; Uriz, A.J.; Moreira, J.C. Analysis and Design of a Microwave Coplanar Sensor for Non-Invasive Blood Glucose Measurements. *IEEE Sens. J.* **2020**, *20*, 10572–1058. [CrossRef]
88. Oloyo, A.A.; Hu, Z. A highly sensitive microwave resonator for non-invasive blood glucose level detection. In Proceedings of the IEEE European Conference on Antennas and Propagation (EuCAP 2018), London, UK, 9–13 April 2018; pp. 1–5.
89. Qin, K.; He, Y.; Pei, Y.; Cai, X.; Luo, Y. A Microwave Biosensor for Non-invasive Blood Glucose Detection with Accuracy Enhancement. In Proceedings of the International Applied Computational Electromagnetics Society Symposium, Nanjing, China, 8–11 August 2019; pp. 1–2.
90. Omer, A.E.; Shaker, G.; Safavi-Naeini, S.; Alquié, G.; Deshours, F.; Kokabi, H.; Shubair, R.M. Non-Invasive Real-Time Monitoring of Glucose Level Using Novel Microwave Biosensor Based on Triple-Pole CSRR. *IEEE Trans. Biomed. Circuits Syst.* **2020**, *14*, 1407–1420. [CrossRef] [PubMed]
91. Morshidi, W.H.W.; Zaharudin, Z.; Khan, S.; Nordin, A.N.; Shaikh, F.A.; Adam, I.; Kader, K.A. Inter-digital sensor for non-invasive blood glucose monitoring. In Proceedings of the IEEE International Conference on Innovative Research and Development (ICIRD), Bangkok, Thailand, 11–12 May 2018; pp. 1–6.
92. Xiao, X.; Li, Q. A Noninvasive Measurement of Blood Glucose Concentration by UWB Microwave Spectrum. *IEEE Antennas Wirel. Propag. Lett.* **2017**, *16*, 1040–1043. [CrossRef]
93. Zhou, Y.; Qing, X.; See, T.S.P.; Chin, F.; Karim, M.F. Transmission characterization of glucose solutions at Ku-band for non-invasive glucose monitoring. In Proceedings of the Progress in Electromagnetics Research Symposium, Singapore, 19–22 November 2017; pp. 2925–2928.
94. Hofmann, M.; Fischer, G.; Weigel, R.; Kissinger, D. Microwave-Based Noninvasive Concentration Measurements for Biomedical Applications. *IEEE Trans. Microw. Theory Tech.* **2013**, *61*, 2195–2204. [CrossRef]
95. Paul, B.; Manuel, M.P.; Alex, Z.C. Design and development of non invasive blood glucose measurement system. In Proceedings of the Physics and Technology of Sensors International Symposium (ISPTS), Pune, India, 7–10 March 2012; pp. 43–46.
96. Choi, H.; Naylon, J.; Luzio, S.; Beutler, J.; Birchall, J.; Martin, C.; Porch, A. Design and In Vitro Interference Test of Microwave Noninvasive Blood Glucose Monitoring Sensor. *IEEE Trans. Microw. Theory Tech.* **2015**, *63*, 3016–3025. [CrossRef]
97. Hofmann, M.; Fersch, T.; Weigel, R.; Fischer, G.; Kissinger, D. A novel approach to non-invasive blood glucose measurement based on RF transmission. In Proceedings of the IEEE International Symposium on Medical Measurements and Applications, Bari, Italy, 30–31 May 2011; pp. 39–42.
98. Satish, K.S.; Anand, S. Design of microstrip sensor for non invasive blood glucose monitoring. In Proceedings of the International Conference on Emerging Trends & Innovation in ICT (ICEI), Pune, India, 3–5 February 2017; pp. 5–8.
99. Jiang, F.; Li, S.; Yu, Y.; Cheng, Q.S.; Koziel, S. Sensitivity optimization of antenna for non-invasive blood glucose monitoring. In Proceedings of the International Applied Computational Electromagnetics Society Symposium (ACES), Suzhou, China, 1–4 August 2017; pp. 1–2.
100. Buford, R.J.; Green, E.C.; McClung, M.J. A microwave frequency sensor for non-invasive blood-glucose measurement. In Proceedings of the IEEE Sensors Applications Symposium, Atlanta, GA, USA, 12–14 February 2008; pp. 4–7.
101. Baghbani, R.; Ashoorirad, M.; Pourziad, A. Microwave sensor for noninvasive glucose measurements design and implementation of a novel linear. *IET Wirel. Sens. Syst.* **2015**, *5*, 51–57. [CrossRef]
102. Freer, B.; Venkataraman, J. Feasibility study for non-invasive blood glucose monitoring. In Proceedings of the IEEE Antennas and Propagation Society International Symposium, Toronto, ON, Canada, 11–17 July 2010; pp. 1–4.
103. Zeising, S.; Kirchner, J.; Khalili, H.F.; Ahmed, D.; Lübke, M.; Thalmayer, A.; Fischer, G. Towards Realisation of a Non-Invasive Blood Glucose Sensor Using Microstripline. In Proceedings of the IEEE International Instrumentation and Measurement Technology Conference (I2MTC), Dubrovnik, Croatia, 25–28 May 2020; pp. 1–6.
104. Raj, S.; Kishore, N.; Upadhyay, G.; Tripathi, S.; Tripathi, V.S. A Novel Design of CSRR Loaded Truncated Patch Antenna for Non-Invasive Blood Glucose Monitoring System. In Proceedings of the 2018 IEEE MTT-S International Microwave and RF Conference (IMaRC), Kolkata, India, 28–30 November 2018; pp. 1–4.

105. Gouzouasis, I.; Cano-Garcia, H.; Sotiriou, I.; Saha, S.; Palikaras, G.; Kosmas, P.; Kallos, E. Detection of varying glucose concentrations in water solutions using a prototype biomedical device for millimeter-wave non-invasive glucose sensing. In Proceedings of the 10th European Conference on Antennas and Propagation (EuCAP), Davos, Switzerland, 10–15 April 2016; pp. 1–4.
106. Saha, S.; Cano-Garcia, H.; Sotiriou, I.; Lipscombe, O.; Gouzouasis, I.; Koutsoupidou, M.; Palikaras, G.; Mackenzie, R.; Reeve, T.; Kosmas, P.; et al. A Glucose Sensing System Based on Transmission Measurements at Millimetre Waves using Micro strip Patch Antennas. *Nat. Sci. Rep.* **2017**, *7*, 6855. [CrossRef] [PubMed]
107. Sreenivas, C.; Laha, S. Compact Continuous Non-Invasive Blood Glucose Monitoring using Bluetooth. In Proceedings of the IEEE Biomedical Circuits and Systems Conference (BioCAS), Nara, Japan, 17–19 October 2019; pp. 1–4.
108. Pullano, S.A.; Greco, M.; Bianco, M.G.; Foti, D.; Brunetti, A.; Fiorillo, A.S. Glucose biosensors in clinical practice: Principles, limits and perspectives of currently used devices. *Theranostics* **2022**, *12*, 493. [CrossRef]
109. Lee, H.; Hong, Y.J.; Baik, S.; Hyeon, T.; Kim, D.H. Enzyme-based glucose sensor: From invasive to wearable device. *Adv. Healthc. Mater.* **2018**, *7*, 1–14. [CrossRef]
110. Wang, T.-T.; Huang, X.-F.; Huang, H.; Luo, P.; Qing, L.-S. Nanomaterial based optical and electrochemical-biosensors for urine glucose detection: A comprehensive review. *Adv. Sens. Energy Mater.* **2022**, *1*, 1–14 [CrossRef]
111. Su, L.; Feng, J.; Zhou, X.; Ren, C.; Li, H.; Chen, X. Colorimetric detection of urine glucose based ZnFe2O4 magnetic nanoparticles. *Anal. Chem.* **2012**, *84*, 5753–5758. [CrossRef]
112. Lin, W.J.; Lin, Y.S.; Chang, H.T.; Unnikrishnan, B.; Huang, C.C. Electrocatalytic CuBr@CuO nanoparticles based salivary glucose probes. *Biosens. Bioelectron.* **2021**, *194*, 113610. [CrossRef] [PubMed]
113. Chung, M.; Fortunato, G.; Radacsi, N. Wearable flexible sweat sensors for healthcare monitoring: A review. *R. Soc. Interface* **2019**, *16*, 20190217. [CrossRef] [PubMed]
114. Cheon, H.J.; Adhikari, M.D.; Chung, M.; Tran, T.D.; Kim, J.; Kim, M.I. Magnetic Nanoparticles-Embedded Enzyme-Inorganic Hybrid Nanoflowers with Enhanced Peroxidase-Like Activity and Substrate Channeling for Glucose Biosensing. *Adv. Healthc. Mater.* **2019**, *8*, 1801507. [CrossRef] [PubMed]
115. Wei, H.; Wang, E. Fe$_3$O$_4$ magnetic nanoparticles as peroxidase mimetics and their applications in H$_2$O$_2$ and glucose detection. *Anal. Chem.* **2008**, *80*, 2250–2254. [CrossRef]
116. Mu, J.; Wang, Y.; Zhao, M.; Zhang, L. Intrinsic peroxidase-like activity and catalase-like activity of Co$_3$O$_4$ nanoparticles. *Chem. Commun.* **2012**, *48*, 2540–2542. [CrossRef]
117. Asati, A.; Santra, S.; Kaittanis, C.; Nath, S.; Perez, J.M. Oxidase-like activity of polymer-coated cerium oxide nanoparticles. *Angew. Chem. Int. Ed. Engl.* **2009**, *121*, 2344–2348. [CrossRef]
118. Wu, N.; Wang, Y.-T.; Wang, X.-Y.; Guo, F.-N.; Wen, H.; Yang, T.; Wang, J.-H. Enhanced peroxidase-like activity of AuNPs loaded graphitic carbon nitride nanosheets for colorimetric biosensing. *Anal. Chim. Acta* **2019**, *1091*, 69–75. [CrossRef]
119. Vivekananth, R.; Babu, R.S.; Prasanna, K.; Lee, C.W.; Kalaivani, R.A. Non-enzymatic glucose sensing platform using self assembled cobalt oxide/graphene nanocomposites immobilized graphite modified electrode. *J. Mater. Sci. Mater. Electron.* **2018**, *29*, 6763–6770. [CrossRef]
120. Mitsumori, M.; Yamaguchi, M.; Kano, Y. A new approach to noninvasive measurement of blood glucose using saliva analyzing system. In Proceedings of the Annual International Conference of the IEEE Engineering in Medicine and Biology Society, Hong Kong, China, 1 November 1998; pp. 1767–1770.
121. Yamaguchi, M.; Mitsumori, M.; Kano, Y. Development of noninvasive procedure for monitoring blood glucose levels using saliva. In Proceedings of the Annual International Conference of the IEEE Engineering in Medicine and Biology Society, Hong Kong, China, 1 November 1998; pp. 1763–1766.
122. Chakraborty, P.; Dhar, S.; Deka, N.; Debnath, K.; Mondal, S.P. Non-enzymatic salivary glucose detection using porous CuO nanostructures. *Sens. Actuators B Chem.* **2020**, *302*, 1–7. [CrossRef]
123. Chakraborty, P.; Deka, N.; Patra, D.C.; Debnath, K.; Mondal, S.P. Salivary glucose sensing using highly sensitive and selective non-enzymatic porous NiO nanostructured electrodes. *Surf. Interfaces* **2021**, *26*, 101324. [CrossRef]
124. Gao, W.; Zhou, X.; Heinig, N.F.; Thomas, J.P.; Zhang, L.; Leung, K.T. Nonenzymatic Saliva-Range Glucose Sensing Using Electrodeposited Cuprous Oxide Nanocubes on a Graphene Strip. *ACS Appl. Nano Mater.* **2021**, *4*, 4790–4799. [CrossRef]
125. Chakraborty, P.; Dhar, S.; Debnath, K.; Majumder, T.; Mondal, S.P. Non-enzymatic and non-invasive glucose detection using Au nanoparticle decorated CuO nanorods. *Sens. Actuators B Chem.* **2019**, *283*, 776–785. [CrossRef]
126. Wang, J.; Xu, L.; Lu, Y.; Sheng, K.; Liu, W.; Chen, C.; Li, Y.; Dong, B.; Song, H. Engineered IrO$_2$@NiO core–shell nanowires for sensitive non-enzymatic detection of trace glucose in saliva. *Anal. Chem.* **2016**, *88*, 12346–12353. [CrossRef]
127. Wang, C.; Yang, X.; Zhu, G.; Wang, T.; Yu, D.; Yu, H. One-Step Synthesis of Copper-Platinum Nanoparticles Modified Electrode for Non-Enzymatic Salivary Glucose Detection. Available online: https://ssrn.com/abstract=4164980 (accessed on 20 August 2022).
128. Alam, F.; Jalal, A.H.; Forouzanfar, S.; Karabiyik, M.; Rabiei Baboukani, A.; Pala, N. Flexible and Linker-Free Enzymatic Sensors Based on Zinc Oxide Nanoflakes for Noninvasive L-Lactate Sensing in Sweat. *IEEE Sens. J.* **2020**, *20*, 5102–5109. [CrossRef]
129. Lin, K.-C.; Muthukumar, S.; Prasad, S. Flex-GO (Flexible graphene oxide) sensor for electrochemical monitoring lactate in low-volume passive perspired human sweat. *Talanta* **2020**, *214*, 120810. [CrossRef] [PubMed]
130. Zhou, L. Molecularly Imprinted Sensor based on Ag-Au NPs/SPCE for Lactate Determination in Sweat for Healthcare and Sport Monitoring. *Int. J. Electrochem. Sci.* **2021**, *16*, 2. [CrossRef]

131. Zhang, Q.; Jiang, D.; Xu, C.; Ge, Y.; Liu, X.; Wei, Q.; Huang, L.; Ren, X.; Wang, C.; Wang, Y. Wearable electrochemical biosensor based on molecularly imprinted Ag nanowires for noninvasive monitoring lactate in human sweat. *Sens. Actuators B Chem.* **2020**, *320*, 128325. [CrossRef]
132. Jia, W.; Bandodkar, A.J.; Valdés-Ramírez, G.; Windmiller, J.R.; Yang, Z.; Ramírez, J.; Chan, G.; Wang, J. Electrochemical tattoo biosensors for real-time noninvasive lactate monitoring in human perspiration. *Anal. Chem.* **2013**, *85*, 6553–6560. [CrossRef]
133. Abrar, M.A.; Dong, Y.; Lee, P.K.; Kim, W.S. Bendable Electro-chemical Lactate Sensor Printed with Silver Nano-particles. *Nat. Sci. Rep.* **2016**, *6*, 30565. [CrossRef]
134. Anderson, K.; Poulter, B.; Dudgeon, J.; Li, S.E.; Ma, X.A. A highly sensitive nonenzymatic glucose biosensor based on the regulatory effect of glucose on electrochemical behaviors of colloidal silver nanoparticles on MoS_2. *Sensors* **2017**, *17*, 1807. [CrossRef]
135. Kim, S.; Jeon, H.J.; Park, S.; Lee, D.Y.; Chung, E. Tear glucose measurement by reflectance spectrum of a nanoparticle embedded contact lens. *Nat. Sci. Rep.* **2020**, *10*, 1–8. [CrossRef] [PubMed]
136. Kheirabadi, Z.A.; Rabbani, M.; Foroushani, M.S. Green Fabrication of Nonenzymatic Glucose Sensor Using Multi-Walled Carbon Nanotubes Decorated with Copper (II) Oxide Nanoparticles for Tear Fluid Analysis. *Appl. Biochem. Biotechnol.* **2022**, *194*, 3689–3705. [CrossRef] [PubMed]
137. Cui, X.; Li, J.; Li, Y.; Liu, M.; Qiao, J.; Wang, D.; Cao, H.; He, W.; Feng, Y.; Yang, Z. Detection of glucose in diabetic tears by using gold nanoparticles and MXene composite surface-enhanced Raman scattering substrates. *Spectrochim. Acta Part A Mol. Biomol. Spectrosc.* **2022**, *266*, 120432. [CrossRef] [PubMed]
138. Jeon, H.J.; Kim, S.; Park, S.; Jeong, I.K.; Kang, J.; Kim, Y.R.; Lee, D.Y.; Chung, E. Optical Assessment of Tear Glucose by Smart Biosensor Based on Nanoparticle Embedded Contact Lens. *Nano Lett.* **2021**, *21*, 8933–8940. [CrossRef]
139. Lee, W.C.; Koh, E.H.; Kim, D.H.; Park, S.G.; Jung, H.S. Plasmonic contact lens materials for glucose sensing in human tears. *Sens. Actuators B Chem.* **2021**, *344*, 130297. [CrossRef]
140. Noviosense. Available online: https://noviosense.com/noviosense/ (accessed on 19 August 2022).
141. Makvandi, P.; Wang, C.; Zare, E.N.; Borzacchiello, A.; Niu, L.; Tay, F.R. Metal-based nanomaterials in biomedical applications: Antimicrobial activity and cytotoxicity aspects. *Adv. Funct. Mater.* **2020**, *30*, 1910021. [CrossRef]
142. Laha, S.S.; Thorat, N.D.; Singh, G.; Sathish, C.I.; Yi, J.; Dixit, A.; Vinu, A. Rare-Earth Doped Iron Oxide Nanostructures for Cancer Theranostics: Magnetic Hyperthermia and Magnetic Resonance Imaging. *Small* **2022**, *18*, 2104855. [CrossRef]
143. Park, W.; Shin, H.; Choi, B.; Rhim, W.-K.; Na, K.; Han, D.K. Advanced hybrid nanomaterials for biomedical applications. *Prog. Mater. Sci.* **2020**, *114*, 100686.
144. Kalaiselvan, C.R.; Laha, S.S.; Somvanshi, S.B.; Tabish, T.A.; Thorat, N.D.; Sahu, N.K. Manganese ferrite ($MnFe_2O_4$) nanostructures for cancer theranostics. *Coord. Chem. Rev.* **2022**, *473*, 1262–1268. [CrossRef]
145. Laha, S.S.; Naik, A.R.; Kuhn, E.R.; Alvarez, M.; Sujkowski, A.; Wessells, R.J.; Jena, B.P. Nanothermometry measure of muscle efficiency. *Nano Lett.* **2017**, *17*, 214809. [CrossRef]
146. Song, Y.; Qu, K.; Zhao, C.; Ren, J.; Qu, X. Graphene oxide: intrinsic peroxidase catalytic activity and its application to glucose detection. *Adv. Mater.* **2010**, *19*, 2206–2210. [CrossRef] [PubMed]
147. Cui, R.; Han, Z.; Zhu, J.J. Helical carbon nanotubes: Intrinsic peroxidase catalytic activity and its application for biocatalysis and biosensing. *Chem. Eur. J.* **2011**, *17*, 9377–9384. [CrossRef] [PubMed]
148. Wu, K.; Li, J.; Zhang, C. Zinc ferrite based gas sensors: A review. *Ceram. Int.* **2019**, *45*, 11143–11157. [CrossRef]
149. Sakhuja, N.; Jha, R.; Laha, S.S.; Rao, A.; Bhat, N. Fe_3O_4 Nanoparticle-Decorated WSe_2 Nanosheets for Selective Chemiresistive Detection of Gaseous Ammonia at Room Temperature. *ACS Appl. Nano Mater.* **2020**, *3*, 11160–11171. [CrossRef]
150. Luaibi, A.Y.; Al-Ghusain, A.J.; Rahman, A.; Al-Sayah, M.H.; Al-Nashash, H.A. Noninvasive blood glucose level measurement using nuclear magnetic resonance. In Proceedings of the Noninvasive blood glucose level measurement using nuclear magnetic resonance, Muscat, Oman, 1–4 February 2015; pp. 1–4.
151. Albalat, A.L.; Alaman, M.B.S.; Diez, M.C.D.; Martinez-Millana, A.; Salcedo, V.T. Non-Invasive Blood Glucose Sensor: A Feasibility Study. In Proceedings of the Annual International Conference of the IEEE Engineering in Medicine and Biology Society (EMBC), Berlin, Germany, 3–6 November 2019; pp. 1179–1182.
152. Nanayakkara, N.D.; Munasingha, S.C.; Ruwanpathirana, G.P. Non-Invasive Blood Glucose Monitoring using a Hybrid Technique. In Proceedings of the Moratuwa Engineering Research Conference (MERCon), Moratuwa, Sri Lanka, 30 May–1 June 2018; pp. 7–12.
153. Periyasamy, R.; Anand, S. A study on non-invasive blood glucose estimation—An approach using capacitance measurement technique. In Proceedings of the International Conference on Signal Processing, Communication, Power and Embedded System (SCOPES), Paralakhemundi, India, 3–5 October 2016; pp. 847–850.
154. Dutta, A.; Chandra Bera, S.; Das, K. A non-invasive microcontroller based estimation of blood glucose concentration by using a modified capacitive sensor at low frequency. *AIP Adv.* **2019**, *9*, 105027. [CrossRef]
155. Suseela, S.; Wahid, P. Non Invasive Monitoring of Blood Glucose Using Saliva as a Diagnostic Fluid. In Proceedings of the Southeast Conference, St. Petersburg, FL, USA, 19–22 April 2018; pp. 1–3.

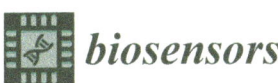

Article

In Silico Investigation of SNR and Dermis Sensitivity for Optimum Dual-Channel Near-Infrared Glucose Sensor Designs for Different Skin Colors

Murad Althobaiti

Biomedical Engineering Department, College of Engineering, Imam Abdulrahman Bin Faisal University, Dammam 31441, Saudi Arabia; mmalthobaiti@iau.edu.sa

Abstract: Diabetes is a serious health condition that requires patients to regularly monitor their blood glucose level, making the development of practical, compact, and non-invasive techniques essential. Optical glucose sensors—and, specifically, NIR sensors—have the advantages of being non-invasive, compact, inexpensive, and user-friendly devices. However, these sensors have low accuracy and are yet to be adopted by healthcare providers. In our previous work, we introduced a non-invasive dual-channel technique for NIR sensors, in which a long channel is utilized to measure the glucose level in the inner skin (dermis) layer, while a short channel is used to measure the noise signal of the superficial skin (epidermis) layer. In this work, we investigated the use of dual-NIR channels for patients with different skin colors (i.e., having different melanin concentrations). We also adopted a Monte Carlo simulation model that takes into consideration the differences between different skin layers, in terms of blood content, water content, melanin concentration in the epidermis layer, and skin optical proprieties. On the basis of the signal-to-noise ratio, as well as the sensitivities of both the epidermis and dermis layers, we suggest the selection of wavelengths and source-to-detector separation for optimal NIR channels under different skin melanin concentrations. This work facilitates the improved design of a compact and non-invasive NIR glucose sensor that can be utilized by patients with different skin colors.

Keywords: bioinstrumentation; dual-channel; glucose; near-infrared; NIR technology; sensors

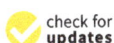

Citation: Althobaiti, M. In Silico Investigation of SNR and Dermis Sensitivity for Optimum Dual-Channel Near-Infrared Glucose Sensor Designs for Different Skin Colors. *Biosensors* **2022**, *12*, 805. https://doi.org/10.3390/bios 12100805

Received: 21 August 2022
Accepted: 26 September 2022
Published: 29 September 2022

Publisher's Note: MDPI stays neutral with regard to jurisdictional claims in published maps and institutional affiliations.

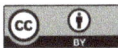

Copyright: © 2022 by the author. Licensee MDPI, Basel, Switzerland. This article is an open access article distributed under the terms and conditions of the Creative Commons Attribution (CC BY) license (https:// creativecommons.org/licenses/by/ 4.0/).

1. Introduction

Diabetes is a long-lasting health condition that impacts the process of turning food into energy in the human body, commonly known as metabolism. Over time, diabetes can lead to serious health issues, such as heart disease, kidney disease, and vision loss. Therefore, the regular monitoring of blood glucose levels is vital for diabetic patients. Over the past few years, scientists and engineers have developed practical invasive and non-invasive techniques that allow patients to regularly monitor their blood glucose level. Invasive electrochemical sensors are considered to be the gold standard for measuring blood glucose [1]. The review article [2] comprehensively investigated recent advancements in non-invasive blood glucose sensors that are optical, electrochemical, and microwave-based sensors. Non-invasive microwave blood glucose sensors have attracted the attention of many researchers due to their high skin penetration depth and low cost. Nevertheless, the sensitivity of microwave-based sensors still needs to be improved to be clinically accepted [2]. Non-invasive electrochemical reaction techniques are currently available, but their accuracy and lifetime are limited [3–5]. Moreover, continuous glucose monitoring (CGM) electrochemical devices are currently in use. CGM devices are minimally invasive techniques based on an implanted needle [6,7]. The article [8] identified 34 non-invasive and 31 minimally invasive glucose monitoring products, and it reviewed their regulatory, technological, and consumer features.

Optical glucose measurement devices are emerging and promising techniques. These techniques have the advantages of being non-invasive, compact, and user-friendly devices [9,10]. Photoacoustic spectroscopy [11], optical coherence tomography [12,13], Raman spectroscopy [14], and near-infrared (NIR) technology are all non-invasive optical techniques that have been investigated for the measurement of glucose. One study [10] reviewed the recent developments of different optical techniques, and their features and limitations were also highlighted. NIR techniques are the most-used and -studied optical techniques, due to their compactness and low cost. They contain three main parts—an NIR source, a tissue sample, and a photodiode—to detect the scattered or attenuated transmitted NIR light. NIR spectroscopy has been utilized in many medical applications, such as neuroimaging [15,16], the detection of breast cancer [17–19], and for blood glucose measurements and monitoring [20–22].

There have been great efforts in the scientific community to tackle the complexity of skin optical measurements. Notably, the article [23] studied the effect of changing the glucose concentration on light transport using a Monte Carlo simulation model. It is evident that, with a single wavelength approach, there is a potential challenge to measure glucose concentration due to the optical complexity of the skin. Another study [24] proposed an optical probe model with two concentric rings to measure the reflected optical signals at two different positions. This allowed estimating the variations in skin optical properties by variations in the blood glucose level. The authors of [25] proposed a technique using Monte Carlo simulation to reduce glucose prediction errors produced by temperature and scattering variations. The authors found that small changes in the temperature or volume fraction of the scattering particle would lead to large glucose prediction errors.

In a previous study [26], we introduced an optimized NIR sensor with two channels for blood glucose measurements. The long channel is utilized to measure the glucose level in the inner skin (dermis) layer. This measured signal carries important information regarding the glucose content. The short channel is used to estimate the interference noise arising from the superficial skin (epidermis) layer. Thus, the long channel signal can be used to determine the glucose content in the dermis layer, and the short channel signal can then be eliminated from the long channel signal. The dual-channel NIR sensor approach uses two sources with different wavelengths. The two wavelengths of the two sources and source–detector separation (SDS) were determined on the basis of a Monte Carlo simulation (MCS) model. The module was specifically investigated for the NIR wavelength range between 1200 and 1900 nm. However, this model does not consider the detailed anatomical features of skin layers, such as blood, water, and melanin concentrations. These parameters are important to consider specifically when investigating the diagnostic window of the NIR spectrum, which ranges between 450 and 1000 nm [16,27,28].

In this manuscript, we systematically studied the effect of the diagnostic window of the NIR wavelength spectrum, the effect of different skin colors (i.e., different skin melanin concentrations), and the source-to-detector separation (SDS) of these wavelength ranges on the optimal selection of the short and long NIR channels. In addition, an improved and more detailed skin model [29–32] was adopted for Monte Carlo simulation (MCS). This model takes into consideration the differences between different skin layers, in terms of the blood volume fraction, water volume fraction, melanin concentrations in the epidermis layer, and optical skin proprieties. The absorption of this NIR range (from 450 to 1050 nm) by the melanin of the epidermis layer and by different dermis layers differs. Therefore, we expect the optimal selections of the short and long NIR channels to be different for different wavelengths and for different skin colors.

2. Methods

Monte Carlo Skin Model

The Monte Carlo simulation (MCS) method was used in this study, which was described in [33,34]. The light source was modeled as a pencil beam light towards the z-direction. A detector with a radius of 2 mm is located at a distance from the source as shown in Figure 1. The photons detection replay mode described in the paper [35] was utilized. In brief, the method, initiated by launching millions of photons (here, 100 million) and the propagation of any launched photon in the skin layers, is calculated on the basis of the optical properties of the tissues.

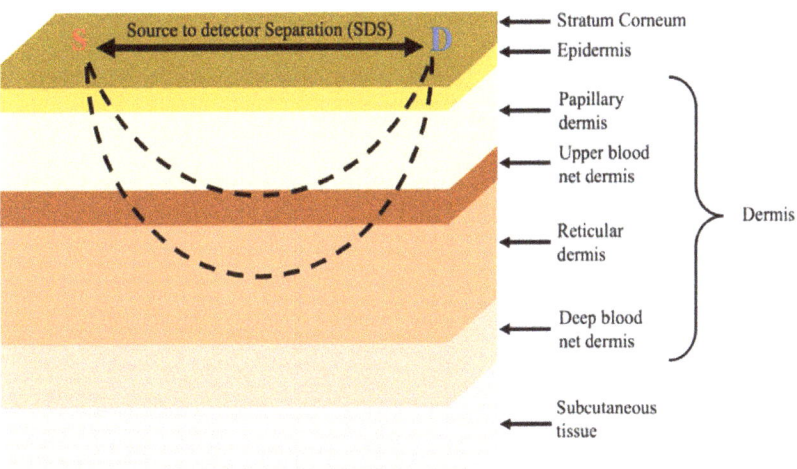

Figure 1. Schematic drawing of the skin model for Monte Carlo simulation. The light propagation distribution, having a "banana shape", is illustrated by the dashed lines between the source (S) and the detector (D).

The skin media are represented as a 3D volume, and each section in the volume is labeled to represent a specific layer of the skin. Therefore, the location of each voxel in the skin layers is pre-identified. At the reflection interface, the reflection coefficient is calculated based on Fresnel's equation. The coefficient is then multiplied by the photon packet weight. For more details, the reader is referred to [33,34]. The history of each propagated photon is tracked with prior knowledge of the optical properties of different skin layers. In the MCS of the tissue, we considered the absorption coefficient (μ_a), scattering coefficient (μ_s), and refractive index (n) of each skin layer. These optical properties are all wavelength-dependent. As a photon travels deeper into the tissue, it loses its energy, which results in a low signal-to-noise ratio (SNR) at the detector side Therefore, with a long SDS, one can measure deeper layers; however, this requires a highly sensitive detector to measure signals with a low SNR. On the other hand, with a short SDS, one can detect photons that are scattered from superficial layers with a good SNR. Therefore, the choice of both the operating source wavelength and the optimal SDS is critical in the design of both the long and short channels for NIR glucose sensors.

For this study, a skin model was built to mimic the propagation of light photons in the NIR diagnostic window, which ranges from 450 to 1050 nm, with an increment of 100 nm. It is also worth noting that, when choosing the operating source wavelengths, [36] was considered for spectral glucose absorptivity. The spectral range 450–1050 nm, known as the "diagnostic window", has attracted the interest of researchers for many different diagnostic applications because water absorption is at its minimum [10,16]. This allows light to penetrate deeper into the tissue. In [36], the authors showed the wavelength-dependent absorptivity of glucose in an aqueous solution and a glassy state. This range is less sensitive for temperature changes on the absorptivity of glucose in comparison to longer wavelengths (>1200 nm).

The anatomical skin model consisted of seven layers, where the layers were optically inhomogeneous. The different skin layers are illustrated in Figure 1.

In this model, according to [29], the absorption coefficients for each dermis layer were calculated considering the differences of important anatomical parameters between different layers:

$$\mu_a^{layer}(\lambda) = (1-S)\gamma V_{blood}\mu_a^{Hb}(\lambda) + S\gamma V_{blood}\mu_a^{HbO_2}(\lambda) + (1-\gamma V_{blood})V_{H_2O}\mu_a^{H_2O}(\lambda) \\ + (1-\gamma V_{blood})(1-V_{H_2O})\mu_a^{other}(\lambda), \quad (1)$$

where V_{blood} and V_{H_2O} are the blood and water volume fractions, respectively; $\mu_a^{H_2O}$, μ_a^{Hb}, and $\mu_a^{HbO_2}$ are the absorption coefficients for water, deoxyhemoglobin, and oxyhemoglobin, respectively; γ is calculated on the basis of the assumption that hemoglobin is only contained in the erythrocytes, which is zero for the stratum corneum and epidermis layers and 0.1 for the dermis layers [29]; μ_a^{other} is the calculated absorption coefficient for hemoglobin-free tissue, which can be estimated as follows [29,37]:

$$\mu_a^{other}(\lambda) = 7.84 \times 10^7 \times \lambda^{-3.25}. \quad (2)$$

According to [29,31], the absorption coefficients (μ_a) for the stratum corneum and the epidermis layers are calculated as follows:

$$\mu_a^{Stratum}(\lambda) = \left(0.1 - 8.3 \times 10^{-4} \times \lambda\right) + 0.125 \times \mu_a^{other}(\lambda), \quad (3)$$

$$\mu_a^{epidermis}(\lambda) = V_{mel}\mu_a^{mel}(\lambda) + V_{H_2O}\mu_a^{HbO_2}(\lambda) + \left(1 - (V_{mel} + V_{H_2O})\right)\mu_a^{other}(\lambda), \quad (4)$$

where μ_a^{mel} is the melanin absorption coefficient, estimated as

$$\mu_a^{mel}(\lambda) = 6.6 \times 10^{10} \times \lambda^{-3.33}. \quad (5)$$

According to the values reported in [38,39] for melanosome volume concentrations (V_{mel}) in the epidermis layer for people having different skin colors, V_{mel} ranges between 1% and 3% for light-skinned Caucasians, from 11% to 16% for Mediterranean people, and from 18% to 43% for darkly pigmented Africans. In this study, we used values of 2%, 10%, 20%, and 30% to study the effect of the melanin concentration on the optimal selection of the NIR channels.

Table 1 summarizes the values utilized in Equation (1) for the estimation of the absorption coefficients of the various skin layers. The values of other optical properties utilized in this model, including the scattering coefficients μ_s and the absorption coefficients for water ($\mu_a^{H_2O}$), deoxyhemoglobin (μ_a^{Hb}), and oxyhemoglobin ($\mu_a^{HbO_2}$), are illustrated in Figure 2. The refractive index values used in this model are 1 for air and 1.4 for tissue [31].

Table 1. Values utilized in Equation (1) for the estimation of the absorption coefficients. The values were taken from [31].

Skin Layer	V_{blood}	V_{H_2O}	Thickness (mm)
Stratum corneum	0	0.05	0.02 mm
Epidermis	0	0.2	0.25 mm
Papillary dermis	0.04	0.5	0.1 mm
Upper blood net dermis	0.3	0.6	0.08 mm
Reticular dermis	0.04	0.7	0.2 mm
Deep blood net dermis	0.1	0.7	0.3 mm
Subcutaneous tissue	0.05	0.7	2 mm

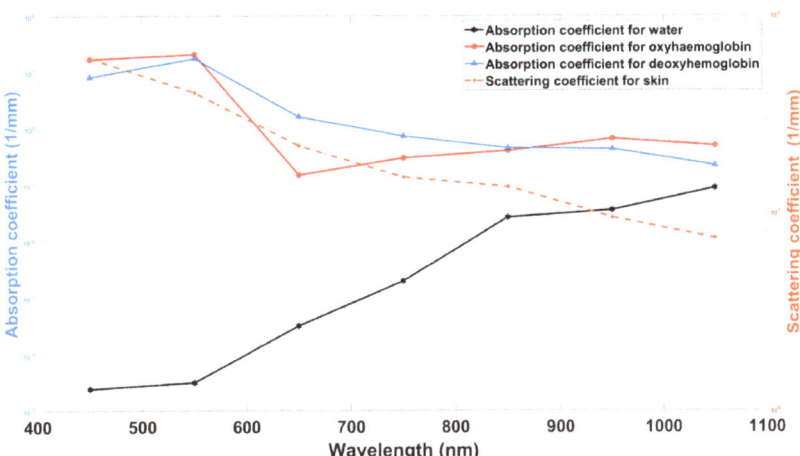

Figure 2. Other optical properties values in the utilized in MCS model: scattering coefficients μ_s and absorption coefficients for water ($\mu_a^{H_2O}$), deoxyhemoglobin (μ_a^{Hb}), and oxyhemoglobin ($\mu_a^{HbO_2}$) [27,31,38].

To systematically assess the performance when changing the wavelength and the SDS in order to choose the optimal NIR channel for measuring glucose content, we previously introduced [26] three metrics. Briefly, the first metric is the epidermis sensitivity, which is the summation of the photon density function (PMDF) for all voxels in the epidermis layer over the summation of all photon density functions (PMDF) in the model:

$$ES = 100 \times \frac{\sum_{Epidermis} PMDF}{\sum_{total} PMDF} \quad (6)$$

The PMDF is computed by taking the voxelwise product of the fluence distribution of the source and the fluence distribution of the detector; details on the computation of the PMDF can be found in [40]. The second metric is the dermis sensitivity, which is calculated similarly to that for the epidermis, as follows:

$$DS = 100 \times \frac{\sum_{Dermis} PMDF}{\sum_{total} PMDF} \quad (7)$$

These metrics can provide an indication of how sensitive a particular NIR channel (with a specific wavelength and SDS) is to the epidermis and the dermis layers, respectively.

The third metric involves the calculation of the SNR for each NIR channel. As the SDS increases, light penetrates deeper into the tissue, i.e., the dermis layer, but the SNR decreases. Therefore, there is a tradeoff between a good SNR and a high depth of light penetration into the tissue. Thus, a balance between high dermis sensitivity and an acceptable SNR should be carefully considered.

By running the MCS for multiple independent seeded simulations, one can calculate the mean (μ) and standard deviation (σ) at each voxel in the model. Thus, one can calculate the SNR (in decibels) as follows [26]:

$$SNR(SD) = 20 log_{10} \frac{\mu(SD)}{\sigma(SD)} \quad (8)$$

The SNR is calculated for all MCS models, i.e., for all different wavelengths and all different ranges of the SDS. To calculate μ and σ, all the voxels in the model are considered. The calculation of the SNR was introduced and detailed [41]. As indicated above, the study was conducted considering various important parameters. First, the simulation was performed for the wavelength range from 450 to 1050 nm with an increment of

100 nm. For each wavelength, the simulation was completed for a range of source-to-detector separations (SDSs); specifically from 0.5 to 8 mm with a step size of 0.5 mm. In a previous study [26], we found that, by running multiple independently seeded MCSs (N = 15 to 30) for each wavelength and SDS, one could achieve an acceptable convergence when calculating the SNR. Here, N = 15 was sufficient for calculating the SNR for longer wavelengths, while N = 20 was sufficient for shorter wavelengths. For consistency, we adopted N = 20 for all MCS runs.

3. Results and Discussion

The calculated sensitivity for the epidermis layer is shown in Figure 3. The epidermis sensitivity was calculated for different melanin concentrations, ranging from 2% (which represents light skin) to 30% (which is for dark skin). The figure also shows the effect of different wavelengths (450 to 1050 nm) and the effect of increasing the SDS from 0.5 to 8 mm. There was a clear reduction in epidermis sensitivity when increasing the melanin concentration from 2% to 10%, but the reduction in epidermis sensitivity was not strong when the melanin concentration was further increased from 20% to 30%. In darker skin, the epidermis layer was very sensitive to wavelengths from 450 to 650 nm for an SDS of up to 2.5 mm. For light skin (2% melanin concentration), the epidermis layer was very sensitive to the same wavelengths from 450 to 650 nm, and the SDS could be up to 4.5 mm.

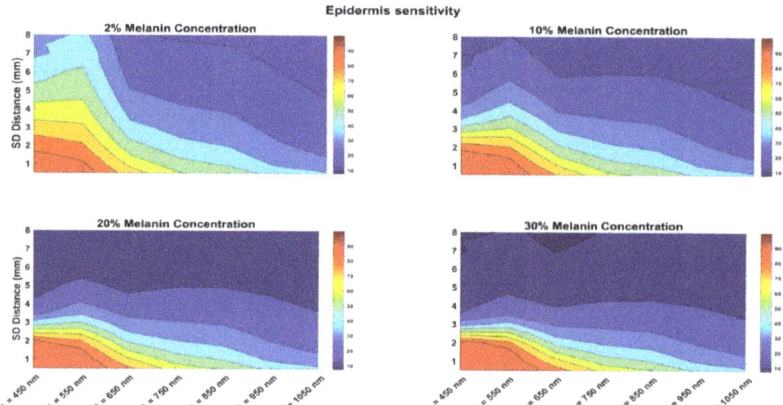

Figure 3. Epidermis sensitivity for various melanin concentrations and with the wavelength ranging between 450 and 1050 nm. Sensitivity also shown for SDS ranging from 0.5 to 8 mm.

Similarly, the calculated sensitivity for the dermis layers is shown in Figure 4. For shorter wavelengths, dermis sensitivity increased as the melanin concentration increased. The SDS from 4 to 8 mm had high dermis sensitivity. However, for a 2% melanin concentration, dermis sensitivity was only 50% when the SDS was longer than 5.5 mm. For darker skin, the wavelengths of 650 and 750 nm had 50% dermis sensitivity when the SDS was longer than 3 mm. For all different melanin concentrations, wavelengths from 450 to 650 nm had the lowest dermis sensitivity (less than 20%) with the SDS less than 2.5 mm. For all wavelengths at all different melanin concentrations, for an SDS of 1.5 mm or less, dermis sensitivity was always less than 30%.

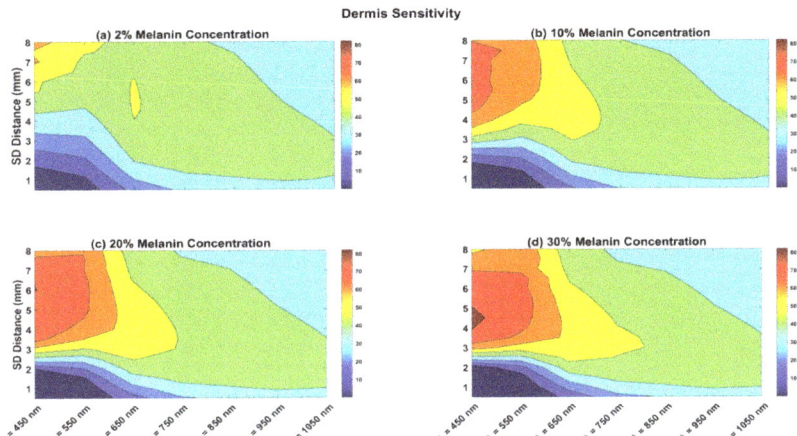

Figure 4. Dermis sensitivity for various melanin concentrations and with the wavelength ranging between 450 and 1050 nm. Sensitivity also shown for SDS ranging from 0.5 to 8 mm.

Figure 5 shows the calculated SNR for all scenarios. As the melanin concentration increased, the SNR clearly deceased. For lighter skin (2% melanin concentration) and wavelengths between 650 and 1050 nm, the SNR was always above 15 dB. As the wavelength increased, the general trend of the SNR increased as well. For wavelengths of 450 and 550 nm, the SNR was almost zero for darker skin when the SDS was longer than 1.5 mm. The SNR was better for light skin at these two wavelengths, where the signal could be measured up to 1.5 mm at 450 nm and up to 4 mm at 550 nm.

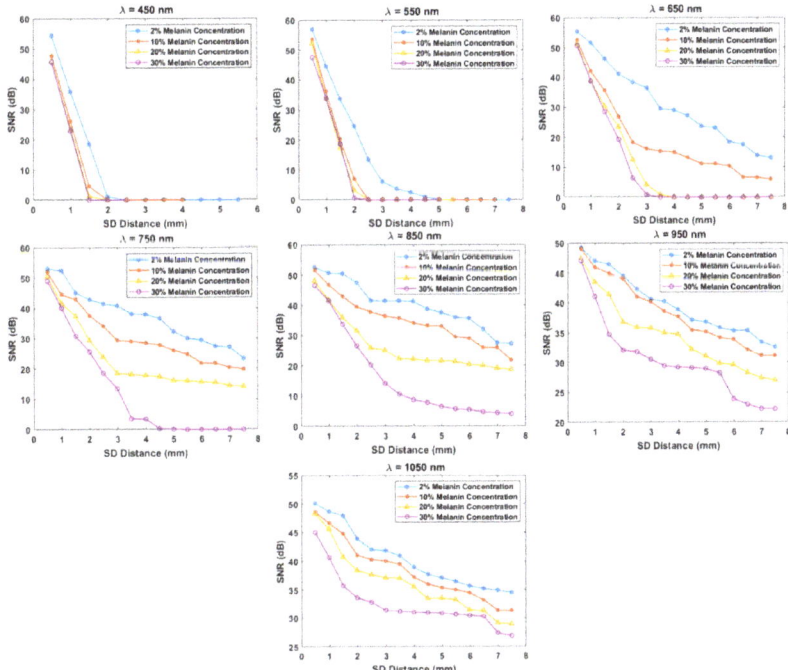

Figure 5. Calculated SNR for all different melanin concentrations, wavelengths, and SDSs.

At a 30% melanin concentration, one needs to go longer than the 750 nm wavelength to have a good SNR with a longer SDS. More specifically, the 850 nm wavelength had an SNR of 5–10 dB with the SDS ranging from 4–7.5 mm. For the same SDS range, a wavelength of 950 nm had a better SNR, of 20–30 dB. Similarly, the SNR was greatly improved for the same SDS range when increasing the wavelength to 1050 nm, to about 25–32 dB.

As the SDS increased, the general trend of the SNR decreased. In comparison to light skin, the SNR in darker skin decreased at a higher rate when the SDS increased. For an SDS of 0.5 to 1 mm, the SNR range was always above 20 dB for all different melanin concentrations and wavelengths.

In the design of dual-channel NIR glucose sensors, epidermis and dermis sensitivity, as well as SNR factors should be considered. From a practical perspective, the channels should have enough source-to-detector separation such that the sensor is easy to design and build. The aim of the short channel is to suppress the noise arising from the superficial epidermis layer. In contrast, the long channel is employed to measure the glucose content confined in the blood-containing inner dermis layer.

For light skin (2% melanin concentration), wavelengths of 450 and 550 nm at an SDS of up to 2.5 mm showed the highest epidermis sensitivity (Figure 3). However, looking at the SNRs of the two wavelengths at the same SDS range, it is clear that a wavelength of 550 nm at a 2.5 mm SDS is a better choice for the short channel. For the long channel, we looked for the highest dermis sensitivity (Figure 4), which was at the long SDS, and the SNR was only good for longer wavelengths. Therefore, the optimal long channel uses the wavelength of 650 nm with an SDS between 4 and 6 mm.

For skin with a 10% melanin concentration, epidermis sensitivity was 80% at 550 nm and 70% at 650 nm at a 2 mm SDS. The SNR at 550 nm was 5 dB, while it was 25 dB at 650 nm at the same SDS. Therefore, the optimal short channel uses the wavelength of 650 nm at a 2 mm SDS. For the long channel, the maximal dermis sensitivity for all wavelengths was between 4.5 and 8 mm SDS. As shown in Figure 4, the dermis sensitivity decreased with increasing wavelength. The optimal long channel uses a wavelength of 650 nm with an SDS between 4.5 and 6 mm.

For darker skin (20% and 30% melanin concentration), the challenge for choosing the short channel was that the SNR was attenuated very quickly with increasing the SDS, specifically for the wavelengths of 450 and 550 nm, which had the highest epidermis sensitivity. Therefore, one must choose a very short SDS, of 1.5 mm or less, at 550 nm. For the long channel, one can choose 750 nm at a 4 to 5 mm SDS. However, for very dark skin (30% melanin concentration), one must assume a longer channel (950 or 1050 nm) to ensure a good SNR. Table 2 summarizes the selections of the wavelengths of the sources and the SDSs for the optimal NIR channels under different skin melanin concentrations.

Table 2. Summary of suggested optimal NIR channels.

Melanin Concentration	Optimal for Short Channel		Optimal for Long Channel	
	Wavelength	SDS	Wavelength	SDS
2%	550 nm	2.5 mm	650 nm	4–6 mm
10%	650 nm	2 mm	650 nm	4–6 mm
20%	550 nm	1.5 mm	750 nm	4–5 mm
30%	550 nm	1.5 mm	950/1050 nm	4–5 mm

4. Conclusions

In this work, we investigated the selection of the optimal dual-NIR channels for glucose measurements under different skin melanin concentrations, specifically for the diagnostic window of the NIR spectrum. The selection was based on the SNR and the sensitivity of both the epidermis and dermis layers considering different skin melanin concentrations. The detailed skin layer model that was adopted through MCS allowed us to take into consideration the differences between different skin layers, in terms of blood volume fraction, water volume fraction, melanin concentration in the epidermis layer, and optical skin proprieties. Since this work focused on the design of the dual-channel and the verifications of its parameters using MC simulation, future work should be experimentally conducted. Future work should also investigate the signal processing for this sensor and may include adopting an estimation model to filter the "noise" measured by the short channel.

Funding: This research received no external funding.

Institutional Review Board Statement: Not applicable.

Informed Consent Statement: Not applicable.

Data Availability Statement: The data presented in this study are openly available in FigShare at https://doi.org/10.6084/m9.figshare.21222452.

Conflicts of Interest: The author declares no conflict of interest.

References

1. Zekri, M.; Dinani, S.; Kamali, M. Regulation of blood glucose concentration in type 1 diabetics using single order sliding mode control combined with fuzzy on-line tunable gain, a simulation study. *J. Med. Signals Sens.* **2015**, *5*, 131–140. [CrossRef] [PubMed]
2. Tang, L.; Chang, S.J.; Chen, C.-J.; Liu, J.-T. Non-Invasive Blood Glucose Monitoring Technology: A Review. *Sensors* **2020**, *20*, 6925. [CrossRef] [PubMed]
3. Wang, J. Electrochemical Glucose Biosensors. *Chem. Rev.* **2008**, *108*, 814–825. [CrossRef] [PubMed]
4. Keenan, D.B.; Mastrototaro, J.J.; Voskanyan, G.; Steil, G.M. Delays in Minimally Invasive Continuous Glucose Monitoring Devices: A Review of Current Technology. *J. Diabetes Sci. Technol.* **2009**, *3*, 1207–1214. [CrossRef]
5. Chen, C.; Xie, Q.; Yang, D.; Xiao, H.; Fu, Y.; Tan, Y.; Yao, S. Recent advances in electrochemical glucose biosensors: A review. *RSC Adv.* **2013**, *3*, 4473–4491. [CrossRef]
6. Ajjan, R.; Slattery, D.; Wright, E. Continuous Glucose Monitoring: A Brief Review for Primary Care Practitioners. *Adv. Ther.* **2019**, *36*, 579–596. [CrossRef]
7. Li, K.; Daniels, J.; Liu, C.; Herrero-Vinas, P.; Georgiou, P. Convolutional Recurrent Neural Networks for Glucose Prediction. *IEEE J. Biomed. Health Inform.* **2020**, *24*, 603–613. [CrossRef]
8. Shang, T.; Zhang, J.Y.; Thomas, A.; Arnold, M.A.; Vetter, B.N.; Heinemann, L.; Klonoff, D.C. Products for Monitoring Glucose Levels in the Human Body With Noninvasive Optical, Noninvasive Fluid Sampling, or Minimally Invasive Technologies. *J. Diabetes Sci. Technol.* **2022**, *16*, 168–214. [CrossRef]
9. Jernelv, I.L.; Milenko, K.; Fuglerud, S.S.; Hjelme, D.R.; Ellingsen, R.; Aksnes, A. A review of optical methods for continuous glucose monitoring. *Appl. Spectrosc. Rev.* **2019**, *54*, 543–572. [CrossRef]
10. Alsunaidi, B.; Althobaiti, M.; Tamal, M.; Albaker, W.; Al-Naib, I. A Review of Non-Invasive Optical Systems for Continuous Blood Glucose Monitoring. *Sensors* **2021**, *21*, 6820. [CrossRef]
11. Sim, J.Y.; Ahn, C.-G.; Jeong, E.-J.; Kim, B.K. In vivo Microscopic Photoacoustic Spectroscopy for Non-Invasive Glucose Monitoring Invulnerable to Skin Secretion Products. *Sci. Rep.* **2018**, *8*, 1059. [CrossRef] [PubMed]
12. Phan, Q.-H.; Lo, Y.-L. Differential Mueller matrix polarimetry technique for non-invasive measurement of glucose concentration on human fingertip. *Opt. Express* **2017**, *25*, 15179–15187. [CrossRef] [PubMed]
13. Chen, T.-L.; Lo, Y.-L.; Liao, C.-C.; Phan, Q.-H. Noninvasive measurement of glucose concentration on human fingertip by optical coherence tomography. *J. Biomed. Opt.* **2018**, *23*, 047001. [CrossRef]
14. Abd Salam, N.A.; Saad, W.H.M.; Manap, Z.; Salehuddin, F. The Evolution of Non-invasive Blood Glucose Monitoring System for Personal Application. *J. Telecommun. Electron. Comput. Eng.* **2016**, *8*, 59–65.
15. Naseer, N.; Hong, K.-S. fNIRS-based brain-computer interfaces: A review. *Front. Hum. Neurosci.* **2015**, *9*, 3. [CrossRef] [PubMed]
16. Althobaiti, M.; Al-Naib, I. Recent Developments in Instrumentation of Functional Near-Infrared Spectroscopy Systems. *Appl. Sci.* **2020**, *10*, 6522. [CrossRef]
17. Vavadi, H.; Mostafa, A.; Zhou, F.; Uddin, K.M.S.; Althobaiti, M.; Xu, C.; Bansal, R.; Ademuyiwa, F.; Poplack, S.; Zhu, Q. Compact ultrasound-guided diffuse optical tomography system for breast cancer imaging. *J. Biomed. Opt.* **2018**, *24*, 21203–21209. [CrossRef]
18. Fang, Q.; Selb, J.; Carp, S.A.; Boverman, G.; Miller, E.L.; Brooks, D.H.; Moore, R.H.; Kopans, D.B.; Boas, D.A. Combined Optical and X-ray Tomosynthesis Breast Imaging. *Radiology* **2011**, *258*, 89–97. [CrossRef]
19. Althobaiti, M.; Vavadi, H.; Zhu, Q. An Automated Preprocessing Method for Diffuse Optical Tomography to Improve Breast Cancer Diagnosis. *Technol. Cancer Res. Treat.* **2018**, *17*, 1533033818802791. [CrossRef]
20. Rachim, V.P.; Chung, W.-Y. Wearable-band type visible-near infrared optical biosensor for non-invasive blood glucose monitoring. *Sens. Actuators B Chem.* **2019**, *286*, 173–180. [CrossRef]
21. Haxha, S.; Jhoja, J. Optical Based Noninvasive Glucose Monitoring Sensor Prototype. *IEEE Photon. J.* **2016**, *8*, 6805911. [CrossRef]

22. Srichan, C.; Srichan, W.; Danvirutai, P.; Ritsongmuang, C.; Sharma, A.; Anutrakulchai, S. Non-invasively accuracy enhanced blood glucose sensor using shallow dense neural networks with NIR monitoring and medical features. *Sci. Rep.* **2022**, *12*, 1769. [CrossRef] [PubMed]
23. Qu, J.Y.; Wilson, B.C. Monte Carlo modeling studies of the effect of physiological factors andother analytes on the determination of glucose concentration in vivoby near infrared optical absorption and scattering measurements. *J. Biomed. Opt.* **1997**, *2*, 319–325. [CrossRef] [PubMed]
24. Kessoku, S.; Maruo, K.; Okawa, S.; Masamoto, K.; Yamada, Y. Influence of blood glucose level on the scattering coefficient of the skin in near-infrared spectroscopy. In Proceedings of the ASME/JSME 2011 8th Thermal Engineering Joint Conference (AJTEC2011), Honolulu, HI, USA, 13–17 March 2011.
25. Tarumi, M.; Shimada, M.; Murakami, T.; Tamura, M.; Shimada, M.; Arimoto, H.; Yamada, Y. Simulation study of in vitro glucose measurement by NIR spectroscopy and a method of error reduction. *Phys. Med. Biol.* **2003**, *48*, 2373–2390. [CrossRef] [PubMed]
26. Althobaiti, M.; Al-Naib, I. Optimization of Dual-Channel Near-Infrared Non-Invasive Glucose Level Measurement Sensors Based On Monte-Carlo Simulations. *IEEE Photon. J.* **2021**, *13*, 3700109. [CrossRef]
27. Jacques, S.L. Optical properties of biological tissues: A review. *Phys. Med. Biol.* **2013**, *58*, R37–R61. [CrossRef]
28. Keiser, G. *Biophotonics: Concepts to Applications*; Springer: Singapore, 2016.
29. Meglinski, I.; Matcher, S. Computer simulation of the skin reflectance spectra. *Comput. Methods Programs Biomed.* **2003**, *70*, 179–186. [CrossRef]
30. Chatterjee, S.; Budidha, K.; Qassem, M.; Kyriacou, P.A. In-silico investigation towards the non-invasive optical detection of blood lactate. *Sci. Rep.* **2021**, *11*, 14274. [CrossRef]
31. Chatterjee, S.; Budidha, K.; Kyriacou, P.A. Investigating the origin of photoplethysmography using a multiwavelength Monte Carlo model. *Physiol. Meas.* **2020**, *41*, 084001. [CrossRef]
32. Petrov, G.I.; Doronin, A.; Whelan, H.T.; Meglinski, I.; Yakovlev, V.V. Human tissue color as viewed in high dynamic range optical spectral transmission measurements. *Biomed. Opt. Express* **2012**, *3*, 2154–2161. [CrossRef]
33. Fang, Q.; Boas, D.A. Monte Carlo Simulation of Photon Migration in 3D Turbid Media Accelerated by Graphics Processing Units. *Opt. Express* **2009**, *17*, 20178–20190. [CrossRef] [PubMed]
34. Yan, S.; Fang, Q. Hybrid mesh and voxel based Monte Carlo algorithm for accurate and efficient photon transport modeling in complex bio-tissues. *Biomed. Opt. Express* **2020**, *11*, 6262–6270. [CrossRef] [PubMed]
35. Yao, R.; Intes, X.; Fang, Q. Direct approach to compute Jacobians for diffuse optical tomography using perturbation Monte Carlo-based photon "replay". *Biomed. Opt. Express* **2018**, *9*, 4588–4603. [CrossRef]
36. Delbeck, S.; Vahlsing, T.; Leonhardt, S.; Steiner, G.; Heise, H.M. Non-invasive monitoring of blood glucose using optical methods for skin spectroscopy—Opportunities and recent advances. *Anal. Bioanal. Chem.* **2019**, *411*, 63–77. [CrossRef] [PubMed]
37. Saidi, I.S. Transcutaneous Optical Measurement of Hyperbilirubinemia in Neonates. Ph.D. Thesis, Rice University, Houston, TX, USA, 1992.
38. Nishidate, I.; Aizu, Y.; Mishina, H. Estimation of melanin and hemoglobin in skin tissue using multiple regression analysis aided by Monte Carlo simulation. *J. Biomed. Opt.* **2004**, *9*, 700–710. [CrossRef]
39. Jacques, S.L.; Glickman, R.D.; Schwartz, J.A. Internal absorption coefficient and threshold for pulsed laser disruption of melanosomes isolated from retinal pigment epithelium. In *SPIE—The International Society for Optical Engineering, Proceedings of the Laser-Tissue Interaction VII, San Jose, CA, USA, 27 January–2 February 1996*; SPIE: Bellingham WA, USA, 1996; Volume 2681. [CrossRef]
40. Brigadoi, S.; Cooper, R. How short is short? Optimum source–detector distance for short-separation channels in functional near-infrared spectroscopy. *Neurophotonics* **2015**, *2*, 025005. [CrossRef] [PubMed]
41. Yuan, Y.; Yu, L.; Doğan, Z.; Fang, Q. Graphics processing units-accelerated adaptive nonlocal means filter for denoising three-dimensional Monte Carlo photon transport simulations. *J. Biomed. Opt.* **2018**, *23*, 121618. [CrossRef]

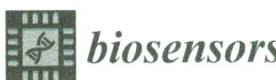

Article

Cu$_2$O-Based Electrochemical Biosensor for Non-Invasive and Portable Glucose Detection

Fabiane Fantinelli Franco [1], Richard A. Hogg [2] and Libu Manjakkal [2,*]

[1] Water and Environment Group, Infrastructure and Environment Division, James Watt School of Engineering, University of Glasgow, Glasgow G12 8LT, UK; fabiane.fantinellifranco@glasgow.ac.uk
[2] Electronic and Nanoscale Engineering, James Watt School of Engineering, University of Glasgow, Glasgow G12 8LT, UK; richard.hogg@glasgow.ac.uk
* Correspondence: libu.manjakkal@glasgow.ac.uk

Abstract: Electrochemical voltammetric sensors are some of the most promising types of sensors for monitoring various physiological analytes due to their implementation as non-invasive and portable devices. Advantages in reduced analysis time, cost-effectiveness, selective sensing, and simple techniques with low-powered circuits distinguish voltammetric sensors from other methods. In this work, we developed a Cu$_2$O-based non-enzymatic portable glucose sensor on a graphene paste printed on cellulose cloth. The electron transfer of Cu$_2$O in a NaOH alkaline medium and sweat equivalent solution at very low potential (+0.35 V) enable its implementation as a low-powered portable glucose sensor. The redox mechanism of the electrodes with the analyte solution was confirmed through cyclic voltammetry, differential pulse voltammetry, and electrochemical impedance spectroscopy studies. The developed biocompatible, disposable, and reproducible sensors showed sensing performance in the range of 0.1 to 1 mM glucose, with a sensitivity of 1082.5 ± 4.7% µA mM^{-1} cm^{-2} on Cu$_2$O coated glassy carbon electrode and 182.9 ± 8.83% µA mM^{-1} cm^{-2} on Cu$_2$O coated graphene printed electrodes, making them a strong candidate for future portable, non-invasive glucose monitoring devices on biodegradable substrates. For portable applications we demonstrated the sensor on artificial sweat in 0.1 M NaOH solution, indicating the Cu$_2$O nanocluster is selective to glucose from 0.0 to +0.6 V even in the presence of common interference such as urea and NaCl.

Keywords: glucose sensor; Cu$_2$O nanomaterial; electrochemical sensor; non-enzymatic sensor

Citation: Franco, F.F.; Hogg, R.A.; Manjakkal, L. Cu$_2$O-Based Electrochemical Biosensor for Non-Invasive and Portable Glucose Detection. *Biosensors* **2022**, *12*, 174. https://doi.org/10.3390/bios12030174

Received: 16 February 2022
Accepted: 12 March 2022
Published: 14 March 2022

Publisher's Note: MDPI stays neutral with regard to jurisdictional claims in published maps and institutional affiliations.

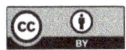

Copyright: © 2022 by the authors. Licensee MDPI, Basel, Switzerland. This article is an open access article distributed under the terms and conditions of the Creative Commons Attribution (CC BY) license (https:// creativecommons.org/licenses/by/ 4.0/).

1. Introduction

Portable sensors are receiving significant and growing interest in healthcare management, especially for monitoring chronic diseases such as diabetes and chronic wounds. It has been noted that one of the major causes of mortality is diabetes related diseases, affecting 537 million people in 2021, a number that is expected to significantly grow in the coming years [1,2]. The increasing glucose levels in the world population denote the importance of developing new sensors which can monitor glucose levels in a cost-effective and simple manner. The present generation of glucose monitoring devices are minimally invasive and measure real-time interstitial fluid glucose levels; however, they still rely on skin piercing, with many patches lasting up to 10 days or less [3]. Other common methods include measurement of blood glucose by finger pricking or blood tests, which is inconvenient and painful [4]. Although these blood-based monitoring systems are well established and frequently used, not all diabetic patients comply with the protocol due to the pain and inconvenience associated with the invasive detection process [5]. As diabetes affects a large share of the population, new non-invasive methods, such as portable or wearable systems, are being extensively researched to increase the level of comfort in patients. As such, market growth for non-invasive glucose-monitoring devices is expected to reach USD 11.35 million between 2021 and 2025 [6]. However, most non-invasive devices incorporate complicated technologies that rely either on spectroscopy or optical techniques specifically tailored to a particular type of diabetes and/or a specific age group [6]. Therefore, cheap and reliable non-invasive techniques are still needed, especially to enhance the viability of routine glucose checkups and other applications in low-income and hard-to-reach areas. In this manner, electrochemical paper-based monitoring devices offer an opportunity for non-invasive detection by using biological fluids other than blood. They have the potential to generate robust, sensitive methods for the detection of metabolic changes in the medium and short term. However, the glucose pathway from blood to sweat has yet to be fully clarified [7]. There are also limitations in accuracy and sensitivity to environmental factors. As a result, the development of proper sampling techniques is urgently needed in order to estimate blood glucose via sweat. Recently, wearable electronics have begun to address these shortcomings with the development of integrated sensor arrays [8–11]. Electrochemical sensors offer the possibility of miniaturized, low-cost, portable sensors that require fewer reagents and no specialized personnel to operate them. Furthermore, the sensing range, cross-sensitivity, and stability can be improved by modifying the sensitive material.

In conventional electrochemical biosensors, the glucose oxidase enzyme is used to detect glucose in physiological pH conditions, since it provides good selectivity and sensitivity. However, enzymes are sensitive to changes in pH, temperature, and humidity, as well as interference from some electro-oxidizable reagents [5]. To overcome the issues due to the enzymatic process, metal and metal-oxide-based glucose sensors have been developed [12–14]. These are usually based on a composition of noble metals (e.g., Au and Pt) [15–17], transition metals (e.g., Cu, Ni, Zn, and Co) [18–20], metal-oxides (e.g., CoO, NiO, and CuO/Cu_2O) [21,22], and their combination with carbon materials [14]. In particular, Cu-based glucose sensors have attracted attention as Cu is a low-cost material and has a wide crustal abundance. Moreover, Cu_2O is a stable Cu oxide, and a p-type semiconducting material with a 2.17 eV bandgap, making it a versatile material for various applications, including solar cells, sensors, and batteries [23–26]. Its low net surface charge prevents the material from being affected by interference from other compounds that commonly affect noble metals [14]. The change of oxidation state from Cu(II) to Cu(III) mediates the electrocatalytic activity of copper nanocomposites, with the possibility of tailoring the synthesis to form nanostructures such as nanoflowers, nanowires, and nanocubes [27–29]. Therefore, Cu_2O is a suitable non-enzymatic alternative for glucose sensing. For the fabrication of single-use biosensors, cellulose-based substrates are non-toxic and provide enhanced biocompatibility and biodegradability [30–32]. It is the most naturally abundant material in the form of wood and cotton, among others [33]. The highly porous structure and large surface area of the cellulose make it a sensible choice as a substrate for electrochemical biosensors.

In this work, a non-invasive, portable sweat-based glucose sensor was fabricated by hand printing graphene paste electrodes on sustainable biodegradable and biocompatible cellulose substrates. Cu_2O nanoclusters were employed as the sensitive material and drop casted on top of the working electrode (WE) to complete the affordable, voltammetric glucose sensors. To study the feasibility of the Cu_2O nanoclusters for glucose sensing, cyclic voltammetry (CV), differential pulsed voltammetry (DPV), and electrochemical impedance spectroscopy (EIS) studies were conducted in 0.1 M sodium hydroxide (NaOH) and artificial sweat/NaOH solutions using Cu_2O a coated glassy carbon electrode (GCE) or graphene paste printed electrodes (PEs). Commercial graphene paste was used for the printed electrodes, Ag/AgCl commercial paste was used for the pseudo-reference electrode (RE), and the WE was further modified with drop casted Cu_2O nanoclusters. The schematic fabrication is shown in Figure 1. As a proof of concept to validate these portable glucose sensors, voltammetric sensors were tested in 0.1 M NaOH and artificial sweat/NaOH solutions with varying concentrations of glucose. X-ray diffraction (XRD) and scanning electron microscopy (SEM) were employed to study the morphology of the Cu_2O nanoclusters and the interface of the sensitive material with the printing pastes and substrate. These biocompatible disposable and reproducible sensors showed good sensing performance in the range of 0.1 to 1 mM glucose, with a sensitivity of $1082.5 \pm 4.7\%$ µA mM^{-1} cm^{-2}

on the GCE and 182.9 ± 8.83% µA mM^{-1} cm^{-2} on graphene PEs, making them a strong candidate for portable, non-invasive sweat glucose monitoring devices.

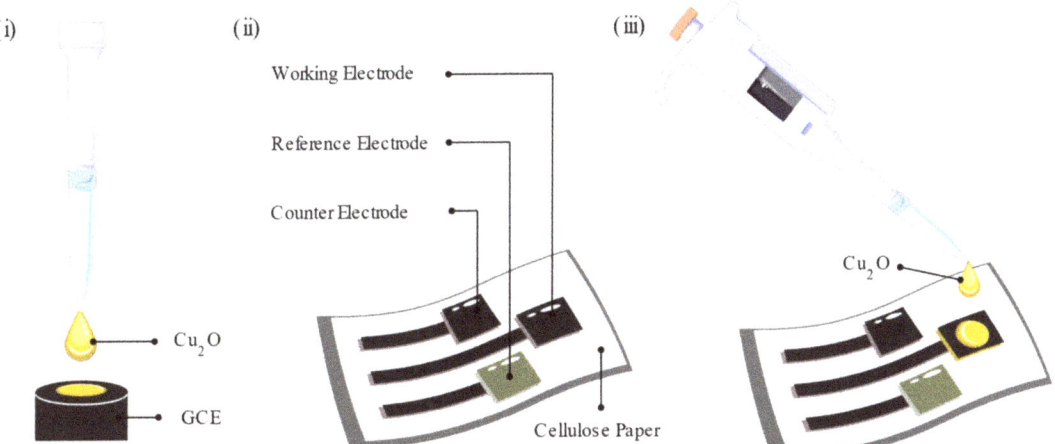

Figure 1. Schematic fabrication of the glucose sensor. (i) Cu$_2$O nanoclusters drop casted on the GCE for material study. (ii) Graphene paste printed on cellulose cloth with a Ag/AgCl RE. (iii) Modified WE with Cu$_2$O on the graphene printed cellulose substrate.

2. Materials and Methods

2.1. Cu$_2$O Synthesis

The Cu$_2$O nanocrystals were synthesized by modifying a previously published work [28]. Briefly, the synthesis consists of an ascorbic acid (C$_6$H$_8$O$_6$) and NaOH reduction route at room temperature. The addition of C$_6$H$_8$O favors the formation of Cu$_2$O, and the concentration of NaOH dictates the nanoparticle shape [34]. The reaction mechanism is as follows [34]:

$$2Cu(OH)_2 + C_6H_8O_6 \rightarrow Cu_2O + C_6H_8O_6 + 3H_2O \quad (1)$$

Firstly, 0.1 mmol of CuCl$_2$ and 0.1 g of polyvinylpyrrolidone were dissolved in 40 mL. After a dropwise addition of 2.5 mL of 0.2 M NaOH aqueous solution, the mixture was stirred for 5 min. Then, 2.5 mL of 0.1 M aqueous ascorbic acid was added dropwise, and the solution was stirred for further 5 min. The Cu$_2$O crystals were recovered by centrifugation and washed two times with ethanol. The crystals were dried and suspended in deionized water (1 mg/mL) to be used for further experiments.

2.2. Sensor Fabrication

For the initial experiments, the sensitive electrode was fabricated on the top of the glassy-carbon electrode (GCE). For this, 5 µL of the Cu$_2$O aqueous solution (1 mg/mL) was drop casted on the GCE and dried at 80 °C for 5 min. For the printed sensor fabrication, first a three-electrode layer was hand printed on top of a cellulose substrate using a graphene paste (JESC-7771G, JE Solutions Consultancy, UK). The RE and the CE were 3 mm × 1.5 cm lines, and the WE consisted of a 3 mm × 2 cm line and a 1 × 0.5 cm rectangle. Among these three electrodes, one was employed as a CE, and the surface of the second electrode was converted to a RE. For RE fabrication, a silver/silver chloride (Ag/AgCl) paste (JESC-7713AgCl, JE Solutions Consultancy, London, UK) was hand printed on the top of graphene electrode and heat treated at 80 °C for 1 h in the oven. Wires were attached to the contact pads using graphene paste and dried at 80 °C for 30 min. Before use, the WEs were further modified by drop casting 20 µL of the Cu$_2$O aqueous solution and dried at 80 °C for a few minutes. Finally, the contact pads were covered with insulative tape, and only the active area of sensor was exposed to the solution.

2.3. Material Characterization

The structural characterization of the sensitive electrode was carried out with an X-Ray diffractometer (XRD, P'Analytical X'Pert with Cu Kα (λ = 1.541 Å)). The morphological characterization and the atomic composition of the electrodes alongside the energy-dispersive X-ray spectroscopy (EDS, Oxford Instruments Energy 250) mapping were performed using a scanning electron microscope (SEM, Philips/FEI XL30 ESEM at 20 kV). The SEM images were analyzed using the ImageJ software.

2.4. Electrochemical Characterization

For electrochemical measurements all reagents were used as received and all solutions were prepared in deionized (DI) water unless otherwise mentioned. The CV, DPV, and EIS analyses of the sensors were carried out using a Gamry potentiostat (Interface 1010E). A three-electrode system, with a commercial glass Ag/AgCl RE, a platinum counter electrode (Pt CE), and a standard GCE, was employed in the initial material studies. A PE with drop casted Cu_2O (as WE) with a commercial RE and CE was used for initial testing of the printed material, and the full printed sensor was employed for the final tests. The experiments were performed under normal ambient conditions. The CV and DPV electrochemical measurements were carried out in 0.1 M NaOH (pH 13) aqueous solution or artificial sweat alkaline solution (15 mM sodium chloride (NaCl), 3 mM potassium chloride, (KCl), and 22 mM urea in 0.1 M NaOH with a final pH of 13) with a glucose concentration varying from 100–1000 µM with a 100 or 300 µM glucose stepwise addition. The limit of detection (LOD) was calculated by using the standard deviation (SD) of the lowest calculation and the calibration slope (S). The equation used was LOD = (SD/S) * 3. The EIS analysis was carried out with 0.1 mM glucose in 0.1 M NaOH from 100 kHz to 0.1 Hz.

3. Results and Discussion

3.1. Material Characterization

The XRD spectra and the SEM images for the Cu_2O materials and PEs are presented in Figure 2. The XRD spectra of the Cu_2O synthesized powder and the Cu_2O coated PE were compared to the simulated Cu_2O spectrum (COD #96-100-0064), shown in Figure 2a. The powder and the Cu_2O coated PE peaks matched the simulated cuprite data, indicating a successful synthesis. The Cu_2O PE peaks were much less intense due to the low amount of drop casted Cu_2O in relation to the surface of the WE. Some peaks were also slightly shifted to the right, indicating a change in microstructure parameters such as crystallite size and strain. This could be due to cuprite interaction with the graphene paste and agglomeration when drop casting. The Cu_2O coated PE XRD spectrum also presented some new peaks from other crystalline materials present in the graphene paste and the substrate. Figure S1a displays the cellulose substrate and the PE with and without the drop casted Cu_2O for comparison. The cellulose contribution is most prominent around $10 < 2\theta < 28°$ due to the influence of its intra- and intermolecular bonding patterns on the cellulose polymer chain [30]. The other intense peaks correspond to the (002) and (004) peaks of graphite in the graphene paste [35].

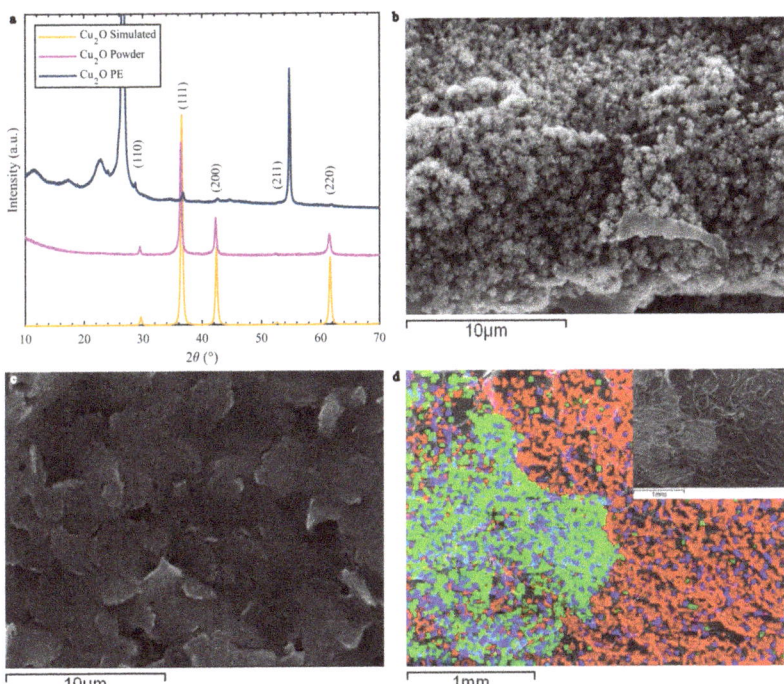

Figure 2. (a) XRD spectrum of simulated Cu_2O, synthesized powder Cu_2O, and WE drop casted with Cu_2O nanoclusters (Cu_2O PE). (b) SEM images of the Cu_2O drop casted on the PEs: (b) Cu_2O nanoclusters, (c) graphene paste and (d) EDS mapping of the interface between Cu_2O and the graphene paste with an inset of the SEM image. Green corresponds to Cu, blue to O, and red to C.

The morphological structure of the Cu_2O nanoclusters drop casted on the PEs can be seen in Figure 2b–d. The Cu_2O nanomaterial appears to form clusters on top of the graphene-paste-based electrode. These clusters are a few micrometers in size and closely dispersed (Figure S2a). The graphene paste adhered well on the cellulose substrate, forming tightly packed layers. This is due to the fibrous, porous structure of cellulose, shown in Figure S2b, which facilitates strong adhesion of materials to its surface. From the EDS mapping (Figure 2d), a clear interface from the drop casted Cu_2O crystals and the graphene paste can be observed, indicating where the cupric material dried and clustered. The EDS spectrum (Figure S2c) showed the presence of Cl, C, O, and Cu on the drop casted site. This could indicate that not all $CuCl_2$ was washed and remained in the final suspension. The graphene paste has odd spots of Cu that could have appeared due to splatters or material run off. On the Cu_2O side, both Cu and O are present, with oxygen sites exposed to the surface. This facilitates the formation of hydroxyl groups and the CuOOH configuration, responsible for the glucose oxidation process [29].

3.2. Cu_2O Nanocluster Study on GCE

Firstly, the Cu_2O nanoclusters were studied with a standard three-electrode configuration by drop casting the material on a commercial GCE. The material was utilized as an enzyme-free glucose detection method, and its electrochemical activity was characterized by CV and DPV on 0.1 M NaOH from 0.0 to +0.6 V, shown in Figure 3. This potential range is commonly employed in the detection of glucose by Cu-based materials [21,29]. The Cu material showed a clear redox response with the addition of glucose, from 100 to 1000 μM. Glucose concentration in sweat is significantly lower than blood glucose, ranging from 10 to 1100 μM [8]. Therefore, the Cu_2O nanoclusters seem suitable for sweat applications. From the DPV (Figure 3b), an increase in peak current can be observed with every 100 µM addition of glucose. By setting the peak current at +0.35 V over three sets of drop casted Cu$_2$O GCEs, a calibration curve was acquired (Figure 3c). A sensitivity of 1082.5 µA mM^{-1} cm^{-2} with a root mean square deviation (RMSD) of ±4.7% and R^2 = 0.959. The upper limit of detection seems to be 1000 µM, where the linear curve starts to stabilize. The calculated LOD was 12 µM.

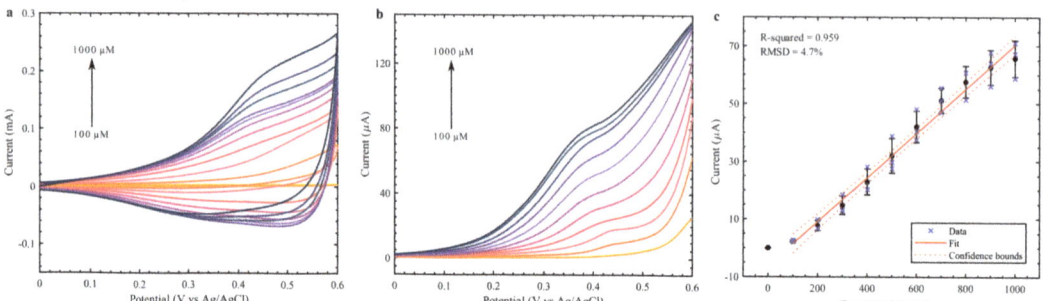

Figure 3. CV (**a**) and DPV (**b**) of Cu$_2$O nanoclusters on GCE with varying glucose concentrations (100–1000 µM) in 0.1 M NaOH. (**c**) Calibration curve at 0.35 V from DPV analysis.

We studied the electron transfer process of the Cu$_2$O nanoclusters with 1 mM of glucose at 0.1 M NaOH by changing the CV scanning rate from 50 to 300 mV/s (Figure S3). The oxidation peak current of glucose increases with faster scanning rates and shifts to slightly more positive potentials. The positive potential shift indicates a slow electron transfer process, while the linear fit of the anodic and cathodic peak currents implies a surface diffusion-limited process [36] due to porous electrode surface as confirmed in SEM image in Figure 2b. This is in line with other literature reports for Cu$_2$O/CuO-based glucose electrocatalysis in alkaline media [37,38]. The mechanism of glucose oxidation on cuprite is not fully understood, but it is assumed that the CuOOH oxidant reagent is responsible for the glucose oxidation into gluconolactone [29,39]. The reaction can be expressed as follows:

$$Cu_2O + 2OH^- + H_2O \rightarrow 2Cu(OH)_2 + 2e^- \quad (2)$$

$$Cu(OH)_2 \rightarrow CuO + H_2O \quad (3)$$

$$CuO + OH^- \rightarrow CuOOH + e^- \quad (4)$$

$$CuOOH + e^- + glucose \rightarrow CuO + OH^- + gluconolactone \quad (5)$$

$$2CuO + H_2O + 2e^- \rightarrow Cu_2O + 2OH^- \quad (6)$$

Equations (2)–(6) show the importance of an alkaline medium in providing the necessary OH$^-$ group for the oxidation process. The cuprite material was also validated in an artificial sweat solution in 0.1 M NaOH (Figure S5). The material presented a similar performance to that of 0.1 M NaOH, indicating that common substances found in sweat (urea, NaCl, KCl) did not affect the oxidation process.

3.3. Printed Glucose Sensor Characterization

The performance of the printed glucose sensors was initially validated using the Cu$_2$O coated PEs with commercial RE and CE. The measured CV and DPV for various concentrations of glucose in 0.1 M NaOH solution are given in Figure 4a,b respectively. We noted that the peaks in CV and DPV were not as clear in the Cu$_2$O coated on PE as compared to the Cu$_2$O coated on top of GCE. Although the peaks were not as clear, the Cu$_2$O PE could still be calibrated at +0.35 V. The calibration curve for three Cu$_2$O PEs is seen in Figure 4c, with a sensitivity of 182.9 ± 8.83% µA mM^{-1} cm^{-2} and R^2 = 0.938 and a calculated LOD of 52.7 µM. As the material was drop casted, it is difficult to calculate the effective area of the electrode, so the total graphene WE area was used in the calculation even though the Cu$_2$O did not cover the whole area. This could underestimate the area sensitivity of the printed electrode, explaining the lower value. The calibration curve was obtained by subtracting the base current without the addition of glucose to each concentration point. Interestingly, this improved the calibration performance of the Cu$_2$O PE but only marginally improved it for the GCE (Figure S4). While the R^2 went from 0.843 to 0.938, and the RMSD from 14.9% to 8.83% for the Cu$_2$O PEs, the GCE only saw a change of 0.01 for the R^2 and 0.09% for the RMSD. This indicates that the baseline current is more significant for the PEs than for the GCE, and a correction is necessary to lower the error between different electrodes.

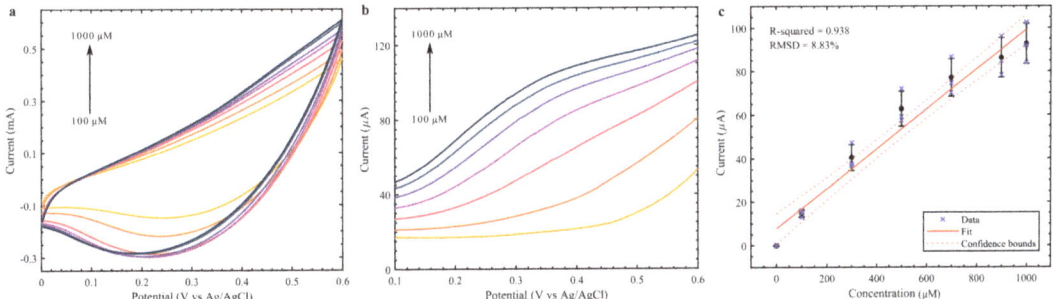

Figure 4. CV (**a**) and DPV (**b**) of Cu$_2$O nanoclusters on printed WE with varying glucose concentrations (100–1000 µM) in 0.1 M NaOH. (**c**) Calibration curve at 0.35 V from DPV analysis.

The measurement shows that both the CV and DPV peaks were not as defined as on the GCE. This variation in performance could be due to the influence of the graphene printed electrode with the solution and less surface area available due to the agglomeration of the Cu$_2$O on the surface of the PE as observed in Figure 2b. Further investigation of the influence of electrodes on the electrochemical Cu$_2$O response was carried out using EIS analysis. Figure 5a shows the complex impedance data of Cu$_2$O coated GCE through the Nyquist and Bode impedance magnitude plot (inset of the Figure 5a) for 0.1 M NaOH with a 100 µM concentration of glucose. For a similar solution, the impedance data plot for Cu$_2$O coated on PE is shown in Figure 5b. The impedance data on the Nyquist plot shows that both GCE- and PE-based electrodes have an almost straight line in low frequency range. This could be due to the diffusion controlled reaction given in Figure S3b. However, we noted that the Cu$_2$O coated GCE has a very high impedance value when compared to the low impedance presented by the PE. It reveals that the electrolyte distribution on the surface of the PE electrode is much better than on the GCE, leading to a lower resistance of the solution reaction with the electrode. Moreover, both the pseudo-capacitance of Cu$_2$O and the electrochemical double layer capacitance from the printed graphene electrode contribute to the electrochemical properties of electrodes. The diffusion of ions in the bulk of the printed electrode can be confirmed from the small semicircle arc in the high frequency range in Figure 5b. In the GCE-based electrode the redox reaction due to the Cu$_2$O material is more prominent, which can be observed by the distinguishable redox reaction in Figure 3a as opposed to the quasi-rectangle CV curve on the PE in Figure 4a. This difference in electrode–electrolyte reaction while coating on GCE or PE causes the variation in sensitivity of both sensors.

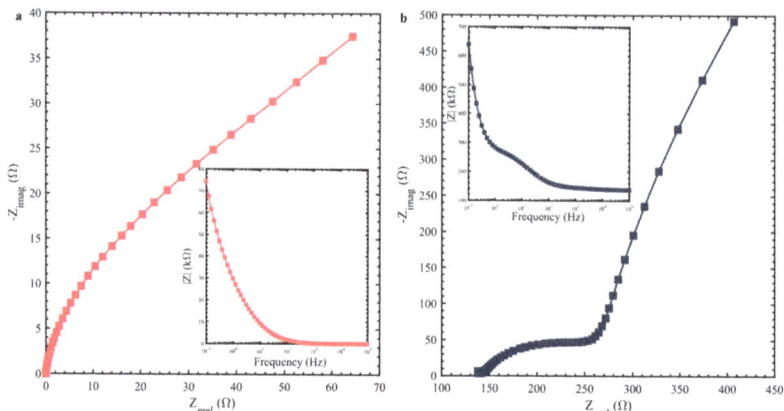

Figure 5. Nyquist plot of 0.1 M NaOH with 100 µM glucose solution of (**a**) Cu$_2$O coated GCE with magnitude of impedance inset and (**b**) Cu$_2$O coated on PE with magnitude of impedance inset.

Finally, for a portable application we tested the performance of fully printed sensors (Figure 1(iii)) in 0.1 M NaOH and artificial alkaline sweat (Figure 6). The CV and DPV for fully printed sensors in 0.1 M NaOH solution with various glucose concentrations are given in Figure 6a,b. The CV and DPV performance of the sensor in artificial sweat with 0.1 M NaOH is given in Figure 6c,d. The preliminary investigation showed an increase in current up to 500 µM in both media. However, the artificial sweat in 0.1 M NaOH presented more defined peaks and stable oxidation peaks, around the same potential as that observed in previous results, while in 0.1 M NaOH solution the peaks shifted to the left. This could be the influence of the pseudo-Ag/AgCl RE, as the artificial sweat solution provides Cl$^-$ ions to replenish the salt layer, while the NaOH does not provide the same favorable conditions. Although the preliminary results are promising, further investigation is needed to fabricate reliable fully printed glucose sensors that can support a wider range of glucose concentrations. The printed sensor performance was compared to other printed CuO/Cu$_2$O-based glucose sensors (Table 1). It can be observed that the fabricated PE-based sensor is comparable to other reported works. Moreover, the low cost of fabrication, biocompatible substrate and electrodes, and biodegradable materials are the major advantages. The sensor size and biodegradable and sustainable textile-based substrate together with its facile fabrication steps facilitate its implementation as a portable glucose sensor.

Table 1. Comparison of CuO/Cu$_2$O-based non-enzymatic electrochemical glucose sensors.

Electrode Material	Substrate	Sensitivity (µA mM^{-1} cm^{-2})	Linear Range (mM)	Applied Potential (V)	LOD (µM)	Reference
CuO nanofibers	GCE	431.3	0.006–2.5	0.4	0.8	[39]
Cu$_2$O nanocubes	SPCE	1040	0.007–4.5	0.7	31	[23]
Cu$_2$O nanocubes/nafion	GCE	2864	0.05–5.65	0.7	1.7	[40]
Cu$_2$O NPs/nafion	GCE	190	0.05–1.1	0.5	47.2	[41]
Cu$_2$O nanowires	Cu foil	4060	0.001–2.0	0.55	0.58	[25]
Cu$_2$O nanowires	Cu foam	6680.7	0.001–1.8	0.5	0.67	[42]
CuO/Cu$_2$O nanosheets	Cu foil	1541	0.001–4	0.6	0.57	[22]
Cu$_2$O nanoclusters	GCE	1082.5	0.1–1	0.35 (DPV)	12	This work
Cu$_2$O nanoclusters	Cellulose PE	182.9	0.1–1	0.35 (DPV)	52.7	This work

SPCE = screen printed carbon electrode; NPs = nanoparticles.

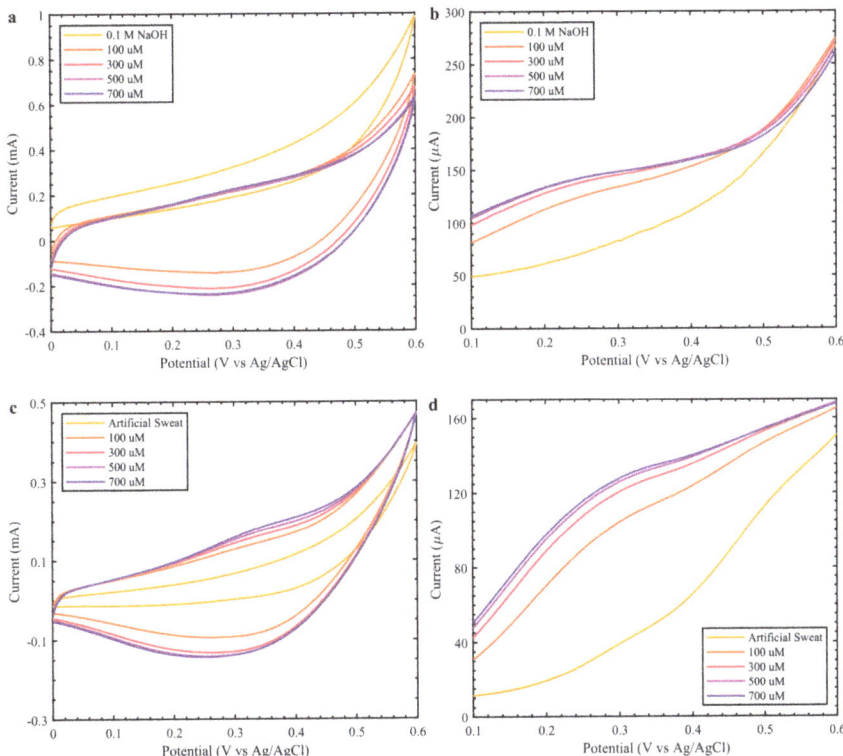

Figure 6. Electrochemical analysis of fully printed Cu_2O-based glucose sensors over a glucose concentration range of 100–700 μM. (**a**) CV and (**b**) DPV in 0.1 M NaOH. (**c**) CV and (**d**) DPV artificial sweat in 0.1 M NaOH.

4. Conclusions

Non-invasive, portable glucose sensors are necessary for increasing the wellbeing of patients living with diabetes. In this paper, we introduce a disposable non-enzymatic Cu_2O-based sensor for portable glucose detection. We synthesized Cu_2O crystals using a simple ascorbic acid reduction route and studied the material performance for glucose detection. The Cu_2O formed nanoclusters and stayed on the surface of the graphene paste, with oxygen exposed to the surface. The Cu_2O nanomaterial showed good performance towards glucose detection in basic medium, with a sensitivity of 1082.5 μA mM^{-1} cm^{-2} on GCE and 182.9 ± 8.83% μA mM^{-1} cm^{-2} at +0.35 V on graphene PEs. The RMSD was comparably low even on the printed sensors, indicating suitability for disposable sensors. Both the Cu_2O on GCE and Cu_2O PEs demonstrated a similar performance in the artificial sweat in 0.1 M NaOH solution, indicating that the Cu_2O nanocluster is selective to glucose from 0.0 to +0.6 V even in the presence of common interference such as urea and NaCl. To assess their suitability for portable glucose detection, fully printed sensors were tested in 0.1 M NaOH and artificial sweat. The sensors showed a similar performance to the Cu_2O PEs, supporting that these cheap, biodegradable sensors can be employed as portable disposable glucose sensors. However, drop casting the Cu_2O material on the printed sensitive electrodes caused a decrease in sensitivity due to poor material dispersion and adhesion. By further improving the Cu_2O nanomaterial and testing new techniques for better adhesion of the sensitive material on the carbon electrode, e.g., screen-printing and inkjet printing, these sensors could be employed in portable glucose sensing and hard-to-reach zones to simplify glucose monitoring.

Supplementary Materials: The following are available online at https://www.mdpi.com/article/10.3390/bios12030174/s1, Figure S1: XRD spectrum of cellulose substrate, graphene paste printed on the cellulose substrate (C-PE), and Cu_2O PE; Figure S2: SEM images of the (a) Cu_2O drop casted on the PEs and (b) cellulose substrate. (c) EDS spectrum of the Cu_2O drop casted on the PE with the SEM image inset; Figure S3: (a) CV curves with changing scan rates (50 to 300 mV/s) of Cu_2O GCE with 1 mM glucose in 0.1 M NaOH. (b) Relationship between peak current and square root of scan rate. Figure S4: Unmodified calibration curves (without subtracting the baseline) of (a) Cu_2O GCEs and (b) Cu_2O PEs; Figure S5: Unmodified calibration curves (without subtracting the baseline) of (a) Cu_2O GCEs and (b) Cu_2O PEs.

Author Contributions: Experimental data—F.F.F.; Printed sensor fabrication—F.F.F. and L.M.; data analysis—F.F.F. and L.M.; writing—original draft preparation, F.F.F.; writing—review and editing, R.A.H., L.M. All authors have read and agreed to the published version of the manuscript.

Funding: This work was supported by the European Commission through the AQUASENSE (H2020-MSCA-ITN-2018-813680) project and NERC discipline hopping activities to tackle environmental challenges project (SEED-2022-317475).

Institutional Review Board Statement: Not applicable.

Informed Consent Statement: Not applicable.

Acknowledgments: We acknowledge Servier Medical Art (https://smart.servier.com), accessed on 25 January 2022, for providing the vectorized micropipettes and arm images.

Conflicts of Interest: The authors declare no conflict of interest.

References

1. Wang, Y.; Wang, J. Diagnostic significance of serum FGD5-AS1 and its predictive value for the development of cardiovascular diseases in patients with type 2 diabetes. *Diabetol. Metab. Syndr.* **2022**, *14*, 20. [CrossRef] [PubMed]
2. Statista International Diabetes Federation. Estimated Number of Diabetics Worldwide in 2021, 2030, and 2045 (In Millions). 2021. Available online: https://www.statista.com/statistics/271442/number-of-diabetics-worldwide/ (accessed on 1 February 2022).
3. Lee, K.; Gunasinghe, S.; Chapman, A.; Findlow, L.A.; Hyland, J.; Ohol, S.; Urwin, A.; Rutter, M.K.; Schofield, J.; Thabit, H.; et al. Real-World Outcomes of Glucose Sensor Use in Type 1 Diabetes—Findings from a Large UK Centre. *Biosensors* **2021**, *11*, 457. [CrossRef] [PubMed]
4. Bihar, E.; Wustoni, S.; Pappa, A.M.; Salama, K.N.; Baran, D.; Inal, S. A fully inkjet-printed disposable glucose sensor on paper. *NPJ Flex. Electron.* **2018**, *2*, 30. [CrossRef]
5. Lee, H.; Hong, Y.J.; Baik, S.; Hyeon, T.; Kim, D. Enzyme-based glucose sensor: From invasive to wearable device. *Adv. Healthc. Mater.* **2018**, *7*, 1701150. [CrossRef]
6. Dixit, K.; Fardindoost, S.; Ravishankara, A.; Tasnim, N.; Hoorfar, M. Exhaled Breath Analysis for Diabetes Diagnosis and Monitoring: Relevance, Challenges and Possibilities. *Biosensors* **2021**, *11*, 476. [CrossRef]
7. Chung, M.; Fortunato, G.; Radacsi, N. Wearable flexible sweat sensors for healthcare monitoring: A review. *J. R. Soc. Interface* **2019**, *16*, 20190217. [CrossRef]
8. Sempionatto, J.R.; Moon, J.-M.; Wang, J. Touch-Based Fingertip Blood-Free Reliable Glucose Monitoring: Personalized Data Processing for Predicting Blood Glucose Concentrations. *ACS Sens.* **2021**, *6*, 1875–1883. [CrossRef]
9. Zhao, J.; Lin, Y.; Wu, J.; Nyein, H.Y.Y.; Bariya, M.; Tai, L.-C.; Chao, M.; Ji, W.; Zhang, G.; Fan, Z.; et al. A Fully Integrated and Self-Powered Smartwatch for Continuous Sweat Glucose Monitoring. *ACS Sens.* **2019**, *4*, 1925–1933. [CrossRef]
10. Lee, H.; Song, C.; Hong, Y.S.; Kim, M.S.; Cho, H.R.; Kang, T.; Shin, K.; Choi, S.H.; Hyeon, T.; Kim, D.-H. Wearable/disposable sweat-based glucose monitoring device with multistage transdermal drug delivery module. *Sci. Adv.* **2017**, *3*, e1601314. [CrossRef]
11. Manjakkal, L.; Yin, L.; Nathan, A.; Wang, J.; Dahiya, R. Energy Autonomous Sweat-Based Wearable Systems. *Adv. Mater.* **2021**, *33*, 2100899. [CrossRef]
12. Adeel, M.; Rahman, M.M.; Caligiuri, I.; Canzonieri, V.; Rizzolio, F.; Daniele, S. Recent advances of electrochemical and optical enzyme-free glucose sensors operating at physiological conditions. *Biosens. Bioelectron.* **2020**, *165*, 112331. [CrossRef] [PubMed]
13. Wei, M.; Qiao, Y.; Zhao, H.; Liang, J.; Li, T.; Luo, Y.; Lu, S.; Shi, X.; Lu, W.; Sun, X. Electrochemical non-enzymatic glucose sensors: Recent progress and perspectives. *Chem. Commun.* **2020**, *56*, 14553–14569. [CrossRef] [PubMed]
14. Thatikayala, D.; Ponnamma, D.; Sadasivuni, K.; Cabibihan, J.-J.; Al-Ali, A.; Malik, R.; Min, B. Progress of Advanced Nanomaterials in the Non-Enzymatic Electrochemical Sensing of Glucose and H_2O_2. *Biosensors* **2020**, *10*, 151. [CrossRef] [PubMed]
15. Zhu, B.; Yu, L.; Beikzadeh, S.; Zhang, S.; Zhang, P.; Wang, L.; Travas-Sejdic, J. Disposable and portable gold nanoparticles modified-laser-scribed graphene sensing strips for electrochemical, non-enzymatic detection of glucose. *Electrochim. Acta* **2021**, *378*, 138132. [CrossRef]

16. Park, S.; Chung, T.D.; Kim, H.C. Nonenzymatic Glucose Detection Using Mesoporous Platinum. *Anal. Chem.* **2003**, *75*, 3046–3049. [CrossRef]
17. Niu, X.H.; Shi, L.B.; Zhao, H.L.; Lan, M.B. Advanced strategies for improving the analytical performance of Pt-based nonenzymatic electrochemical glucose sensors: A minireview. *Anal. Methods* **2016**, *8*, 1755–1764. [CrossRef]
18. Wu, W.; Yu, B.; Wu, H.; Wang, S.; Xia, Q.; Ding, Y. Synthesis of tremella-like CoS and its application in sensing of hydrogen peroxide and glucose. *Mater. Sci. Eng. C* **2017**, *70*, 430–437. [CrossRef]
19. Deepalakshmi, T.; Tran, D.T.; Kim, N.H.; Chong, K.T.; Lee, J.H. Nitrogen-Doped Graphene-Encapsulated Nickel Cobalt Nitride as a Highly Sensitive and Selective Electrode for Glucose and Hydrogen Peroxide Sensing Applications. *ACS Appl. Mater. Interfaces* **2018**, *10*, 35847–35858. [CrossRef]
20. Su, L.; Feng, J.; Zhou, X.; Ren, C.; Li, H.; Chen, X. Colorimetric Detection of Urine Glucose Based $ZnFe_2O_4$ Magnetic Nanoparticles. *Anal. Chem.* **2012**, *84*, 5753–5758. [CrossRef]
21. Wang, M.; Ma, J.; Chang, Q.; Fan, X.; Zhang, G.; Zhang, F.; Peng, W.; Li, Y. Fabrication of a novel ZnO–CoO/rGO nanocomposite for nonenzymatic detection of glucose and hydrogen peroxide. *Ceram. Int.* **2018**, *44*, 5250–5256. [CrossRef]
22. Lv, J.; Kong, C.; Xu, Y.; Yang, Z.; Zhang, X.; Yang, S.; Meng, G.; Bi, J.; Li, J.; Yang, S. Facile synthesis of novel CuO/Cu_2O nanosheets on copper foil for high sensitive nonenzymatic glucose biosensor. *Sens. Actuators B Chem.* **2017**, *248*, 630–638. [CrossRef]
23. Espro, C.; Marini, S.; Giusi, D.; Ampelli, C.; Neri, G. Non-enzymatic screen printed sensor based on Cu_2O nanocubes for glucose determination in bio-fermentation processes. *J. Electroanal. Chem.* **2020**, *873*, 114354. [CrossRef]
24. Zhan, G.; Zeng, H.C. Topological Transformations of Core–Shell Precursors to Hierarchically Hollow Assemblages of Copper Silicate Nanotubes. *ACS Appl. Mater. Interfaces* **2017**, *9*, 37210–37218. [CrossRef] [PubMed]
25. Van Dat, P.; Viet, N.X. Facile synthesis of novel areca flower like Cu_2O nanowire on copper foil for a highly sensitive enzyme-free glucose sensor. *Mater. Sci. Eng. C* **2019**, *103*, 109758. [CrossRef]
26. Luo, Z.; Fu, L.; Zhu, J.; Yang, W.; Li, D.; Zhou, L. Cu_2O as a promising cathode with high specific capacity for thermal battery. *J. Power Sources* **2020**, *448*, 227569. [CrossRef]
27. Zhang, L.; Li, Q.; Xue, H.; Pang, H. Fabrication of Cu_2O-based Materials for Lithium-Ion Batteries. *ChemSusChem* **2018**, *11*, 1581–1599. [CrossRef]
28. Valentini, F.; Biagiotti, V.; Lete, C.; Palleschi, G.; Wang, J. The electrochemical detection of ammonia in drinking water based on multi-walled carbon nanotube/copper nanoparticle composite paste electrodes. *Sens. Actuators B Chem.* **2007**, *128*, 326–333. [CrossRef]
29. Chatterjee, S.; Pal, A.J. Introducing Cu_2O Thin Films as a Hole-Transport Layer in Efficient Planar Perovskite Solar Cell Structures. *J. Phys. Chem. C* **2016**, *120*, 1428–1437. [CrossRef]
30. Kamel, S.; Khattab, T.A. Recent Advances in Cellulose-Based Biosensors for Medical Diagnosis. *Biosensors* **2020**, *10*, 67. [CrossRef]
31. Manjakkal, L.; Dang, W.; Yogeswaran, N.; Dahiya, R. Textile-based potentiometric electrochemical pH sensor for wearable applications. *Biosensors* **2019**, *9*, 14. [CrossRef]
32. Manjakkal, L.; Dervin, S.; Dahiya, R. Flexible potentiometric pH sensors for wearable systems. *RSC Adv.* **2020**, *10*, 8594–8617. [CrossRef]
33. Thakur, V.K.; Voicu, S.I. Recent advances in cellulose and chitosan based membranes for water purification: A concise review. *Carbohydr. Polym.* **2016**, *146*, 148–165. [CrossRef] [PubMed]
34. Vivas, L.; Chi-Duran, I.; Enríquez, J.; Barraza, N.; Singh, D.P. Ascorbic acid based controlled growth of various Cu and Cu_2O nanostructures. *Mater. Res. Express* **2019**, *6*, 065033. [CrossRef]
35. Ain, Q.T.; Haq, S.H.; Alshammari, A.; Al-Mutlaq, M.A.; Anjum, M.N. The systemic effect of PEG-nGO-induced oxidative stress in vivo in a rodent model. *Beilstein J. Nanotechnol.* **2019**, *10*, 901–911. [CrossRef]
36. Elgrishi, N.; Rountree, K.J.; McCarthy, B.D.; Rountree, E.S.; Eisenhart, T.T.; Dempsey, J.L. A Practical Beginner's Guide to Cyclic Voltammetry. *J. Chem. Educ.* **2018**, *95*, 197–206. [CrossRef]
37. Avinash, B.; Ravikumar, C.R.; Kumar, M.R.A.; Nagaswarupa, H.P.; Santosh, M.S.; Bhatt, A.S.; Kuznetsov, D. Nano CuO: Electrochemical sensor for the determination of paracetamol and d-glucose. *J. Phys. Chem. Solids* **2019**, *134*, 193–200. [CrossRef]
38. Lu, C.; Li, Z.; Ren, L.; Su, N.; Lu, D.; Liu, Z. In Situ Oxidation of Cu_2O Crystal for Electrochemical Detection of Glucose. *Sensors* **2019**, *19*, 2926. [CrossRef]
39. Wang, W.; Zhang, L.; Tong, S.; Li, X.; Song, W. Three-dimensional network films of electrospun copper oxide nanofibers for glucose determination. *Biosens. Bioelectron.* **2009**, *25*, 708–714. [CrossRef]
40. Liu, W.; Zhao, X.; Dai, Y.; Qi, Y. Study on the oriented self-assembly of cuprous oxide micro-nano cubes and its application as a non-enzymatic glucose sensor. *Colloids Surf. B Biointerfaces* **2022**, *211*, 112317. [CrossRef]
41. Li, S.; Zheng, Y.; Qin, G.W.; Ren, Y.; Pei, W.; Zuo, L. Enzyme-free amperometric sensing of hydrogen peroxide and glucose at a hierarchical Cu_2O modified electrode. *Talanta* **2011**, *85*, 1260–1264. [CrossRef]
42. Lu, W.; Sun, Y.; Dai, H.; Ni, P.; Jiang, S.; Wang, Y.; Li, Z.; Li, Z. Direct growth of pod-like Cu_2O nanowire arrays on copper foam: Highly sensitive and efficient nonenzymatic glucose and H_2O_2 biosensor. *Sens. Actuators B Chem.* **2016**, *231*, 860–866. [CrossRef]

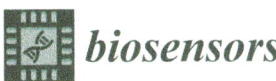

Review

The Ketogenic Diet: Breath Acetone Sensing Technology

Omar Alkedeh and Ronny Priefer *

Department of Pharmaceutical Sciences, Massachusetts College of Pharmacy and Health Sciences University, Boston, MA 02115, USA; oalke1@stu.mcphs.edu
* Correspondence: ronny.priefer@mcphs.edu

Abstract: The ketogenic diet, while originally thought to treat epilepsy in children, is now used for weight loss due to increasing evidence indicating that fat is burned more rapidly when there is a low carbohydrate intake. This low carbohydrate intake can lead to elevated ketone levels in the blood and breath. Breath and blood ketones can be measured to gauge the level of ketosis and allow for adjustment of the diet to meet the user's needs. Blood ketone levels have been historically used, but now breath acetone sensors are becoming more common due to less invasiveness and convenience. New technologies are being researched in the area of acetone sensors to capitalize on the rising popularity of the diet. Current breath acetone sensors come in the form of handheld breathalyzer devices. Technologies in development mostly consist of semiconductor metal oxides in different physio-chemical formations. These current devices and future technologies are investigated here with regard to utility and efficacy. Technologies currently in development do not have extensive testing of the selectivity of the sensors including the many compounds present in human breath. While some sensors have undergone human testing, the sample sizes are very small, and the testing was not extensive. Data regarding current devices is lacking and more research needs to be done to effectively evaluate current devices if they are to have a place as medical devices. Future technologies are very promising but are still in early development stages.

Keywords: breathalyzer; acetone; ketogenic diet; semi-conductor metal oxides

Citation: Alkedeh, O.; Priefer, R. The Ketogenic Diet: Breath Acetone Sensing Technology. *Biosensors* **2021**, *11*, 26. https://doi.org/10.3390/bios11010026

Received: 14 December 2020
Accepted: 12 January 2021
Published: 19 January 2021

Publisher's Note: MDPI stays neutral with regard to jurisdictional claims in published maps and institutional affiliations.

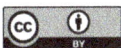

Copyright: © 2021 by the authors. Licensee MDPI, Basel, Switzerland. This article is an open access article distributed under the terms and conditions of the Creative Commons Attribution (CC BY) license (https://creativecommons.org/licenses/by/4.0/).

1. Introduction

A ketogenic diet has many variations in micronutrients, timing, portion size, frequency of meals, and caloric restriction, but the main tenet is reduced carbohydrate intake. A precursor to the modern ketogenic diet was first introduced for epileptic children in 1911 where physicians in France used starvation as a method of controlling seizures and noted positive progress, although without quantifiable evidence [1]. Subsequent studies have shown that there may be some benefit, specifically with a low carbohydrate diet in controlling children's epilepsy [2,3]. At the Mayo Clinic, RM Wilder coined the term "ketogenic diet" after he observed the increased ketone levels in the patients that had reduced carbohydrate intake [4]. The modern ketogenic diet has now become a popular method of weight loss, and has lost favor in seizure control, due to more advanced antiepileptic medications. Many people struggle with obesity because of the prevalence of highly carbohydrate dense meals, including ingredients such as high fructose corn syrup. The ketogenic diet has been shown to aid with weight loss when combined with exercise [5–7]. With this popularity, the ketogenic diet, including supplements, foods, education, and devices has a market of around $10 billion and a projection of $15 billion by 2027 [8].

The human breath contains hundreds of volatile organic compounds (VOCs) [9,10] as first noted by Linus Pauling in 1971 [11]. The most recognizable of these markers is ethanol through the use of alcohol breathalyzers [12]. While ethanol in the breath dictates the same compound in the blood, acetone is not present in the blood in a significant quantity but is rather a metabolic step in the breakdown of fatty acids. This breakdown yields three compounds of interest with respect to the ketogenic diet: specifically, βhydroxybutyrate (BHB), acetoacetate (AcAc), and acetone [13]. These ketone bodies are markers of a ketogenic state in which the body is not using glucose for energy, but rather free fatty acids. The term "ketogenic diet" or "ketodiet" is a derivation of ketone-genesis, or the making of ketones. This state of ketosis is hypothesized to assist in weight loss by increasing the rate of lipolysis [5–7,14,15]. The breaking down of fatty acids leads to AcAc production in the blood, which is then further metabolized into BHB and acetone. The majority of acetone is formed when AcAc is enzymatically decarboxylated via acetoacetate decarboxylase located in various tissues throughout the body (Figure 1). This process is dependent on blood glucose levels, with a higher level of glucose correlating with lower levels of acetone production, while lower levels of glucose correlate with higher acetone production [13]. In states of starvation, or low glucose, the body needs energy in the form of ATP and this lipolysis is essential in supplying the ketone bodies needed to produce it. It is hypothesized that by measuring the levels of either AcAc, BHB, or acetone, an estimated level of ketosis can be gauged [2,5,7,14,16–23].

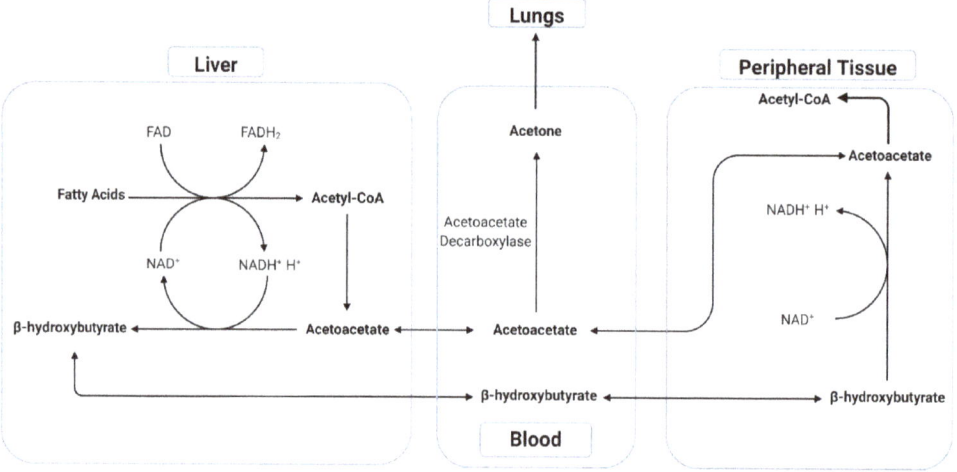

Figure 1. Human ketone metabolic pathways summary.

Acetone specifically can be measured in the breath and has been shown to correlate with the level of ketosis such as BHB detection in the blood [2,17]. Other VOCs have been explored as biomarkers for the diagnosis and management of disease states and monitoring of lifestyle. These can range from epilepsy [2,3], various cancers [24,25], diabetes [17,26], lactose intolerance [27] exposure to pollutants [9], and ketogenic diets where the level of acetone measured in exhaled air has been reported to correlate with the degree of ketosis [2,3,5–7,14,18,28,29]. This is of interest to those on a ketogenic diet because it indicates "how well" their diet is working and if adjustments are needed. It is important for dieters to know where they are along the axis to help guide their decisions and for type 1 diabetics to avoid ketoacidosis, a severe ketogenic state characterized by extremely high ketone levels and very low blood glucose which could result in a coma [30].

This zone of ketogenesis that has been suggested to be optimal is in the range of 1.5–3.0 mmol/L of BHB, if measuring blood ketones, and 2–40 ppm of acetone if measuring in the breath [14]. Falling within this range would inform dieters if they are in a state of ketosis. Breath acetone (BrAce) and BHB have been positively correlated showing R^2 values ranging from 0.7 [18] to 0.9 [2,5]. Blood BHB is routinely measured in clinics across the country as a normal laboratory assay. BrAce has only recently come into popularity due to emerging technologies. Early renditions of acetone breathalyzers used similar redox reactions as their ethanol counterparts in the hopes of crossover, but ultimately lacked specificity. Modern renditions of the breathalyzers have adopted newer technologies to increase sensitivity and specificity. Many current approaches employ the use of semiconductor metal oxides as a reactive sensor [31–35]. These can take many forms, with respect to the metal used and physicochemical arrangements. A small portion of BrAce meters on the market utilize photoionization detectors which detect acetone's absorbance under different wavelengths to determine the concentration present in the breath [36]. Future technologies currently in development mostly revolve around development of novel metal oxides to increase specificity, sensitivity, and durability.

2. Current Technology

Current ketone sensing technologies employ mass spectrometry, photoionization, gas chromatography, light-addressable potentiometric sensors, quantum cascade lasers, and semiconductor metal oxides [26]. These approaches can be used to detect ketones in the urine, breath, and blood. Previous technologies predominately involved the use of mass spectrometry and gas chromatography. However, these technologies are limited due to their cost and bulk. Tests would need to be ordered with the patient's samples being sent to the lab which would take time to receive results. Because of the cost and inconvenience, these tests were not routinely done. The current standard of care for diabetics is to check glycated hemoglobin and blood glucose levels using a blood test to mostly monitor high levels of glucose. Ketone sensing technology has been proposed as a supplemental diagnostic tool for high levels of ketones [26].

Current trends in ketone sensing technologies revolve around handheld breath acetone detectors. These devices are capable of detecting levels of acetone in the breath usually in ppm levels and report it to the user. Utility of this with respect to the ketogenic diet comes from linking the degree of ketosis to BrAce. Some key factors need to be identified before confidently accepting the breathalyzer's readout. These include the patient health, the device has high sensitivity and specificity for acetone, the dieter has not ingested anything that could interfere with the signal, and the timing between meals and exercise. Additionally, there are some identified factors that affect BrAce readout, some of which are; exercise, obesity, garlic ingestion, disulfiram, and variability in body temperatures [7]. Exercise has been shown to increase BrAce in adults because energy in the form of glucose has been depleted and the body moves to metabolize fat stores [37]. Obese individuals have been shown to have lower levels of BrAce. This mechanism is not fully understood and may be related to insulin resistance where fat oxidation is limited [21]. Garlic ingestion has been shown to moderately increase BrAce by possibly inhibiting acetone metabolism [38]. Disulfiram, a drug used to treat alcohol dependence, may also increase BrAce through its acetaldehyde dehydrogenase inhibition. Temperature extremes also have effects on overall metabolic rate in humans and variations may correlate with BrAce changes [39]. These factors are important to consider when using single point measurements of BrAce. Repeated measurements over a day provide ketone exposure rather than immediate ketosis status which may be more useful for long term dieters.

The majority of current devices use semiconductor metal oxide (SMO) sensors to detect BrAce. This is due to the cheap manufacturing cost, portability, low energy input, and the wide range of evidence supporting their accuracy [26,40–43]. Many SMOs are available with sensitivity and specificity to acetone. A number of current commercially available devices are generic versions with no patent that have been rebranded by multiple companies [35]. This makes it difficult to determine their exact makeup, technology, and reliability.

Evidence for currently available commercial ketone breathalyzers is lacking. Many studies have assessed the utility of novel sensors in the ketogenic diet [25,41–68], but very few have evaluated currently available devices. The BIOSENSE™ device is a breathalyzer with published clinical trial data detailing its efficacy. However, the data reported in this trial should be taken lightly because an independent reviewer was not present and the sample size was very small. The parent company, Readout Health, has published prospective observational cohort study of 21 subjects using the BIOSENSE™ and Precision Xtra devices. The Precision Xtra is an FDA cleared device from Abbot Laboratories, Inc., Abbot Park, IL, USA that measures blood ketones and glucose [69]. The subjects recruited were majority female (81%), described as ethnically diverse, and divided between a ketogenic diet and standard diet. They self-reported daily values for blood ketones and BrAce. Values were measured five times throughout the day and subjects were adherent at a rate of 100%, 93%, and 63% to three, four, and fives daily tests, respectively. A total of 1214 measurements comparing BrAce and blood ketones were run in a linear regression analysis and obtain the coefficient of determination to be $R^2 = 0.57$ ($p < 0.0001$) [70]. Additionally, measurements from each individual were plotted separately for each day giving a total of 248 total subject days and used to examine the daily ketone exposure (DKE). The value derived from the area under the curve (AUC) of ketone concentration over time [70]. This DKE value for both BrAce and blood BHB was analyzed and another linear regression was calculated giving $R^2 = 0.80$ [70].

This Readout Health study produced valuable results with respect to DKE. The authors demonstrated that ketone levels throughout the day are highly variable, thus limiting the utility of single point measurements. By measuring multiple times throughout the day, a DKE calculation can be obtained to give overall ketone exposure. More data is needed to determine the utility of DKE calculations in comparison to single point readings. The BIOSENSE™ device measures single point readings, but a mobile application also determines a DKE calculation called a "Ketone Score" [70].

However, the utility of the BIOSENSE™ device cannot be accurately assessed. There are many limitations to the study and not enough data. The sample size of the device is only 21 which is very low for a clinical trial. The subjects' baseline characteristics were never described in the study and only mentioned to be ethnically diverse which limits the generalizability of the results. There was a lack of gender distribution with 80% of the subjects being female. The DKE calculation was determined using days that had four or five readings and those readings had adherences of 93% and 63%, respectively which again limits the sample size and generalizability. The specific build of the device was only mentioned as a metal oxide semiconductor with no details beyond that. The subjects' diet was also not monitored even though the authors recognized that certain factors and drugs can influence BrAce. This study was also conducted by the same company that produced the BIOSENSE™ device with no data handling by a third party, so accuracy of the data is questionable.

Another reported device is the METRON disposable acetone sensor. This device is not currently commercially available but has a mechanism unique to other acetone sensors. The device is described by US Patent 8,871,521 [71] as a hollow tube with a liquid and powder component. The subject would break a seal and combine the two components and then blow through the device. A reaction between sodium nitroprusside (SNP) and an ammonium salt would occur facilitated by acetone in the breath. The level of BrAce would correlate with reaction extent via colorimetric spectroscopy. A purple color would be observed with 1.4 mg/dL of BrAce, or a "positive" result. This device is no longer commercially available.

The INVOY breathalyzer contains a liquid nanoparticle sensor as detailed in US Patent 9,486,169 [72]. The specific metal oxide was not mentioned, and no studies have evaluated its effectiveness. It is described in the patent as containing liquid cartridges that can react with BrAce and produce a colorimetric change that is detected by a camera and relayed to a sensing system which then gives an approximate BrAce level.

The Ketoscan device developed by Sentech GMI corp. in Korea uses a photoionization detector calibrated for acetone, as described in its patent application [73]. There is no published data describing its specificity or sensitivity or use in a ketogenic diet. The Ketoscan company has posts on its website claiming of undergoing clinical trials; however, there are no published results in any scientific journal and only simple results comparing the detected fat lost with the device to actual fat lost are indicated; however, this data is not currently verifiable.

Other ketone breathalyzers listed in Table 1 have very limited data on their functionality, build, and effectiveness. Some can be assumed to be SMO containing due to similar user steps and build, but no data is currently available evaluating these devices. Their accuracy with respect to specificity and sensitivity is questionable and may or may not be provided. More studies are needed to evaluate current available ketone sensing systems. FDA status is also indicated in the table because it may indicate the intentions of the manufacturer and quality of the device.

End-tidal breath or the last air out of a breath is noted to contain the true concentration of acetone [74]. What this means for sensors is that a sustained breath is needed to accurately detect the breath acetone level. Currently available sensors do not indicate they have a specific mechanism for this, but most direct the user to exhale for around 10 s which gets around the end-tidal volume of air for healthy people.

Table 1. Current commercially available breath acetone sensing devices.

Brand	Technology	FDA Status	Strengths	Limits
METRON [71]	SNP [c], ammonium sulfate powder	N/A [b]	Disposable	Off Market
INVOY [72,75]	Liquid Cartridges with Metal Oxide [d]	Registered Class 1	Available through a nutrition program	Disposable cartridges
Ketoscan [36,73]	Photoionization Detector	Registered Class 1	Undergoing trials	Limited data
House of Keto [35]	Metal Oxide Detector	N/A [b]	Cheap cost	Generic build, Limited data
Ketonix [76]	N/A [a]	Registered Class 1	Cheap cost	Limited data
Qetoe [34]	Metal Oxide Detector	N/A [b]	Cheap cost	Generic build, Limited data
Lencool [33]	Metal Oxide Detector	N/A [b]	Cheap cost	Generic build, Limited data
Lexico health [32]	Metal Oxide Detector	N/A [b]	Cheap cost	Generic build, Limited data
KetoPRX [77]	N/A [a]	N/A [b]	Cheap cost	Generic build, Limited data
Keyto [78]	N/A [a]	N/A [b]	Easy use	Limited data
LEVL [79]	N/A [a]	Registered Class 1	Clinician coaching included	Expensive, limited data
Biosense [31,70]	Metal Oxide Detector	Registered Class 1	Data available	expensive

[a] Technology in use was not publicly available. [b] The device listed is not registered with the FDA or the status could not be determined. [c] Sodium Nitroprusside (SNP). [d] Specific details regarding composition of liquid and the metal oxide was not listed.

3. Future Technologies

The main sensors presented here are metal oxides and light-based sensors. Semiconductor metal oxides at their basic level detect resistance changes along their surface when exposed to the different gases. Oxygen is present on their surface which is reduced, and that electron changes the resistance of the sensor. These sensors are no longer plain metal oxides but consist of many different nano-arrangements and can also be doped with other metals, changing their porosity and overall function. The challenge many researchers have is to find the right ratio of metals to combine, an adequate nano-arrangement, and a cheap and simple process for development [80]. Light based sensors are also presented as an alternative to the bulk gas chromatography and mass spectrometry. They emit light that is then picked up by a sensor and in between the emitter and sensor is the gas. Certain gases affect the light differently and this can be calibrated into the sensors to find the exact gas concentration present [43].

3.1. Metal Oxides and Organic Based Sensors

Many sensors in development are utilizing metal oxides as its base and experimenting with augmentations to the metal in an effort to increase the sensitivity, specificity, efficiency, and durability. Plain metal oxides have some utility in sensors, but do not have the sensitivity and selectivity of the novel augmented sensors being researched today. Other metals in certain nano conformations, such as nanosheets, nanoparticles, and nanotubes are being researched to allow for more VOC and oxygen adsorption to their surface and increase selectivity toward acetone. One variation between the sensors seen is the operating temperature. This is the temperature that the researchers have selected for the device to operate at in order to achieve maximum response. This temperature is not sustained but exists for a small amount of time in the sensor. A lower operating temperature would be ideal because a lower power consumption and higher temperature tend to lower stability of the sensors. Here we explore some BrAce sensors utilizing metal oxides and discuss their effectiveness and utility. A summary of highlighted data is provided on Table 2.

3.1.1. Zinc Oxide, Cadmium Based

Graphene quantum dots (GQD) are nanostructures with use in many different applications including gas sensing. Liu et al. [54] have developed a GQD-functionalized three-dimensional ordered mesoporous (3DOM) ZnO sensor for acetone detection. The goal was to improve upon basic ZnO sensors and demonstrate a manufacturing process for assembling the sensor. First polymethyl methacrylate (PMMA) spheres were permeated with $ZnO(NO_3)_2$ and underwent a calcination process to remove volatiles, yielding a 3DOM ZnO structure. GQDs were made by dispersing graphite powder with strong acids. This solution was subsequently washed, dried, and heated to produce the GQDs. The 3DOM ZnO were spin-coated with the GQDs to produce the sensor backbone and tested on various gases. Operating temperature of this sensor was lower than other 3DOM ZnO sensors (320 °C vs. 380 °C) which is crucial since there is a concern of decomposition of the GQDs at temperatures greater than 350 °C. The addition of the GQD yielded faster response and recovery times (at 1 ppm of acetone GQD 3DOM ZnO (9/16 s) vs. 3DOM ZnO (16/27 s). The incorporation of the GQD sensor also led to a lower detection limit of 50 ppb vs. 200 ppb with the 3DOM ZnO sensor. With regards to selectivity, the GQD 3DOM ZnO sensor exhibited poor response to water and was highly selective to acetone compared to other gases (R_{air}/R_{gas} = 15.2 at 1 ppm). NO_2, H_2S, NH_3, toluene, ethanol, methanol, isopropanol, and NO were tested with values lower than 4.1. As for stability, the sensor was measured to have lost 3% weight when subjected to temperatures from 50–200 °C. This weight loss was attributed to the decomposition of water present in the samples by the authors. The authors described that this sensor has potential utility as a diabetic diagnostic tool to detect high ketones in the breath, but the same concept can be applied to a ketogenic diet [54].

Researchers at Shenzhen University in China have developed two ZnO based sensors which are Au or Pd doped to enhance the acetone sensing capabilities [53]. The sensor was prepared using microwave assisted solvothermal reactions. The Au doped sensors achieved a maximum response of R_{air}/R_{gas} = 102 at 150 °C with 2.0 wt% Au, while the Pd doped sensor achieved a maximum response of R_{air}/R_{gas} = 69 at 150 °C with 1.5 wt% Pd. Selectivity for acetone was compared to ethanol, methanol, H_2, NH_3, and SO_2. Both sensors displayed selectivity, with the Au doped sensor being more selective to acetone. The response and recovery times of the Au doped sensor was 8 and 5 s, respectively, while the plain ZnO sensor was 9 and 7 s, respectively. Sensor stability was noted to be excellent by the authors with only slight variation in response at 150 °C [53].

Table 2. All discussed semiconductor metal oxide (SMOs) and organic based sensors.

Technology	Operating Temp (°C)	Detection Limit (ppb)	Response/Recovery Time (s)	Maximum Response (R_{air}/R_{gas}) [a]	Reference	Selectivity (Max Response/2nd Best Response)	Relative Humidity Tested	Tested on Human Breath? (Y/N)
MgNi$_2$O$_3$	200	500	25/250 (40 ppm)	2.3 (10 ppm)	Lavanya et al. [59]	~1.87	N/A	N
NiTa$_2$O$_6$	600	200	9/18 (2 ppm)	N/A	Liu et al. [61]	~1.5	20–98%	Y
PtCu/WO$_3$·H$_2$O HS	280	10	3.4/7.5 (50 ppm)	204.9 (50 ppm)	Deng et al. [56]	~5.4	N/A	N
PdAu/SnO$_2$	250	45	5/4 (2 ppm)	6.5 (2 ppm)	Li at al. [48]	~2.1	40–70%	N
Cr/WO$_3$	250	298	N/A	71.52 (100 ppm)	Ding et al. [52]	~4.3	25–90%	N
Apo-Pt@HP WO$_3$NFs	350	N/A	N/A	88.04 (5 ppm)	Kim et al. [42]	~2.95	90%	Y
ZnO QDs	430	100	N/A	N/A	Jung et al. [43]	N/A	N/A	Y
3DOM ZnO	320	8.7	9/16 (1 ppm)	15.2 (1 ppm)	Liu et al. [54]	~3.75	25–90%	Y
Au (2%)/ZnO nanorod	150	5	8/5 (100 ppm)	102 (100 ppm)	Huang et al. [53]	~3.4	N/A	N
Pd (1.5%)/ZnO nanorod	150	5	9/7 (100 ppm)	69 (100 ppm)	Huang et al. [53]	~2.6	N/A	N
CdTe/PPY	24	5	155/270–310 (5 ppm)	N/A	Šetka et al. [50]	N/A	30%	N
Bi$_{0.9}$La$_{0.1}$FeO$_3$	260	50	15/13 (50 ppb)	40 (100 ppm)	Peng et al. [47]	5.71	55–90%	N
ZnO nanoplates	450	45	23/637 (50 ppm)	20 (125 ppm)	Van Duy et al. [66]	2.22	10–80%	N
Pt-PH-SO$_2$	400	200	7/(N/A)	44.83 (5 ppm)	Cho et al. [63]	~3.57	90%	N
Si:WO$_3$	350	20	14/36 (100 ppb)	N/A	Righettoni [49]	18	0–90%	Y
Catalytic enhanced Si:WO$_3$	400	50	55/100 (500 ppb)	4.3 (1 ppm)	Weber et al. [81]	250	90%	Y

[a] Maximum response recorded without humidity or other interfering gases.

Šetka et al. developed a new sensor capable of working at room temperature using cadmium telluride/polypyrrole (CdTe/PPy) nanocomposites which were integrated into Love mode surface acoustic wave (L SAW) sensors [50]. This new sensor achieved high specificity and selectivity for VOCs, including acetone. The sensor was made up of two components, the first being PPy, which is a conductive polymer, and the second being CdTe. The PPy was meant to overcome weaknesses associated with plain conductive polymers such as high working temperature, poor selectivity, or low response speed [50]. By incorporating a metal in the form of CdTe, these limitations could be overcome. The CdTe quantum dots (QD) were first formed using $CdCl_2$, tri-sodium citrate dihydrate, and mercaptopropionic acid (MPA). The pH was adjusted, and sodium tellurite and sodium borohydride were added. The solution was mixed and heated to form the CdTe QDs which were combined with the polypyyrole by mixing the solutions and then spin coating. CdTe and PPY were combined in two different concentrations (CdTe/PPy 1:10 and 1:2) and another sensor was left with only PPy. The 1:10 CdTe/PPy sensor showed the highest response while the 1:2 CdTe/PPy sensor showed the lowest. The PPy sensor had sensitivity to acetone (652 Hz/ppm), while the 1:10 CdTe/PPy sensor was improved with approximately 1.2× greater sensitivity. Overall, this technique and new sensor is promising; however, human testing needs to be conducted to assess its function once exposed to the hundreds of VOCs found within the human breath. A positive attribute to this sensor is the ability to operate at room temperature with low energy requirement.

Researchers in Vietnam have synthesized ultrathin porous ZnO nanoplates via a urea mediated synthesis [66]. These nanoplates are 2D structures which are hypothesized to have excellent sensitivity due to their exposed planes. The nanoplates were synthesized via a hydrothermal method. A scanning electron microscope was used to observe the structures and demonstrate their ultrathin and porous structure which is thought to contribute to their gas sensing ability. The sensor was tested with acetone, ethanol, methanol, toluene, and NH_3 gases at temperatures ranging from 350 to 450 °C. The sensor was found to be temperature dependent with a decrease in temperature leading to decreased response. At 125 ppm of acetone, the sensor had a response of 20 (R_{air}/R_{gas}). The response and recovery time for the sensor were calculated from transient resistance versus time when flow was switched from air to gas and back to air. The sensor had response and recover times at acetone concentration of 50 ppm, of 23 and 637 s, respectively and at concentrations of 50–125 ppm, of 7 and 550 s, respectively. Compared to the aforementioned GQD 3DOM ZnO [53] and the CdTe/PPy [50] sensors, the response/recovery time is very high. The operating temperature of 450 °C is also very high and would require a greater energy input. Despite the high temperature, the sensor displayed excellent stability over 10 exposures to acetone over 10,000 s with little variation in response.

A miniaturized gas chromatographic column utilizing ZnO QD was developed by researchers in the Republic of Korea [43]. These QDs were synthesized using a: Zn acetate, N,N-dimethylformamide, and tetramethylammonium hydroxide then laid on the sensor. A patient would breathe into a sampling loop, and a pump would slowly push 1 mL of the sample through a packed column. The acetone was then detected on the ZnO QDs based on changes in the resistance of the sensor. Using this method, the gasses are physically separated before to ensure greater accuracy. Responses were recorded in terms of ($\Delta \log(R)$) and were positively correlated with stock acetone gas in ppm with an R^2 of 0.9915. The device was tested on three subjects with one undergoing a ketogenic diet. It was noted there was an increased response correlating with higher BrAce in the subject undergoing the ketogenic diet. The correlation is very strong at $R^2 = 0.9915$ [43]; however, the sample size of 3 is very small with only a few data points, and thus not enough to draw conclusions about the device's utility.

3.1.2. Iron Oxides

La_xFeO_3 based sensors have rising popularity with researchers looking to optimize and enhance current sensors. La_xFeO_3 has stability at high temperatures and can be formed into specific crystal arrangements to allow ultralow detection limits of acetone. Chen et al. in China have developed nano-LaFeO$_3$ thick-films in an attempt to reach ppb levels of acetone detection [41]. To make their sensor, lanthanum nitrate, ferric nitrate, and citric acid were mixed and formulated using the sol-gel method, then heated in an oven and mixed with water to make a paste to spread onto the sensor plate. The sensor was determined to have the highest response when annealed at 800 °C. The sensor exhibited different responses depending on the concentration of acetone. For acetone concentrations of 0.5 ppm, 1 ppm, 5 ppm, 10 ppm, the responses were 2.068, 3.245, 5.195, and 7.925 (R_{air}/R_{gas}), respectively. Ethanol and acetone were compared at 5 ppm and ethanol had a higher response, 2.44 vs. 1.936 showing poor selectivity. Compared to other gases such as HCHO, NH$_3$, and methanol, the sensor had greater selectivity for acetone. Optimal operating temperature was determined to be 260 °C with response times from 37–51 s and recovery times of 82–155 s.

A $Bi_{1-x}La_xFeO_3$ (x = 0–0.2) sensor was developed by Peng at al. in China [47]. The authors' goal was ultralow levels of acetone detection. A sol-gel method was used to make the sensor using: $Bi(NO_3)_3 \cdot 5H_2O$, $Fe(NO_3)_3 \cdot 9H_2O$, and $La(NO_3)_3 \cdot 6H_2O$ mixed in acids and then heated to yield the final powder, which was cast on a gold sensor plate. Using $Bi_{1-x}La_xFeO_3$ (x = 0.1) at 50 ppb acetonitrile, tetrahydrofuran, N-hexane, CHCl$_3$, CH$_2$Cl$_2$, NH$_3$, and xylene were tested alongside acetone and there was no detectable response, while with acetone there was a response of 8 (R_{air}/R_{gas}). The highest response achieved was 40 (R_{air}/R_{gas}) at 100 ppm of acetone and 260 °C. The sensor was tested in 55%, 70%, and 90% RH with response decreasing as the RH was increased and acetone test gas concentration decreased. The lowest response was 2.8 (R_{air}/R_{gas}) at 90% RH and 50 pbb of acetone and the highest was around 16 (R_{air}/R_{gas}) at 55% RH and 1000 ppb. Response/recovery time was exceptional at 260 °C and 15 and 13 s, respectively. The sensors were tested for stability over 4 weeks and found little variation in response when tested at 50, 600, and 1000 ppb of acetone. This sensor was not tested on human subjects, but has been proposed as a diabetic or ketogenic diet device [47].

3.1.3. Tin Oxides

Li et al. in China incorporated Pd and Au onto SnO$_2$ nanosheets (NSs) for another sensor. This sensor was made to compare the effects of Pd and Au on enhancing the gas sensing performance of SnO$_2$ nanosheets. To make the sensor, a hydro-solvothermal method was used to produce SnO$_2$ nanosheets. Pd and Au were then added along with ascorbic acid to produce the doped nanosheets. Two separate sensors with only either Pd or Au on the SnO$_2$ nanosheets were also made for comparison. The Pd/Au SnO$_2$ sensor outperformed bother sensors in all categories and required a lower operating temperature. The sensor was not tested on humans, but the authors noted that under 94% RH the sensor performed well. It exhibited a 45 ppb detection limit which is very low compared to other sensors and had a response of 6.5 (R_{air}/R_{gas}) at 2 ppm of acetone under an operating temperature of 250 °C and very fast response/recovery times of 5/4 s possibly owing the fast times to a highly exposed surface area and porosity from the unique nanosheet structure. This sensor was made as an enhancement of a basic SnO$_2$ sensor to demonstrate how Pd and Au can improve the sensor. Compared to a basic SnO$_2$ sensor, the PdAu/SnO$_2$ sensor has over three times the response to acetone at 1 ppm. Stability over 40 days was tested and a response reduction of 3–5% was detected when measuring at 250 °C [48].

Similarly, another SnO$_2$ sensor was developed by Cho et al. [63] to maximize gas sensing performance by increasing porosity. This was done by using SnO$_2$ spheres made via a novel electrostatic spraying method which also incorporated Pt into the nanostructures resulting in Pt-pore-loaded hierarchical SnO$_2$ (Pt-PH-SnO$_2$) spheres. These were compared to PH-SnO$_2$ spheres and hierarchical SnO$_2$ spheres. The benefit of the new Pt-PH-SnO$_2$ spheres as compared to previous sensors is the pores which allow for about a 20% enhanced gas sensing response. This sensor also demonstrated a novel electrostatic spraying technique which allows an easier and more robust method of SMO sensor synthesis. The maximum response of the Pt-PH-SnO$_2$ sensor was 44.83 (R_{air}/R_{gas}) at 5 ppm compared to a much lower 6.61 (R_{air}/R_{gas}) from the PH-SnO$_2$ sensor. The operating temperature is on the higher end at 400 °C. The detection limit is 200 ppb which is intermediate compared to other sensors discussed. The response time of the Pt-PH-SnO$_2$ sensor was noted to be 7 s, but no acetone concentration was given [63]. The recovery time was noted to be fast; however, no value was mentioned. This sensor was evaluated in 90% RH and exhibited similar performance with or without humidity. Stability of the sensor was noted to be great. Measurements were taken at 18 months and the response was reduced to 34.18 at 5 ppm. No human tests were conducted and more data on this sensor is needed, such as complete response and recovery times and accuracy compared to other sensors.

3.1.4. Tungsten Oxides

Tungsten Oxides are very popular in current BrAce sensor research. Ding et al. have developed a WO$_3$ sensor and compared its functionality when doped with chromium [52]. This sensor follows the process of Cr doping from research in 2008 to form a similar sensor [82]. The sensors were not tested on humans but was tested in 40% RH. The sensor had a low detection limit of 298 ppb, an operating temperature of 250 °C, and a response of 71.52 (R_{air}/R_{gas}) at 100 ppm. The plain WO$_3$ sensor was noted to have a response three times lower than the chromium doped one. Through thorough investigation by Ding et al., tungsten annealed at 450 °C and 100 mg of chromium were determined to give the best response [52]. Tungsten oxide was also used in another sensor made and tested by Kim et al. in Korea and the United States. WO$_3$ nanofibers incorporated with Pt nanoparticles were encapsulated in a protein cage and then heat treated to give the desired dispersion of Pt nanoparticles. The sensor was tested under varying RH up to 90%, but not tested on humans. The response/recovery times and detection limits were not addressed by the researchers. A response of 88.04 (R_{air}/R_{gas}) at 5 ppm was noted. This sensor utilizes a novel method of a sacrificial template in the form of a protein which allows for a different method of dispersing nanoparticles on a medium [42].

Platinum and palladium have been historically used in their pure form as electrodes for various electronic application. Current uses, with respect to breath acetone sensors, involve the addition of Pt or Pd in the sensor to enhance its functionality. One such sensor has been developed by Deng et al. in China where WO$_3$·H$_2$O hollow spheres were modified with 0.02% PtCu nanocrystals to improve response by up to 9.5 times [56]. Deng at al.'s sensor exhibited maximum response of 204.9 (R_{air}/R_{gas}) with 0.02% PtCu at a temperature of 280 °C using a stock 50 ppm acetone sample [56]. Their sensor also demonstrated good selectivity for acetone when compared to other gases, including the following: methylbenzene, ethanol, formaldehyde, methanol, benzene, ammonia, and hydrogen with acetone achieving a response 4 times greater than any of the aforementioned gases, but was not tested for in humid conditions nor tested on humans [56]. An early tungsten-based sensor from 2012 was developed by researchers from Switzerland and Austria using Si-doped WO$_3$ nanostructured films [49]. This sensor has limited data on its capabilities such as maximum response. The fast response and recovery times of 10 and 35 s, respectively, and very low detection limit of 20 ppb seem very promising. Revisiting this sensor may be warranted to possibly optimize it and further test with humans. It was tested on five healthy male participants in 2012 with limited data regarding the tests. It seemed to exhibit very high selectivity when comparing the acetone response to the second best response of ethanol with a value of around 18. This may not accurately represent the sensor as a whole due to only testing against ethanol in the 2012 study. This sensor was further tested in 2013 on 8 healthy subjects to correlated glucose levels and breath components and found a strong correlation of 0.98 after overnight fasting [82]. Further testing of this sensor on 20 volunteers in 2017 on fat metabolism showed that the elevated breath acetone post exercise was correlated with elevated blood BHB and that the sensor is suitable as an exercise monitor [83]. A year later in 2018, this sensor was tested again with a ketogenic diet and 11 volunteers and found that a ketogenic diet raised ketone levels. The breath acetone level was compared to blood BHB and the levels were in agreement. The authors noted that the sensor could be suitable for tracking a ketogenic diet along with ketosis status of an epileptic patient. Further research on this sensor incorporated it into a sensing array for human detection in collapsed buildings. The array would include this Si:WO_3 sensor, a Si:MoO_3 sensor, and a Ti:ZnO sensor. This array was set to detect acetone, ammonia, and isoprene concentrations at 19, 21, and 3 ppb respectively. This was a unique approach to using breath acetone monitoring [84]. Lastly in 2020, the sensor was enhanced with a catalytic filter made of Al_2O_3 nanoparticles which was heated to 135 °C before the sensor was heated to 400 °C. This allows it to have an enhanced selectivity of over 250 against many analytes including alcohols, aldehydes, aromatics, isoprene, ammonia, hydrogen gas, and carbon monoxide. Stability was excellent with responses staying constant when subjected to 145 days at 90% relative humidity [81].

3.1.5. Nickel Oxides

Nickel containing sensors have some popularity in gas sensors and a current research exists to try and find optimal chemical and physical configurations. Liu et al. in China have developed a nickel-based sensor using stabilized zirconia and $NiTa_2O_6$. Their sensor had a detection range of 0.2–200 ppm of acetone, sensitivity of $-11/-27$ (mV/decade), response and recovery times in seconds of 9 and 18, respectively. The selectivity was not great with ethanol and methanol achieving around half of the response to acetone under various conditions. The response of the sensor fluctuated between -2.5–1.5 mV in relative humidity ranges of 20–98%, which demonstrates good applicability for human breath. The operating temperature of 600 °C was quite high; however, the sensor demonstrated good stability over repeated use [61]. Another nickel-based sensor was developed by researchers from India and Italy using $MgNi_2O_3$ nanoparticles. The sensor did not have a linear response for detecting acetone concentration, but a calibration was possible to determine a concentration based on previous known values. The sensor has an operating temperature of 200 °C, which is much lower compared to the aforementioned $NiTa_6O_6$ sensor. The response to acetone at 10 ppm was 2.3 (R_{air}/R_{gas}). A detection limit was extrapolated to be 0.3 ppm with values only measuring down to 0.5 ppm. The response and recovery times were 25 and 250 s, respectively. The sensor was also proposed to be able to directly measure blood glucose levels. The long-term stability of the sensor was not discussed; however, the sensor was noted to be stable over the fluctuations of the test with a constant response. This sensor was not tested in humid conditions nor tested on human subjects [59].

3.2. Light Based

New sensors are under development utilizing light absorbance and diffraction. Lasers are often used for these applications due to their precision and stability which allows for more accurate measurements [85–89]. Schwarm et al. have developed a laser sensor that has been tested on subjects undergoing a ketogenic diet [37]. The sensor follows classic Beer–Lambert law by measuring absorbance of a gas and comparing it to known levels of acetone to determine the concentration present in exhaled breath. The sensor has an array of fiber optic cables and mirrors to lay out the laser path. This sensor uses an 8.2 μm region which was determined to give the least interference. Accuracy has only been tested against known concentrations of acetone in N_2 gas in a testing chamber and not compared with gas chromatography or mass spectroscopy in humans. Human testing was done to determine if the sensor can detect changes in BrAce but not for accuracy. Five subjects were enrolled out of UCLA medical center and underwent a ketogenic diet. They had baseline BrAce measured before the diet and began a 36-h ketogenic diet. All subjects demonstrated elevated BrAce from baseline for the duration of the diet and 3 h post diet. The sensor was the exclusive BrAce measuring device used and accuracy of the results are not clear. This sensor is in the early stages and seems promising if more human testing is done.

Another light-based sensor from the UK uses direct Ultraviolet (UV) absorbance to measure acetone [45]. Acetone of known concentrations were measured using the sensor and gas chromatography. The sensor was tested on 10 healthy human subjects against gas chromatography and showed a linear correlation with an R = 0.971 [45]. The human breath samples were collected into Tedlar® bags and not directly measured with either gas chromatography or the sensor to obtain more consistent results. This sensor also had a detection limit of 0.7 ppm. Being a light-based sensor, the values governing the sensors are different than the SMOs and a direct comparison may be difficult. The largest advantage of this sensor is the use of cheap UV LEDs which also have a low energy requirement compared to traditionally employed lasers.

3.3. Comparisons

Certain metal oxides are used because of their cheap cost and are easy to work with such as zinc and iron, which can be acquired cheaply. Tungsten is sought after as a sensor because of its unique ability to be formed in complex crystalline and nanoparticle morphologies. Current research does not include bare metal oxides and most sensors are doped with other metals such as Cr, Pd, Pt, Au, and Si in hopes of enhancing their abilities. The versatility of these metal oxides comes at a price, however. Historically, these bare metal oxides had poor stability with repeated exposure to humidity and the various analytes. Progress has been made to enhance stability, but there is a limit to this because the sensor will always be in direct contact with the analytes and humidity. Light based sensors can be beneficial because of this, and allow for a closed loop system to protect the sensors and offer long term stability such as Li et al.'s [45].

The more prominent sensors discussed here are the semiconductor metal oxides. They differ in their material, operating temperature, output data (selectivity, sensitivity, response), and the extensiveness of their testing. Humidity is necessary to test in because human breath is very humid and before human testing can begin, the sensor must be validated in humid conditions. Many sensors test in humid conditions and even test long term stability in humid conditions which is very valuable such as Weber et al.'s sensor [82]. More than half the sensors discussed here were not tested on humans. In the early stages of development this is acceptable, but to further pursue them as commercial devices, they should undergo the testing. The selectivity of the sensors is very important to differentiate between different VOCs. The highest selectivity (250) was seen with Weber et al.'s sensor [81]. This is due to the catalytic process added to eliminate other analytes before they reach the sensor. The maximum response was also noted for each sensor and the highest was noted with Deng et al.'s sensor with a response of 204 (R_{air}/R_{gas}) at 50 ppm. The maximum response is important because it needs to be significant enough to be detected, but also it needs to vary from other analytes to have good selectivity. The response and recovery times are also crucial because it allows for convenience and ease of use. A sensor with a long response or recovery time might not see commercial success. The lowest times reported were with Li et al.'s sensor 5/4 s response and recovery times respectively at 2 ppm of acetone. The operating temperature is another crucial parameter. A high operating temperature can be dangerous and thus requires significant power to use the sensor. A lower temperature is preferred to also keep the sensor stable.

For a manufacturer to decide on the use of the different technologies, it comes down to their needs. A high operating temperature sensor may be suitable if it is cheap and the company can afford the excess power needed in a new power delivery system. A sensor with low selectivity may find success with a company that then adds a step before it to reduce other analytes such as Weber et al.'s design with the catalytic step prior [81]. There is not a sensor that is best all around, but there are certainly sensors that have valuable traits.

4. Conclusions

The rising popularity of the ketogenic diet is expanding the use of acetone breathalyzers owing to, in part, the data demonstrating the possible benefit of the diet with respect to diabetes management and weight loss. This popularity has founded a new market for acetone breathalyzers. Many breathalyzers are currently on the market, but there is a lack of scientific evaluation of these sensors. Most sensors do not have any data regarding their utility for use in a ketogenic diet. Novel sensors being developed provide some of the data and testing, but more is still needed. Novel sensors have been developed utilizing SMOs, lasers, UV light, nanoparticles, and organic scaffolds. SMO sensors typically containing basic metal oxides such as zinc, iron, and tungsten, however, are being phased out in favor of sensors doped with other metals such as gold, platinum, and palladium and/or nanoparticles. There is a significant body of research on these sensors regarding their sensitivity, selectivity, efficiency, and durability. Many of these novel technologies report high responses to acetone; however, many of these have not undergone human testing and may show conflicting results compared to simulated breath in the lab. Selectivity is especially an area of concern because the sensors need to differentiate between the different analytes. Some sensors have not reported selectivity data and others have only reported against a few analytes which does not adequately simulate real world applications. To more adequately compare the various sensors on the market and in development, more rigorous testing is needed which can pave the way for more FDA registered devices.

Funding: This research received no external funding.

Acknowledgments: The authors wish to thank the School of Pharmacy at the Massachusetts College of Pharmacy and Health Sciences University for financial support of this project.

Conflicts of Interest: The authors declare no conflict of interest.

References

1. Marie, L.D.A. La Lutte Contrjz L'épilepsie Par La Rééducation Alimentaire. *Epilepsia* **1911**, *A2*, 265–273. [CrossRef]
2. Musa-Veloso, K.; Likhodii, S.S.; Rarama, E.; Benoit, S.; Liu, Y.-M.C.; Chartrand, D.; Curtis, R.; Carmant, L.; Lortie, A.; Comeau, F.J.; et al. Breath acetone predicts plasma ketone bodies in children with epilepsy on a ketogenic diet. *Nutrition* **2006**, *22*, 1–8. [CrossRef] [PubMed]
3. Musa-Veloso, K.; Rarama, E.; Comeau, F.; Curtis, R.; Cunnane, S. Epilepsy and the Ketogenic Diet: Assessment of Ketosis in Children Using Breath Acetone. *Pediatr. Res.* **2002**, *52*, 443–448. [CrossRef] [PubMed]
4. Wilder, R. The effects of ketonemia on the course of epilepsy. *Mayo Clin. Proc.* **1921**, *2*, 307–308.
5. Musa-Veloso, K.; Likhodii, S.S.; Cunnane, S.C. Breath acetone is a reliable indicator of ketosis in adults consuming ketogenic meals. *Am. J. Clin. Nutr.* **2002**, *76*, 65–70. [CrossRef]
6. Saslow, L.R.; Kim, S.; Daubenmier, J.J.; Moskowitz, J.T.; Phinney, S.D.; Goldman, V.; Murphy, E.J.; Cox, R.M.; Moran, P.; Hecht, F.M. A Randomized Pilot Trial of a Moderate Carbohydrate Diet Compared to a Very Low Carbohydrate Diet in Overweight or Obese Individuals with Type 2 Diabetes Mellitus or Prediabetes. *PLoS ONE* **2014**, *9*, e91027. [CrossRef]
7. Anderson, J.C. Measuring breath acetone for monitoring fat loss: Review. *Obesity* **2015**, *23*, 2327–2334. [CrossRef]
8. Ketogenic Diet Market to Reach US$ 15,640.6 Mn at CAGR of 5.5% in 2027. The Insight Partners. Available online: https://www.theinsightpartners.com/reports/ketogenic-diet-market (accessed on 4 November 2020).
9. Pleil, J.D.; Lindstrom, A.B. Collection of a single alveolar exhaled breath for volatile organic compounds analysis. *Am. J. Ind. Med.* **1995**, *28*, 109–121. [CrossRef] [PubMed]
10. Schnabel, R.; Fijten, R.; Smolinska, A.; Dallinga, J.W.; Boumans, M.L.; Stobberingh, E.; Boots, A.W.; Roekaerts, P.M.H.J.; Bergmans, D.C.J.J.; Van Schooten, F.-J. Analysis of volatile organic compounds in exhaled breath to diagnose ventilator-associated pneumonia. *Sci. Rep.* **2015**, *5*, 17179. [CrossRef]
11. Pauling, L.; Robinson, A.B.; Teranishi, R.; Cary, P. Quantitative Analysis of Urine Vapor and Breath by Gas-Liquid Partition Chromatography. *Proc. Natl. Acad. Sci. USA* **1971**, *68*, 2374–2376. [CrossRef]
12. Lachenmeier, D.W.; Godelmann, R.; Steiner, M.; Ansay, B.; Weigel, J.; Krieg, G. Rapid and mobile determination of alcoholic strength in wine, beer and spirits using a flow-through infrared sensor. *Chem. Central J.* **2010**, *4*, 5. [CrossRef] [PubMed]
13. Kalapos, M.P. On the mammalian acetone metabolism: From chemistry to clinical implications. *Biochim. Biophys. Acta* **2003**, *1621*, 122–139. [CrossRef]
14. Crofford, O.B.; Mallard, R.E.; Winton, R.E.; Rogers, N.L.; Jackson, J.C.; Keller, U. Acetone in breath and blood. *Trans. Am. Clin. Climatol. Assoc.* **1977**, *88*, 128–139. [PubMed]
15. Samudrala, D.; Lammers, G.; Mandon, J.; Blanchet, L.; Schreuder, T.H.A.; Hopman, M.T.E.; Harren, F.J.; Tappy, L.; Cristescu, S.M. Breath acetone to monitor life style interventions in field conditions: An exploratory study. *Obesity* **2014**, *22*, 980–983. [CrossRef] [PubMed]
16. Laffel, L.M. Ketone bodies: A review of physiology, pathophysiology and application of monitoring to diabetes. *Diabetes Metab. Res. Rev.* **1999**, *15*, 412–426. [CrossRef]
17. Saasa, V.; Beukes, M.; Lemmer, Y.; Mwakikunga, B.W. Blood Ketone Bodies and Breath Acetone Analysis and Their Correlations in Type 2 Diabetes Mellitus. *Diagnostics* **2019**, *9*, 224. [CrossRef]

18. Amlendu, P.; Ashley, Q.; Di, W.; Haojiong, Z.; Mirna, T.; David, J.; Xiaojun, X.; Francis, T.; Nongjian, T.; Forzani, E.S. Breath Acetone as Biomarker for Lipid Oxidation and Early Ketone Detection. *Glob. J. Obes. Diabetes Metab. Syndr.* **2014**, *1*, 012–019. [CrossRef]
19. Seidelmann, S.B.; Claggett, B.; Cheng, S.; Henglin, M.; Shah, A.; Steffen, L.M.; Folsom, A.R.; Rimm, E.B.; Willett, W.C.; Solomon, S.D. Dietary carbohydrate intake and mortality: A prospective cohort study and meta-analysis. *Lancet Public Health* **2018**, *3*, e419–e428. [CrossRef]
20. Bazzano, L.A.; Hu, T.; Reynolds, K.; Yao, L.; Bunol, C.; Liu, Y.; Chen, C.-S.; Klag, M.J.; Whelton, P.K.; He, J. Effects of Low-Carbohydrate and Low-Fat Diets. *Ann. Intern. Med.* **2014**, *161*, 309–318. [CrossRef]
21. Gemmink, A.; Schrauwen, P.; Hesselink, M.K.C. Exercising your fat (metabolism) into shape: A muscle-centred view. *Diabetologia* **2020**, *63*, 1453–1463. [CrossRef]
22. Veech, R.L. The therapeutic implications of ketone bodies: The effects of ketone bodies in pathological conditions: Ketosis, ketogenic diet, redox states, insulin resistance, and mitochondrial metabolism. *Prostaglandins Leukot. Essent. Fat. Acids* **2004**, *70*, 309–319. [CrossRef] [PubMed]
23. Shai, I.; Schwarzfuchs, D.; Henkin, Y.; Shahar, D.R.; Witkow, S.; Greenberg, I.; Golan, R.; Fraser, D.; Bolotin, A.; Vardi, H.; et al. Weight Loss with a Low-Carbohydrate, Mediterranean, or Low-Fat Diet. *N. Engl. J. Med.* **2008**, *359*, 229–241. [CrossRef] [PubMed]
24. Van Keulen, K.E.; Jansen, M.E.; Schrauwen, R.W.M.; Kolkman, J.J.; Siersema, P.D. Volatile organic compounds in breath can serve as a non-invasive diagnostic biomarker for the detection of advanced adenomas and colorectal cancer. *Aliment. Pharmacol. Ther.* **2019**, *51*, 334–346. [CrossRef]
25. Mitrayana; Apriyanto, D.K.; Satriawan, M. CO_2 Laser Photoacoustic Spectrometer for Measuring Acetone in the Breath of Lung Cancer Patients. *Biosensors* **2020**, *10*, 55. [CrossRef] [PubMed]
26. Saasa, V.; Malwela, T.; Beukes, M.; Mokgotho, M.P.; Liu, C.-P.; Mwakikunga, B.W. Sensing Technologies for Detection of Acetone in Human Breath for Diabetes Diagnosis and Monitoring. *Diagnostics* **2018**, *8*, 12. [CrossRef]
27. Rezaie, A.; Buresi, M.; Lembo, A.; Lin, H.; McCallum, R.; Rao, S.; Schmulson, M.; Valdovinos, M.; Zakko, S.; Pimentel, M. Hydrogen and Methane-Based Breath Testing in Gastrointestinal Disorders: The North American Consensus. *Am. J. Gastroenterol.* **2017**, *112*, 775–784. [CrossRef]
28. Jones, A. Breath-Acetone Concentrations in Fasting Healthy Men: Response of Infrared Breath-Alcohol Analyzers. *J. Anal. Toxicol.* **1987**, *11*, 67–69. [CrossRef]
29. Paoli, A.; Bosco, G.; Camporesi, E.M.; Mangar, D. Ketosis, ketogenic diet and food intake control: A complex relationship. *Front. Psychol.* **2015**, *6*, 27. [CrossRef]
30. Clarke, W.L.; Jones, T.; Rewers, A.; Dunger, D.; Klingensmith, G.J. Assessment and management of hypoglycemia in children and adolescents with diabetes. *Pediatr. Diabetes* **2009**, *10*, 134–145. [CrossRef]
31. Biosense. Readout Health, Biosense™. Available online: https://mybiosense.com/ (accessed on 5 November 2020).
32. Lexico Health. Keto Breath Analyzer. Available online: https://www.lexicohealth.com/ketone-breath-analyzer (accessed on 5 November 2020).
33. Lencool. Available online: https://www.amazon.com/Ketosis-breathalyzer-Testing-ketosis-Mouthpieces/dp/B07RXX9Q1Z (accessed on 5 November 2020).
34. Qetoe Ketone Breath Meter. Available online: https://www.qetoe.com/ (accessed on 5 November 2020).
35. House of Keto Monitor™. Available online: https://www.houseofketo.com/ (accessed on 5 November 2020).
36. KETOscan. Available online: https://ketoscan.com/ketoscan-technology/ (accessed on 5 November 2020).
37. Schwarm, K.K.; Strand, C.L.; Miller, V.A.; Spearrin, R.M. Calibration-free breath acetone sensor with interference correction based on wavelength modulation spectroscopy near 8.2 μm. *Appl. Phys. A* **2020**, *126*, 9. [CrossRef]
38. Taucher, J.; Hansel, A.; Jordan, A.; Lindinger, W. Analysis of Compounds in Human Breath after Ingestion of Garlic Using Proton-Transfer-Reaction Mass Spectrometry. *J. Agric. Food Chem.* **1996**, *44*, 3778–3782. [CrossRef]
39. Landsberg, L.; Young, J.B.; Leonard, W.R.; Linsenmeier, R.A.; Turek, F.W. Is obesity associated with lower body temperatures? Core temperature: A forgotten variable in energy balance. *Metabolism* **2009**, *58*, 871–876. [CrossRef]
40. Gaffney, E.M.; Lim, K.; Minteer, S.D. Breath biosensing: Using electrochemical enzymatic sensors for detection of biomarkers in human breath. *Curr. Opin. Electrochem.* **2020**, *23*, 26–30. [CrossRef]
41. Chen, Y.; Qin, H.; Wang, X.; Li, L.; Hu, J. Acetone sensing properties and mechanism of nano-LaFeO3 thick-films. *Sens. Actuators B Chem.* **2016**, *235*, 56–66. [CrossRef]
42. Kim, D.-H.; Jang, J.-S.; Koo, W.-T.; Choi, S.-J.; Kim, S.-J.; Kim, I.-D. Hierarchically interconnected porosity control of catalyst-loaded WO_3 nanofiber scaffold: Superior acetone sensing layers for exhaled breath analysis. *Sens. Actuators B Chem.* **2018**, *259*, 616–625. [CrossRef]
43. Jung, H.; Cho, W.; Yoo, R.; Lee, H.-S.; Choe, Y.-S.; Jeon, J.Y.; Lee, W. Highly selective real-time detection of breath acetone by using ZnO quantum dots with a miniaturized gas chromatographic column. *Sens. Actuators B Chem.* **2018**, *274*, 527–532. [CrossRef]
44. Jo, Y.-M.; Lim, K.; Choi, H.J.; Yoon, J.W.; Kim, S.Y.; Yoon, J.-W. 2D metal-organic framework derived co-loading of Co_3O_4 and PdO nanocatalysts on In_2O_3 hollow spheres for tailored design of high-performance breath acetone sensors. *Sens. Actuators B Chem.* **2020**, *325*, 128821. [CrossRef]
45. Li, J.; Smeeton, T.; Zanola, M.; Barrett, J.; Berryman-Bousquet, V. A compact breath acetone analyser based on an ultraviolet light emitting diode. *Sens. Actuators B Chem.* **2018**, *273*, 76–82. [CrossRef]

46. Sachdeva, S.; Agarwal, A.; Agarwal, R. A Comparative Study of Gas Sensing Properties of Tungsten Oxide, Tin Oxide and Tin-Doped Tungsten Oxide Thin Films for Acetone Gas Detection. *J. Electron. Mater.* **2019**, *48*, 1617–1628. [CrossRef]
47. Peng, S.; Ma, M.; Yang, W.; Wang, Z.; Wang, Z.; Bi, J.; Wu, J. Acetone sensing with parts-per-billion limit of detection using a BiFeO3-based solid solution sensor at the morphotropic phase boundary. *Sens. Actuators B Chem.* **2020**, *313*, 128060. [CrossRef]
48. Li, G.; Cheng, Z.; Xiang, Q.; Yan, L.; Wang, X.; Xu, J. Bimetal PdAu decorated SnO_2 nanosheets based gas sensor with temperature-dependent dual selectivity for detecting formaldehyde and acetone. *Sens. Actuators B Chem.* **2019**, *283*, 590–601. [CrossRef]
49. Righettoni, M.; Tricoli, A.; Gass, S.; Schmid, A.; Amann, A.; Pratsinis, S.E. Breath acetone monitoring by portable Si:WO_3 gas sensors. *Anal. Chim. Acta* **2012**, *738*, 69–75. [CrossRef] [PubMed]
50. Šetka, M.; Bahos, F.; Chmela, O.; Matatagui, D.; Gràcia, I.; Drbohlavová, J.; Vallejos, S. Cadmium telluride/polypyrrole nanocomposite based Love wave sensors highly sensitive to acetone at room temperature. *Sens. Actuators B Chem.* **2020**, *321*, 128573. [CrossRef]
51. Modi, N.; Priefer, R. Effectiveness of mainstream diets. *Obes. Med.* **2020**, *18*, 100239. [CrossRef]
52. Ito, K.; Kawamura, N.; Suzuki, Y.; Maruo, Y.Y. Colorimetric detection of gaseous acetone based on a reaction between acetone and 4-nitrophenylhydrazine in porous glass. *Microchem. J.* **2020**, *159*, 105428. [CrossRef]
53. Ding, Q.; Wang, Y.; Guo, P.; Li, J.; Chen, C.; Wang, T.; Sun, K.; He, D. Cr-Doped Urchin-Like WO_3 Hollow Spheres: The Cooperative Modulation of Crystal Growth and Energy-Band Structure for High-Sensitive Acetone Detection. *Sensors* **2020**, *20*, 3473. [CrossRef] [PubMed]
54. Huang, J.; Zhou, J.; Liu, Z.; Li, X.; Geng, Y.; Tian, X.; Du, Y.; Qian, Z. Enhanced acetone-sensing properties to ppb detection level using Au/Pd-doped ZnO nanorod. *Sens. Actuators B Chem.* **2020**, *310*, 127129. [CrossRef]
55. Liu, W.; Zhou, X.; Xu, L.; Zhu, S.; Yang, S.; Chen, X.; Dong, B.; Bai, X.; Lu, G.; Song, H. Graphene quantum dot-functionalized three-dimensional ordered mesoporous ZnO for acetone detection toward diagnosis of diabetes. *Nanoscale* **2019**, *11*, 11496–11504. [CrossRef] [PubMed]
56. Aghaei, S.; Aasi, A.; Farhangdoust, S.; Panchapakesan, B. Graphene-like BC6N nanosheets are potential candidates for detection of volatile organic compounds (VOCs) in human breath: A DFT study. *Appl. Surf. Sci.* **2021**, *536*, 147756. [CrossRef]
57. Deng, L.; Bao, L.; Xu, J.; Wang, X.; Wang, X. Highly sensitive acetone gas sensor based on ultra-low content bimetallic PtCu modified $WO_3 \cdot H_2O$ hollow sphere. *Chin. Chem. Lett.* **2020**, *31*, 2041–2044. [CrossRef]
58. Kohli, N.; Hastir, A.; Kumari, M.; Singh, R.C. Hydrothermally synthesized heterostructures of In_2O_3/MWCNT as acetone gas sensor. *Sens. Actuators A Phys.* **2020**, *314*, 112240. [CrossRef]
59. Fan, X.; Xu, Y.; Ma, C.; He, W. In-situ growth of Co_3O_4 nanoparticles based on electrospray for an acetone gas sensor. *J. Alloys Compd.* **2021**, *854*, 157234. [CrossRef]
60. Lavanya, N.; Leonardi, S.G.; Marini, S.; Espro, C.; Kanagaraj, M.; Reddy, S.L.; Sekar, C.; Neri, G. MgNi2O4 nanoparticles as novel and versatile sensing material for non-enzymatic electrochemical sensing of glucose and conductometric determination of acetone. *J. Alloys Compd.* **2020**, *817*, 152787. [CrossRef]
61. Liu, T.; Guan, H.; Wang, T.; Liang, X.; Liu, F.; Liu, F.; Zhang, C.; Lu, G. Mixed potential type acetone sensor based on GDC used for breath analysis. *Sens. Actuators B Chem.* **2021**, *326*, 128846. [CrossRef]
62. Liu, F.; Wang, J.; Li, B.; You, R.; Wang, C.; Jiang, L.; Yang, Y.; Yan, X.; Sun, P.; Lu, G. Ni-based tantalate sensing electrode for fast and low detection limit of acetone sensor combining stabilized zirconia. *Sens. Actuators B Chem.* **2020**, *304*, 127375. [CrossRef]
63. Liu, B.; Wang, S.; Yuan, Z.; Duan, Z.; Zhao, Q.; Zhang, Y.; Su, Y.; Jiang, Y.; Xie, G.; Tai, H. Novel chitosan/ZnO bilayer film with enhanced humidity-tolerant property: Endowing triboelectric nanogenerator with acetone analysis capability. *Nano Energy* **2020**, *78*, 105256. [CrossRef]
64. Cho, H.-J.; Choi, S.-J.; Kim, N.-H.; Kim, I.-D. Porosity controlled 3D SnO_2 spheres via electrostatic spray: Selective acetone sensors. *Sens. Actuators B Chem.* **2020**, *304*, 127350. [CrossRef]
65. Chuang, M.-Y.; Lin, Y.-T.; Tung, T.-W.; Chang, L.-Y.; Zan, H.-W.; Meng, H.-F.; Lu, C.-J.; Tao, Y.-T. Room-temperature-operated organic-based acetone gas sensor for breath analysis. *Sens. Actuators B Chem.* **2018**, *260*, 593–600. [CrossRef]
66. Hussain, T.; Sajjad, M.; Singh, D.; Bae, H.; Lee, H.; Larsson, J.A.; Ahuja, R.; Karton, A. Sensing of volatile organic compounds on two-dimensional nitrogenated holey graphene, graphdiyne, and their heterostructure. *Carbon* **2020**, *163*, 213–223. [CrossRef]
67. Van Duy, L.; Van Duy, N.; Hung, C.M.; Hoa, N.D.; Dich, N.Q. Urea mediated synthesis and acetone-sensing properties of ultrathin porous ZnO nanoplates. *Mater. Today Commun.* **2020**, *25*, 101445. [CrossRef]
68. Hanh, N.H.; Van Duy, L.; Hung, C.M.; Van Duy, N.; Heo, Y.-W.; Van Hieu, N.; Hoa, N.D. VOC gas sensor based on hollow cubic assembled nanocrystal Zn2SnO4 for breath analysis. *Sens. Actuators A Phys.* **2020**, *302*, 111834. [CrossRef]
69. Kołodziejczak-Radzimska, A.; Jesionowski, T. Zinc Oxide—From Synthesis to Application: A Review. *Materials* **2014**, *7*, 2833–2881. [CrossRef] [PubMed]
70. Precision Xtra Blood Glucose & Ketone Monitoring System. Available online: https://abbottstore.com/diabetes-management/precision-brand/precision-brand/precision-xtra-blood-glucose-ketone-monitoring-system-1-pack-9881465.html (accessed on 9 November 2020).
71. Suntrup, D.J., III; Ratto, T.V.; Ratto, M.; McCarter, J.P. Characterization of a high-resolution breath acetone meter for ketosis monitoring. *PeerJ* **2020**, *8*, e9969. [CrossRef] [PubMed]
72. Akers, R.F. Breath Ketone Detector. U.S. Patent 8871521B2, 28 October 2014.

73. Lubna, A. Ketone Measurement System and Related Method with Accuracy and Reporting Enhancement Features. U.S. Patent 9486169B1, 8 November 2016.
74. Herbig, J.; Titzmann, T.; Beauchamp, J.; Kohl, I.; Hansel, A. Buffered end-tidal (BET) sampling—A novel method for real-time breath-gas analysis. *J. Breath Res.* **2008**, *2*, 037008. [CrossRef]
75. Yoo, D.J. Measuring Device for Amount of Body Fat Burned. U.S. Patent 16/619358, 7 May 2020.
76. Invoy. Available online: https://www.invoy.com/how-it-works/ (accessed on 5 November 2020).
77. Ketonix. KETONIX Breath Ketone Analyzer. Available online: https://www.ketonix.com/ (accessed on 5 November 2020).
78. Keto PRX. Available online: https://www.amazon.com/PRX-Ketone-Breath-Testing-Mouthpieces/dp/B0814H9J89 (accessed on 5 November 2020).
79. Keyto. Available online: https://getkeyto.com/ (accessed on 5 November 2020).
80. Evans, M.; Cogan, K.E.; Egan, B. Metabolism of ketone bodies during exercise and training: Physiological basis for exogenous supplementation. *J. Physiol.* **2017**, *595*, 2857–2871. [CrossRef]
81. LEVLcare. Available online: https://levlcare.com/science/ (accessed on 5 November 2020).
82. Weber, I.C.; Braun, H.P.; Krumeich, F.; Güntner, A.T.; Pratsinis, S.E. Superior Acetone Selectivity in Gas Mixtures by Catalyst-Filtered Chemoresistive Sensors. *Adv. Sci.* **2020**, *7*, 2001503. [CrossRef]
83. Hanson, R.K. Applications of quantitative laser sensors to kinetics, propulsion and practical energy systems. *Proc. Combust. Inst.* **2011**, *33*, 1–40. [CrossRef]
84. Wang, C.; Yin, L.; Zhang, L.; Xiang, D.; Gao, R. Metal Oxide Gas Sensors: Sensitivity and Influencing Factors. *Sensors* **2010**, *10*, 2088–2106. [CrossRef]
85. Righettoni, M.; Schmid, A.; Amann, A.; Pratsinis, E.S. Correlations between blood glucose and breath components from portable gas sensors and PTR-TOF-MS. *J. Breath Res.* **2013**, *7*, 037110. [CrossRef]
86. Wang, L.; Teleki, A.; Pratsinis, S.E.; Gouma, P.I. Ferroelectric WO_3 Nanoparticles for Acetone Selective Detection. *Chem. Mater.* **2008**, *20*, 4794–4796. [CrossRef]
87. Güntner, A.T.; Sievi, N.A.; Theodore, S.J.; Gulich, T.; Kohler, M.; Pratsinis, S.E. Noninvasive Body Fat Burn Monitoring from Exhaled Acetone with Si-doped WO_3-sensing Nanoparticles. *Anal. Chem.* **2017**, *89*, 10578–10584. [CrossRef] [PubMed]
88. Güntner, A.T.; Kompalla, J.F.; Landis, H.; Theodore, S.J.; Geidl, B.; Sievi, N.A.; Kohler, M.; Pratsinis, S.E.; Gerber, P. Guiding Ketogenic Diet with Breath Acetone Sensors. *Sensors* **2018**, *18*, 3655. [CrossRef] [PubMed]
89. Güntner, A.T.; Pineau, N.J.; Mochalski, P.; Wiesenhofer, H.; Agapiou, A.; Mayhew, C.A.; Pratsinis, S.E. Sniffing Entrapped Humans with Sensor Arrays. *Anal. Chem.* **2018**, *90*, 4940–4945. [CrossRef] [PubMed]

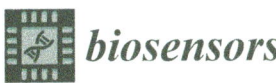

Article

Real-Time Cuffless Continuous Blood Pressure Estimation Using 1D Squeeze U-Net Model: A Progress toward mHealth

Tasbiraha Athaya [1] and Sunwoong Choi [2,*]

[1] Department of Computer Science, University of Central Florida, Orlando, FL 32816, USA
[2] School of Electrical Engineering, Kookmin University, Seoul 02707, Korea
* Correspondence: schoi@kookmin.ac.kr

Abstract: Measuring continuous blood pressure (BP) in real time by using a mobile health (mHealth) application would open a new door in the advancement of the healthcare system. This study aimed to propose a real-time method and system for measuring BP without using a cuff from a digital artery. An energy-efficient real-time smartphone-application-friendly one-dimensional (1D) Squeeze U-net model is proposed to estimate systolic and diastolic BP values, using only raw photoplethysmogram (PPG) signal. The proposed real-time cuffless BP prediction method was assessed for accuracy, reliability, and potential usefulness in the hypertensive assessment of 100 individuals in two publicly available datasets: Multiparameter Intelligent Monitoring in Intensive Care (MIMIC-I) and Medical Information Mart for Intensive Care (MIMIC-III) waveform database. The proposed model was used to build an android application to measure BP at home. This proposed deep-learning model performs best in terms of systolic BP, diastolic BP, and mean arterial pressure, with a mean absolute error of 4.42, 2.25, and 2.56 mmHg and standard deviation of 4.78, 2.98, and 3.21 mmHg, respectively. The results meet the grade A performance requirements of the British Hypertension Society and satisfy the AAMI error range. The result suggests that only using a short-time PPG signal is sufficient to obtain accurate BP measurements in real time. It is a novel approach for real-time cuffless BP estimation by implementing an mHealth application and can measure BP at home and assess hypertension.

Keywords: blood pressure (BP); Squeeze U-net; photoplethysmogram (PPG); mHealth; real time; deep learning

Citation: Athaya, T.; Choi, S. Real-Time Cuffless Continuous Blood Pressure Estimation Using 1D Squeeze U-Net Model: A Progress toward mHealth. *Biosensors* **2022**, *12*, 655. https://doi.org/10.3390/bios12080655

Received: 8 July 2022
Accepted: 16 August 2022
Published: 18 August 2022

Publisher's Note: MDPI stays neutral with regard to jurisdictional claims in published maps and institutional affiliations.

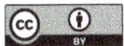

Copyright: © 2022 by the authors. Licensee MDPI, Basel, Switzerland. This article is an open access article distributed under the terms and conditions of the Creative Commons Attribution (CC BY) license (https://creativecommons.org/licenses/by/4.0/).

1. Introduction

Fluctuations in blood pressure (BP) correlate strongly with vital organ damage in the case of high BP or hypertension [1]. Early detection and control of hypertension problems are crucial, but they rely on precise and accessible measurements [2]. According to statistics from the World Heart Federation (WHF), almost half of cardiac strokes are the reason for hypertension [3]. It also raises your chances of having a hemorrhagic stroke, cardiac failure, a heart attack, or chronic renal diseases [3,4]. By the time of 2025, the number of persons suffering from hypertension is intended to reach almost 1.5 billion. Any healthcare system would be overburdened by the consequences of this sickness [2]. Epidemiological studies reveal that hypertension prevalence and control have plateaued in developed countries since the middle of the 2000s [5,6]. As a result, proper blood pressure regulation is essential for preventing both primary and secondary coronary heart diseases; thus, introducing a reliable and comfortable method to measure BP values is mandatory.

The first and most reliable process of measuring continuous BP is the invasive or direct way, also called the invasive arterial BP (ABP). In order to monitor real-time continuous BP, a catheter is placed inside an artery for invasive ABP measurement. In this process, BP can be measured in every cardiac cycle, and variations in blood pressure can be tracked in a more precise way. Hence, it is widely regarded as the gold standard in the field of BP measurement methods [7]. However, this method requires arterial puncture. The kits used are non-reusable and have a high risk of complications and infections. Moreover, the measurement needs to be performed by trained professionals; thus, this method is only used for critically ill patients. The difficulties associated with the invasive methods initiate the necessity of introducing noninvasive measurement methods.

Traditionally and most commonly, noninvasive cuff-based auscultatory and oscillometric measurements are used to check BP. The measured results are expressed as systolic BP (SBP) and diastolic BP (DBP). To measure BP, cuff-based equipment is widely used in houses and hospitals [8]. Even a wireless cuff-based BP measurement device with a smartphone was also proposed [9]. However, the measurement process is discontinuous and takes a long time, and the result varies for different cuff sizes. Furthermore, continuous BP measurement is impossible because repetitive cuff inflation causes discomfort. With technological advancement, research has been conducted widely to measure BP more accurately at a low cost. Almost everyone has a smartphone in their hand. Wearable devices are becoming increasingly popular. So, signals acquired using different sensors for accurate BP measurement are nowadays a wide research topic. It also paves the way for real-time continuous BP measurements.

Recently, an increase in interest has been observed in the prediction of cuffless real-time BP values to enable an easy and comfortable way of predicting BP in real time by using features of different easily measurable biosignals. Several noninvasive cuffless BP estimation methods have been proposed using photoplethysmogram (PPG) and electrocardiogram (ECG) signals, including ultrasound-based [10], pulse transit time (PTT)-based [11–15], and feature-based approaches [8,16–19].

The ultrasound-based technique was developed for continuous real-time BP measurement; however, higher complexity existed [19]. Reviewing the complexities, a comparably lower complex PTT-based approach [11–15] was studied extensively for a long time. PTT is the time needed for the pulse pressure waveform of the artery to reach a peripheral site (e.g., fingertip) from the semilunar valves. Usually, it is measured from the start of the R-wave on the ECG signal to the arrival of the PPG signal at the fingertip [20]. Thus, the time can be calculated by using two channels of biosignals, and frequent calibrations are needed to ensure prediction accuracy [12].

Furthermore, feature-based approaches [8,16–19,21] have been proposed to improve the PTT-based BP estimation methods. In a feature-based approach, multiple features that influence BP are extracted from the ECG and PPG signals and merged to obtain BP values with improved accuracy. Different machine-learning models, such as the random forest, support vector machine, and neural networks, are used to predict BP values by using the extracted features. However, two channels of biosignals are required for most of these methods. Feature-based models using one-channel ECG [18] or PPG [22] signals exhibit an inferior performance. Moreover, additional sensors are needed to acquire ECG signals that are impossible to acquire by using smartphones. Feature-based methods need complicated feature extraction and selection processes that urge high-quality waveforms to extract proper features [23]. Moreover, it is difficult to get a generalized model by using a definite number of features. A study also used different BP and bodily parameters to predict BP values by using different machine learning models and ensemble methods [24]. However, they obtained very low accuracy.

Deep learning (DL) approaches can automatically learn useful features. Based on this property of DL, S. Baker et al. proposed continuous BP estimation by using raw ECG and PPG signals [25], and K. Qin et al., G. Slapničar et al., and T. Athaya et al. proposed that estimation techniques using only raw PPG signals can be actualized [23,26,27]. Using a one-channel raw PPG signal is more suitable than using two channels of biosignals to estimate continuous BP by using smartphones and wearable devices [28]. G. Slapničar et al. proposed a complex GRU-based spectro-temporal deep neural network by using both derivatives and information of PPG signal frequency domain information with lower accuracy [26]. K. Qin et al. and T. Athaya et al. predicted BP waveform by using raw PPG signal, and from the predicted BP waveform, SBP, DBP, and ABP values were predicted [23,27].

However, T. Athaya et al. used the U-net model, which needs many parameters and is thus unsuitable for real-time mHealth applications [27]. Furthermore, K. Qin et al. used regularized deep autoencoder (RDAE), which provides lower accuracy [23]. Moreover, the model is not generalized for every BP value, and calibration is needed to obtain a better performance. Although continuous methods are proposed in these studies, none of the methods ensures real-time BP estimation.

Unlike the abovementioned methods, herein, the prediction of real-time continuous BP values and implementation using a smartphone application are proposed. A real-time application-friendly Squeeze U-net model was used to predict the BP values by directly feeding a one-channel raw PPG signal as the model input. The proposed model ensures a user-friendly and generalized system to measure BP values ubiquitously and unobtrusively without calibration to obtain accurate results. The proposed architecture of the model provides low computational complexity and higher efficiency to estimate BP. The main contributions herein are as follows:

- Real-time BP values are estimated by using a single-channel raw PPG signal as the input of the mobile application-friendly modified 1D Squeeze U-net model.
- This study is a novel approach to implementing a DL 1D Squeeze U-net model in an mHealth application, using PPG signals without any feature selection to generate BP values with high accuracy and at no cost.

The rest of the study is organized as follows: Section 2 describes the used materials and proposed methodology. Section 3 shows the results from using the chosen materials and methods. Section 4 discusses the implications of the proposed approach. Finally, Section 5 concludes the study.

2. Materials and Methods

2.1. Data Acquisition

DL works best when huge amounts of data are utilized to train, validate, and test the models. The invasive ABP and fingertip PPG signals were needed herein. The first step of Figure 1 is data collection. The signals are acquired from two publicly available popular databases containing health-related data. The databases contain simultaneous recordings of the fingertip PPG, ABP, one or more ECG, pulmonary arterial pressure, and central venous pressure signals. The databases are as follows:

- Multiparameter Intelligent Monitoring in Intensive Care (MIMIC) database [29].
- Medical Information Mart for Intensive Care III (MIMIC-III) waveform database [30,31].

2.2. Data Preparation

The next step in Figure 1 is data preparation. The Squeeze U-net was used for predicting BP values. As the Squeeze U-net is the SqueezeNet type of the U-net model, the data preparation for training and validation of the model is the same as the process used for the U-net model [27]. First, the PPG signal acquired from the two databases is filtered by using an Equiripple FIR bandpass filter using a cutoff frequency of 0.5–8 Hz. Frequencies of less than 0.5 Hz and higher than 8 Hz are considered to be noise and are, thus, filtered out.

In the databases, the ABP signals are obtained from the brachial artery, and the PPG signals are obtained from the digital artery. As blood enters first in the brachial artery and then in the digital artery, a phase difference is shown between the two signals, even if they are recorded simultaneously. To remove the delay between the two signals measured from different sources, the filtered PPG signals are phase matched with the respective ABP signals, using the cross-correlation technique for properly replicating the output ABP signals, using PPG signals as the input. Afterward, the phase-matched signals are divided into segments of 256 samples.

Next, the segments are checked for artifacts and divided into two classes: acceptable and unacceptable signals. The unacceptable segments with artifacts are removed from the final dataset by using a random forest machine-learning model [32]. In Reference [32], real-time artifact detection of PPG signals is shown. As our system is also in real time, we used the approach. As much variation of the PPG signal as possible was maintained in the final dataset to enable the generalization of the trained model.

Next, the data were shuffled for unbiased training of the model. Finally, the acquired signals were normalized by using Equation (1) to nullify the variation of PPG and ABP signal values for different individuals [27,33].

$$x_{norm(i)} = \frac{(x_i - x_{min})}{x_{max} - x_{min}}, \quad (1)$$

where x_i refers to the ith signal segment, and x_{max} and x_{min} are the highest and lowest values of all segmented signals, respectively. Note that $x_{max} = 2.9$ mV and $x_{min} = -2.4$ mV for PPG and $x_{max} = 192.24$ mmHg and $x_{min} = 50.33$ mmHg for ABP.

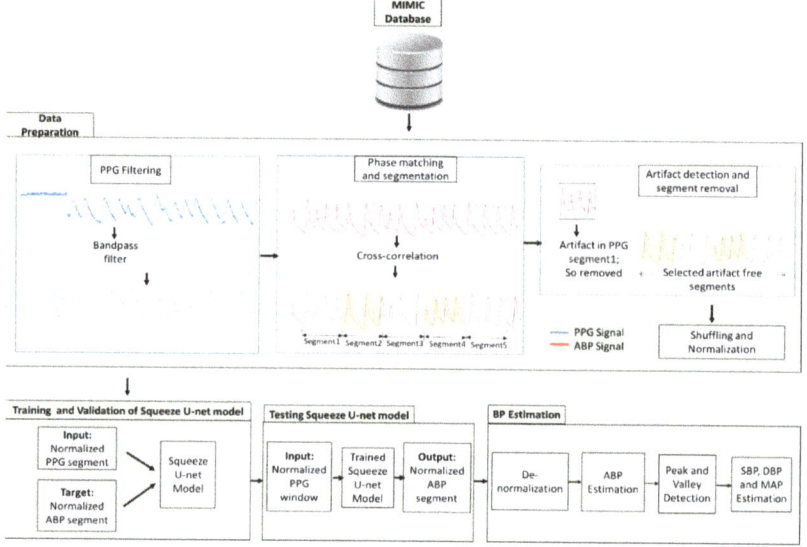

Figure 1. Proposed methodology to train, validate, and test the proposed Squeeze U-net model.

Herein, 45 individuals of the MIMIC-I dataset and a subset of 55 individuals of the MIMIC-III waveform dataset comprising fingertip PPG and ABP signals with a 125 Hz sampling rate were used. Finally, recordings of 100 individuals were acquired for the whole experiment.

2.3. Proposed Architecture of Squeeze U-Net Model

The second step of Figure 1 is the training and validation of the proposed Squeeze U-net model. The proposed model is modified to one-dimensional (1D) convolutional blocks despite comprising 2D convolutional blocks such as the original one. Inspired by the SqueezeNet type of the U-net model for biomedical image segmentation, the proposed model has been presented to ease the development of deep neural networks on embedded systems, while minimizing the computational and memory requirements, especially for real-time smartphone applications [34].

The SqueezeNet fire module [35] architecture was introduced in both the contracting and expansion paths while designing the proposed model. Note that the convolution blocks of the fire modules were changed to 1D for our proposed modified model. The initial depth-wise convolution of the fire module reduces the number of channels, and this is compensated by two parallel convolutions in the expansion units, with each convolution having half the number of output channels of that of the squeeze unit. Both parallel convolutions support avoiding feature loss and vanishing gradients, which can occur when the number of channels is reduced [36].

The fire module (Figure 2) comprises a squeeze, two expansion convolution units, and a concatenate unit. The squeeze unit has a 1×1 convolution filter. The output of this unit expands the convolution units of 1×1 filters (left) and 3×1 filters (right) in parallel. The convolution filters in the 1×1 squeeze unit, 1×1 expansion unit, and 3×1 expansion unit are denoted as $s_{1\times 1}$, $e_{1\times 1}$, and $e_{3\times 1}$, respectively. While using fire modules, $s_{1\times 1}$ is set less than ($e_{1\times 1} + e_{3\times 1}$) to limit the number of input samples. In CNN, to decrease the number of parameters, it is necessary to minimize the number of input samples. Thus, the output of the expansion units goes to the concatenate unit to give ($e_{1\times 1} + e_{3\times 1}$) filters. The result of the concatenate unit is the output of the fire module.

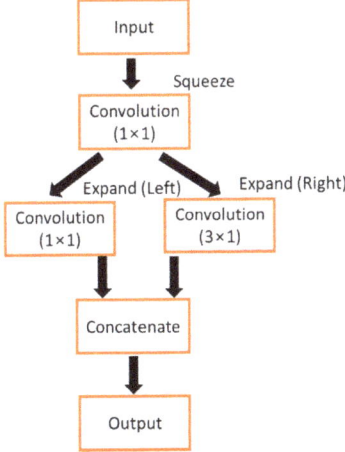

Figure 2. Structure of the proposed fire module of Squeeze U-net.

The proposed 1D Squeeze U-net model is illustrated in Figure 3. The model has contracting and expansion paths on the left and right sides, respectively. The contracting and expansion paths comprise several contraction blocks (CBs) and expansion blocks (EBs), as the U-net does. The numeral on the left side of the blocks illustrates the size of the input vector or sample. The numeral on the right side of every output unit illustrates the size of the feature vector.

2.3.1. Contracting Path

In the first contraction block (CB1) of the proposed model, the PPG segment of 256 samples was used as the input. The input is passed to the 3×1 convolution unit with stride 2 in CB1. Striding helps decrease the number of samples to 128 and increases the model's expressiveness. The feature vectors are 64 after the 3×1 convolution operation with stride 2 in CB1. In CB2, the output of the convolution unit of CB1 goes to the 2×1 max-pooling layer. No convolution operation is performed in CB2. Max-pooling halves the samples from 128 to 64, and the number of feature vectors remains the same. The CB2 output is passed into two fire modules and one 2×1 max-pooling in CB3.

In the Squeeze U-net network, fire modules are introduced for down-sampling units in the contracting path. The fire modules are used to reduce the total parameter number for the model. After passing the first fire module, the number of feature vectors doubles and remains the same after the next fire module and max-pooling operation. The fire modules of CB3 have 16 squeeze filters ($s_{1\times 1}$) and 64 expand filters ($e_{1\times 1}$ and $e_{3\times 1}$). Then the 4th block (CB4) of the contracting path comes, which has a similar structure as CB3. The fire modules of CB4 have 32 $s_{1\times 1}$, 128 $e_{1\times 1}$, and $e_{3\times 1}$, making the number of feature vectors 256 after two consecutive fire modules. The last block (CB5) of the contracting path is max-pooled and passes four fire modules. The first two fire modules have 48 $s_{1\times1}$, 192 $e_{1\times1}$, and $e_{3\times1}$. The other two fire modules have 64 $s_{1\times1}$, 256 $e_{1\times1}$, and $e_{3\times1}$. Next, the dropout is performed, and the output is passed into a 1D convolution transpose unit with stride 1. The output of this block is concatenated with the output of the second fire module of block CB5. The concatenated output goes to a fire module. This fire module has 48 $s_{1\times1}$, 192 $e_{1\times1}$, and $e_{3\times1}$. The output of this fire module again passes into the 2 × 1 1D convolution transpose unit with stride 1. The output of this block is concatenated with the input of the first fire module of CB5, and the concatenated result is passed into a fire module. This fire module has 32 $s_{1\times1}$, 128 $e_{1\times1}$, and $e_{3\times1}$. At the end of CB5, the number of feature vectors becomes 256. Similar to the structure of U-net, this Squeeze U-net network uses the Leaky ReLU activation function in every convolution unit.

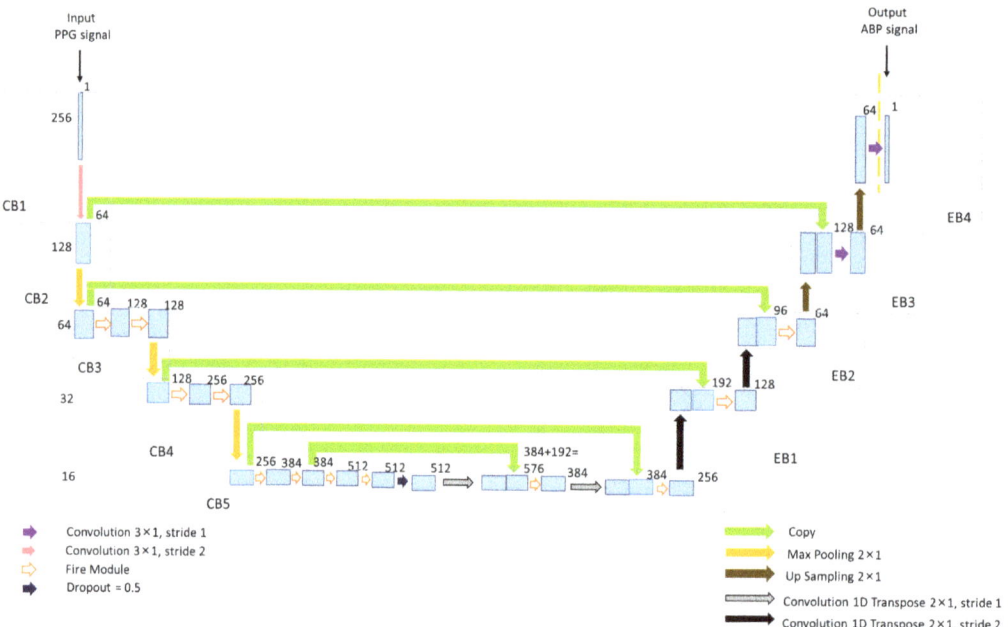

Figure 3. The proposed architecture of one-dimensional (1D) Squeeze U-net DL model.

2.3.2. Expansion Path

The expansion path has four expansion blocks, which are denoted as EB1, EB2, EB3, and EB4. Each EB1 and EB2 block comprises a 2 × 1 1D convolution transpose unit with stride 2. The output of the convolution transpose unit is passed into the concatenation units. After passing the concatenation units, in EB1 and EB2, the number of feature vectors becomes 192 and 96, respectively. The EB1 and EB2 blocks of the expansion path also have fire modules. The outputs of the concatenation units go to these fire modules. The EB1 fire module of the expansion path has 16 $s_{1\times1}$, 64 $e_{1\times1}$, and $e_{3\times1}$, and EB2 has 16 $s_{1\times1}$, 32 $e_{1\times1}$, and $e_{3\times1}$. After passing the fire modules in EB1 and EB2, the number of feature vectors becomes 128 and 64, respectively. Each EB3 and EB4 block has a 2 × 1 up-sampling unit. The output of the up-sampling unit of EB3 is concatenated with the input layer of CB2. The output of the concatenated unit passes into a 3 × 1 convolution unit of stride 1 in EB3. The EB3 output goes through a 2 × 1 up-sampling unit in EB4. The output of the EB4 up-sampling unit again passes to the 3 × 1 convolution unit in EB4 and gives the output ABP window of 256 samples.

2.4. Training and Testing of Squeeze U-Net Model

The normalized PPG signals are used as the input of the 1D Squeeze U-net model to obtain the normalized ABP-like signals in the testing phase (Figure 1). Of the overall pre-processed data, 70% were used to train the network, 15% to validate, and the left 15% to test. The training, validating, and testing data were totally different from each other. The network is trained and tested by using Keras. The training data are needed for iterative model training until the maximum number of epochs is reached to obtain a generalized model with the highest performance. The network performance is monitored dynamically. The validation is performed to fine-tune the hyperparameters and stop the training process when no improvement is seen to generalize the network. Then the testing was performed by using the highest-performing network structure with the test dataset.

The Adam optimizer was used to train the network, and the chosen loss function was mean squared error. For the Squeeze U-net model, the learning rate was set at 10^{-4}, and the batch size was set to 10. The learning rate and batch size of the network were both determined through experimentation. When there was no improvement in the consecutive six epochs, early stopping was applied, and the Squeeze U-net model's training was ended after 33 epochs. The epoch performance in reduced validation loss was automatically saved for each epoch in this training method. An NVIDIA GTX 1080 Ti 10 GB graphics card with a GPU server and 257 GB RAM was used in this experiment. Python language was used to write all the codes.

2.5. BP Estimation

In the final step, the BP values are estimated as depicted in Figure 1. The obtained signal was denormalized by using the stored denormalization factors of the training phase. Next, a standard peak detection algorithm [37] was used to estimate the SBP and DBP values. From these values, the mean arterial pressure (MAP) was estimated by using Equation (2) [38].

$$MAP = \frac{1}{3}SBP + \frac{2}{3}DBP \qquad (2)$$

3. Results

3.1. Performance of Squeeze U-Net Model

The dataset for performance evaluation is distributed from different BP values of all ranges. The data summary is displayed in Table 1. We tried making a dataset comprising all kinds of BP values for proper result evaluation.

Table 1. Summary of data used for testing network performance.

BP Values	Min (mmHg)	Max (mmHg)	Mean (mmHg)	STD (mmHg)
SBP	75.69	192.24	130.05	23.79
DBP	50.33	111.23	64.66	13.28
MAP	62.69	130.74	84.08	15.61

Different performance matrices have been used in different studies to show the performance of the model. We tried incorporating all performance matrices to evaluate the performance of the proposed model for real-time BP estimation. The mean error (ME), mean absolute error (MAE), standard deviation (STD), root mean square error (RMSE), and Pearson's correlation coefficient (r) evaluation factors were used [39].

The performance details of the proposed Squeeze U-net model to estimate the real-time SBP, DBP, and MAP values are presented in Table 2. In all three cases, the evaluation factors provide good values, indicating that the network can be used to estimate SBP, DBP, and MAP accurately. The real-time SBP, DBP, and MAP estimation results using the Squeeze U-net model are illustrated in Figure 4. The figure shows the similarity between the predicted and actual values.

Table 2. Performance detail of Squeeze U-net models for systolic blood pressure (SBP), diastolic blood pressure (DBP), and mean arterial pressure (MAP) values measurement.

BP Values	ME (mmHg)	MAE (mmHg)	STD (mmHg)	RMSE (mmHg)	r
SBP	−1.002	4.42	4.78	6.50	0.970
DBP	0.019	2.25	2.98	3.73	0.964
MAP	−0.315	2.56	3.21	4.10	0.971

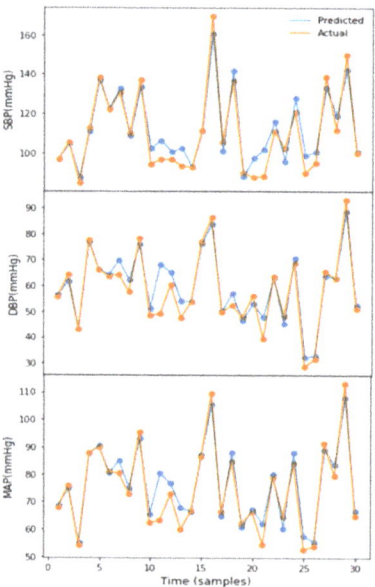

Figure 4. An example of real-time systolic blood pressure (SBP), diastolic blood pressure (DBP), and mean arterial pressure (MAP) estimation.

Figure 5 shows the histogram plots of the prediction error, using the 1D Squeeze U-net model for SBP, DBP, and MAP values. For three cases, the error values lie at zero, indicating an accurate prediction of most values. The prediction accuracy of MAP is the highest.

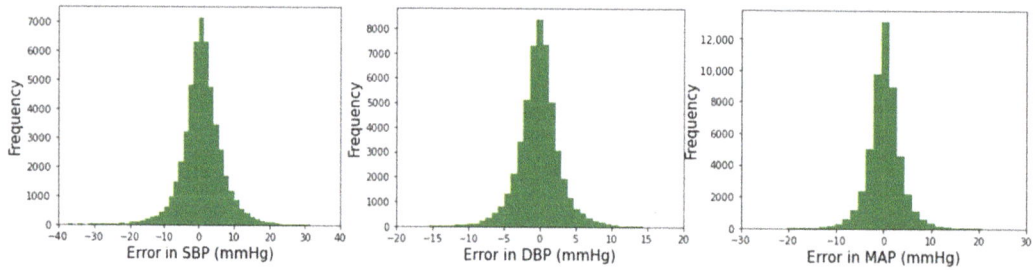

Figure 5. Histograms of error for estimated real-time SBP, DBP, and MAP values.

Figure 6 shows that the proposed network performs well in all four BP stages: normal, prehypertension, hypertension stage-1, and hypertension stage-2 [40]. In the normal stage, the SBP and DBP estimation accuracy rates are 93.94% and 99.24%, with the latter being the highest. The SBP prediction accuracy is better in the prehypertension stage than that of DBP. For hypertension stage-1, the percentage of prediction accuracy is low for both SBP and DBP. For SBP 30.36% and DBP 31.8%, the values are inaccurately predicted as prehypertension stage. Despite minor variations in predicting hypertension stage-1, the prediction accuracy for hypertension stage-2 is fairly good. For a vast amount of data, relatively fewer values are discovered in a deviation area of more than 20 mmHg, which is trivial.

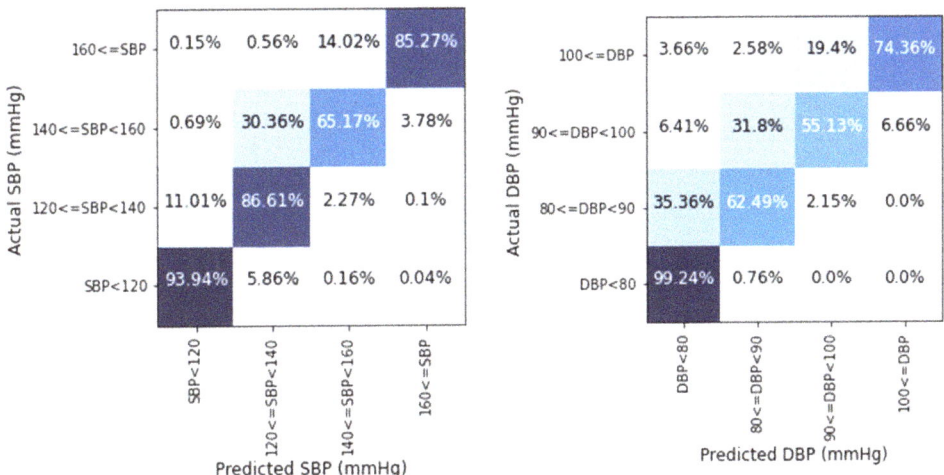

Figure 6. Prediction accuracy of SBP and DBP values in four BP stages.

Figure 7 depicts the scatter plots of our anticipated outcome vs. the actual SBP, DBP, and MAP values. It has been demonstrated that the acquired result yields a linear relation, demonstrating that the anticipated outcome is largely correct, except in some situations.

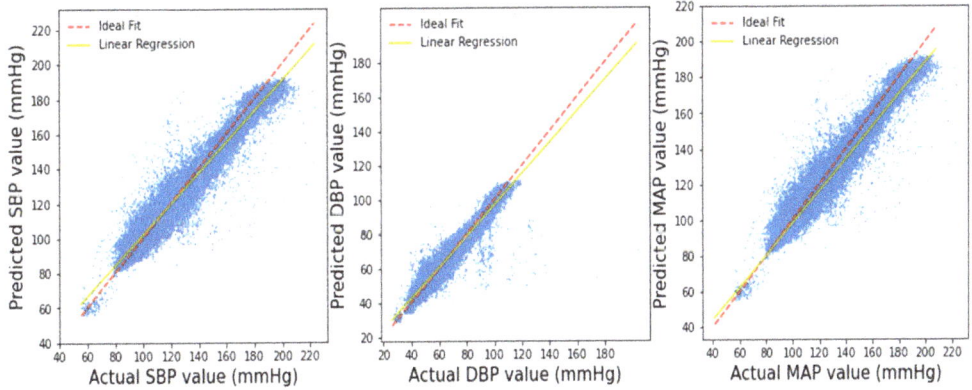

Figure 7. Linear regression plot for SBP, DBP, and MAP results.

The Bland–Altman analysis for the proposed deep learning model is displayed in Figure 8 according to the AAMI norm [41]. No Bland–Altman plot exists for MAP in the AAMI norm. The x-axis shows SBP pressures ranging from 80 to 190 mmHg and DBP pressures ranging from 30 to 140 mmHg. The y-axis represents inaccuracies ranging from 30 to +30 mmHg. From 15 to +15 mmHg, reference horizontal dotted lines are provided at 5 mmHg intervals. The mean of each actual BP and its related projected BP is represented by a point across their difference. Differences more than 30 mmHg are shown at 30 mmHg, and differences less than 30 mmHg are plotted at 30 mmHg. Most SBP and DBP discrepancies are between ±5 mmHg in both scenarios.

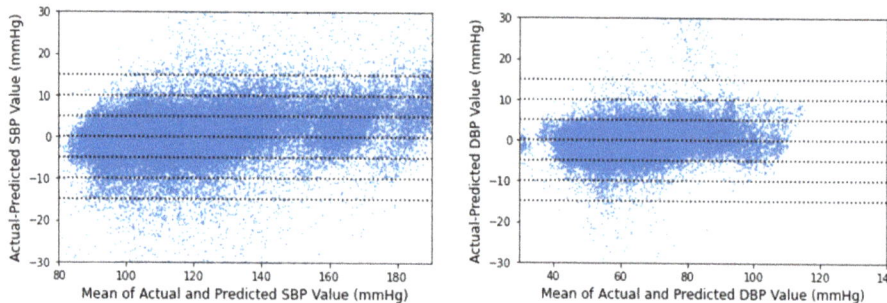

Figure 8. Bland–Altman analysis for real-time SBP and DBP values.

3.2. Result Evaluation and Comparison

Although several studies are found in the web of science that can estimate BP or continuous BP, few studies predicted BP values in real time. The results were compared with recent works that predicted continuous BP or real-time BP. Furthermore, the comparison of the obtained results was actualized by using two established standards: AAMI [42] and British Hypertension Society (BHS) standards [43].

To satisfy the AAMI error range, the testing device used to measure BP values must have ME $\leq$ 5 mmHg and STD $\leq$ 8 mmHg, with above 85 subjects. Table 3 compares our results based on the AAMI standard. In References [25,44], it is observed that calculating the ME gives incorrect estimations, as a lower ME may result in a higher MAE. Herein, both ME and MAE were included in all papers. The standard norm for AAMI is passed for all three BP values using our 1D Squeeze U-net model. Our results obtained a comparatively better MAE and STD than all other papers.

Table 3. Comparison with related works based on AAMI standard.

Works	BP Values	MAE	ME	STD	Result
AAMI [42]	BP		$\leq$5	$\leq$8	Passed
[17]	SBP	6.726	4.638	14.505	Failed
	DBP	2.516	3.155	6.442	Passed
	MAP	-	-	-	-
[18]	SBP	7.10	−0.11	9.99	Failed
	DBP	4.61	−0.03	6.36	Passed
	MAP	4.66	−0.01	6.29	Passed
[19]	SBP	6.13	1.62	7.76	Failed
	DBP	4.54	1.49	5.52	Passed
	MAP	4.81	1.53	6.03	Passed
[25]	SBP	4.41	-	6.11	Failed
	DBP	2.91	-	4.23	-
	MAP	2.77	-	3.88	-
[23]	SBP	7.945	1.447	10.375	Failed
	DBP	4.114	−0.417	5.504	Passed
	MAP	3.834	0.204	5.130	Passed
[27]	SBP	3.68	-	4.42	-
	DBP	1.97	-	2.92	-
	MAP	2.17	-	3.06	-
This work	SBP	4.42	−1.002	4.78	Passed
	DBP	2.25	0.019	2.98	Passed
	MAP	2.56	−0.315	3.21	Passed

The testing device is divided into three grades (A, B, or C) based on the conditions of the BHS grading standard [43] (Table 4). The criterion of a device to satisfy the BHS standard error range is that it must reach the minimum Grade B in estimating the SBP and DBP values. According to the BHS grading standard criteria, the proposed model obtained grade A in predicting SBP and DBP values. The SBP, DBP, and MAP results are shown in Table 4 according to the BHS standard. References [17–19] obtained grade B in predicting the SBP value. Reference [23] obtained grade C for SBP prediction without calibration. Since a generalized model is desired, calibration-free results are considered. Only References [25,27] obtained grade A for SBP prediction. All papers obtained grade A in predicting the DBP values, indicating that DBP correlates strongly with the PPG and ECG signals. Compared to the other models, our work obtained grade A for all three values, indicating the superiority of our results over those in References [17–19,23], according to the BHS standard.

Table 4. Comparison with related works based on British Hypertension Society (BHS) protocol.

Works	BP Values	Cumulative Error (%)			Grade
		≤5 mmHg	≤10 mmHg	≤15 mmHg	
BHS standard	-	60.00%	85.00%	95.00%	A
	-	50.00%	75.00%	90.00%	B
	-	40.00%	65%	85%	C
[17]	SBP	59.46%	79.97%	88.85%	B
	DBP	76.95%	95.72%	99.97%	A
	MAP	-	-	-	-
[18]	SBP	50.07%	76.40%	90.39%	B
	DBP	65.66%	89.77%	96.63%	A
	MAP	65.14%	89.58%	96.61%	A
[19]	SBP	51.00%	81.00%	94.00%	B
	DBP	62.00%	92.00%	99.00%	A
	MAP	60.00%	90.00%	98.00%	A
[25]	SBP	67.66%	89.82%	96.82%	A
	DBP	82.79%	96.12%	99.09%	A
	MAP	84.21%	97.38%	99.58%	A
[23]	SBP	46.30%	72.10%	85.20%	C
	DBP	73.20%	91.90%	97.00%	A
	MAP	76.00%	92.30%	96.90%	A
[27]	SBP	76.21%	93.66%	97.71%	A
	DBP	93.51%	98.70%	99.46%	A
	MAP	-	-	-	-
This work	SBP	64.20%	87.85%	95.26%	A
	DBP	95.58%	99.35%	99.67%	A
	MAP	90.80%	98.61%	99.51%	A

Comparisons based on real-time BP measurement, methodology, dataset, RMSE, and Pearson's correlation coefficient (r) with recent papers are presented in Table 5. Y.-H. Li et al. [17] proposed the BiLSTM network that uses ECG and PPG features to predict SBP and DBP values in real time. They showed an implementation of their real-time algorithm in the MATLAB interface. ResNet with a bidirectional LSTM was used by F. Miao et al. [18]. The 50-layered networks are combined to extract features from preprocessed signals. The BP values were estimated by using the features. The study showed no device implementation of their real-time algorithm. In contrast, F. Miao et al. used a multi-sensor regression algorithm with their self-made database, using both ECG and PPG signals from multiple sensors [19]. They used a USB port to send the digital signal to show it on a personal computer in real time. Unlike the feature-based works, S. Baker et al. combined the CNN and LSTM models with raw PPG and ECG signals to predict continuous BP [25]. However, their method is not in real time, and the correlation coefficient is comparatively low. The abovementioned studies either used a combination of two signals or ECG signals. However, as mentioned before, the ECG signal is complicated and cost ineffective. The signal cannot be obtained by using smartphones or smartwatches. To acquire the ECG signal, additional sensors are needed.

Table 5. Comparison with related works based on real-time BP estimation.

Works	Method	Database	Input	RMSE	Pearson r	Real Time	Device Demonstration
[17]	BiLSTM	MIMIC-II	ECG, PPG (Features)	SBP: 8.051 DBP: 3.998 MAP: N/A	-	Yes	Yes
[18]	ResLSTM	MIMIC-III	ECG (Features)	-	SBP: 0.88 DBP: 0.71 MAP: 0.85	Yes	No
[19]	Multi-instance regression algorithm	Self-made	ECG, PPG (Features)	-	SBP: 0.90 DBP: 0.84 MAP: 0.88	Yes	Yes
[25]	CNN–LSTM	MIMIC-III	ECG, PPG (Raw)	-	SBP: 0.80 DBP: 0.85 MAP: 0.86	No	No
[23]	RDAE	MIMIC-II	PPG	-	-	No	No
[27]	U-net	MIMIC-I and MIMIC-III	PPG (Raw)	SBP: 5.75 DBP: 3.52 MAP: 3.75	SBP: 0.97 DBP: 0.96 MAP: N/A	No	No
This work	1D Squeeze U-net	MIMIC-I and MIMIC-III	PPG (Raw)	SBP: 6.50 DBP: 3.73 MAP: 4.10	SBP: 0.97 DBP: 0.96 MAP: 97	Yes	Yes

Unlike in these works, K. Qin et al. and T. Athaya et al. used raw PPG signals, using regularized convolution-based deep autoencoder (RDAE) and U-net models, respectively, to obtain continuous BP values [23,27]. The result of Reference [23] was unsatisfactory and needs calibration for improvement. However, the performance of Reference [27] was good, but it needs several parameters, operations, and prediction time (Table 6) to make it unsuitable for real-time implementation. Both works cannot measure BP in real time.

Table 6. Quantitative comparison between U-net and Squeeze U-net regarding model size, number of operations, and prediction time.

Model	#Parameters	Size (MB)	#Float Operations	Time/Prediction (ms)
U-net [27]	10,812,682	126.91	162,176,642	2.00
Squeeze U-net	819,921	101.44	1,637,678	0.32
Reduction Factor	13×	1.3×	99×	6.1×

Different from the stated methods, our 1D Squeeze U-net method can predict BP values in real time by using raw PPG signals, with comparatively better accuracy and lower computational complexity; it is also suitable for mHealth application implementation. Table 6 showed the number of parameters, model size, number of operations, and prediction time of the proposed model which is comparatively lower to get better accuracy. As we used the proposed system to implement in an android device, keeping the computational complexity lower is very important.

3.3. mHealth Application

The computationally efficient Squeeze U-net model was used to calculate the real-time continuous BP, using an android application. Note that no other related works used an android application to predict real-time BP values, as per our knowledge. All stages of prior signal processing are performed in the android studio platform. The trained Squeeze U-net model is loaded by using TensorFlow Lite [45]. This model is used to predict SBP, DBP, and MAP values for new subjects.

For the implementation phase, the filtering process differs from the training phase. The PPG data are recorded by using the back camera of an android smartphone. A real-time Equiripple FIR bandpass filter is used in the implementation phase to estimate the BP values in real time. The real-time implementation process is shown in Figure 9. Placing the fingertip in the back camera, frames are acquired from the camera. Each time, a signal sample is calculated from the frame by taking the average of the red channel. The sampling frequency of the recorded signal using an android back camera is 30 Hz. The sampling frequency of the recorded signals must match the trained model; thus, linear interpolation [46] is performed with the recorded PPG signals [32]. Real-time Equiripple FIR bandpass filtering is performed on the red channel of the PPG signal by using the same filter coefficients used in the training phase. A single sample of the filtered PPG signal is taken in a 256 fixed-size queue. The segment is then normalized and used as the input of the trained Squeeze U-net model to get the predicted signal of 256 samples. Then the denormalization, peak detection, and estimation of BP values are performed sequentially.

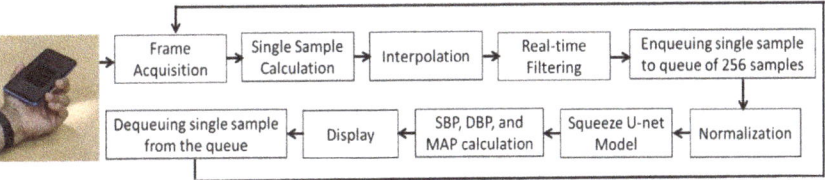

Figure 9. Implementation of real-time PPG signal filtering and BP values estimation.

The step-by-step real-time BP measurement process using this smartphone application is shown in Figure 10. By placing the index finger lightly on the camera, the PPG signal is acquired by using the rear camera of the smartphone to see the BP values in real time. To obtain accurate measurement results, neither the finger nor camera should not be moved until the measurement is completed. The graphs and BP values (Figure 10) are updated every second.

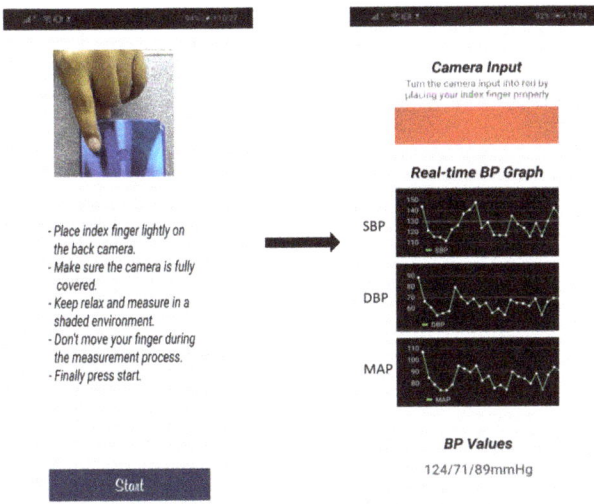

Figure 10. Real-time BP measurement using mHealth application.

4. Discussion

The analysis of the results evidently provides comparable performances for real-time SBP, DBP, and MAP predictions. Mobile health diagnosis has been proven to be successful and scalable in identifying and managing chronic diseases. By utilizing the optical and computational power of smartphones, physiological information may be assessed from the shape of pulse waves, and, hence, it can estimate BP without using a cuff. So, the proposed Squeeze U-net model that uses a smartphone application can easily measure real-time BP values without any cost and replace cuff-based devices. However, individual variations present unique challenges to the robustness and generalized prediction ability of the prediction model. Thus, the application needs to be tested with the data of persons of different ages, BP levels, and genders, and then it can be commercially used.

Note that PPG signals can have different kinds of artifacts, and the signal quality varies from person to person based on the muscle layer's volume and thickness, dermal and epidermal layers of skin, and volume of subcutaneous fats in a cross-section of the skin. The estimation result varies for the difference in finger pressure because the PPG signal is sensitive to finger pressure [47]. These parameters affect the estimation result. Although our study tried accumulating all kinds of PPG signals for a generalized model, some uncertainties still remain that might result in a high error level. Thus, the preliminary target of this application is for home use. However, if the proposed model is calibrated for each person, it should provide higher accuracy in real-time BP prediction, as the individual calibration process includes uncertain parameters.

In this study, the data from ICU patients were used. Because of different diseases, ICU patients exhibit abnormal PPG signals; thus, more normal subjects need to be included in the study in order to obtain more reliable predictions. Furthermore, the model's response to the sudden change in BP values has not yet been explored, which is a challenging topic that can be explored in further studies. In the future, the model can be trained with an equal amount of data from patients in the four BP stages shown in Figure 6. Individual calibration can be added to remove the uncertainty of individual parameters and to control the sudden change in BP values. We will also perform research to set up a system so that the finger movement can be controlled. This can help the system to be used not only at home but also in hospitals and medical settings for regular and accurate prediction.

5. Conclusions

Herein, a novel 1D Squeeze U-net model that is efficient for android smartphones was proposed to predict real-time continuous BP, using a raw PPG signal, with simple preprocessing. The performance of the DL model was tested on 100 individuals of MIMIC and MIMIC-III waveform databases and provided promising results in real-time BP estimation. When checking the compliance of our model with the standards defined by the healthcare organizations AAMI and BHS, our network achieved impressive performance. The computationally efficient model was implemented in an android application that can measure BP in real time. After performing certain tests, we have determined that the application can be a useful tool for detecting hypertension in various circumstances, such as low-income nations, where smartphones are widely available and access to healthcare is limited, as they can have access to this application without any cost. Overall, our results show convincing evidence that the proposed Squeeze U-net model that uses a raw PPG signal can be reliably used for real-time BP estimation, thus incorporating real-time continuous BP value prediction in mHealth applications.

Author Contributions: Conception, T.A.; methodology, T.A.; software, T.A.; validation, T.A. and S.C.; formal analysis, T.A. and S.C.; investigation, T.A. and S.C.; resources, T.A.; data curation, T.A.; writing—original draft preparation, T.A.; writing—review and editing, T.A. and S.C.; visualization, T.A. and S.C.; supervision, S.C.; project administration, S.C.; funding acquisition, S.C. All authors have read and agreed to the published version of the manuscript.

Funding: This work was supported by the National Research Foundation of Korea (NRF) Grant, funded by the Korean Government (MSIT) (Nos. 2016R1A5A1012966 and 2021R1F1A1062285).

Data Availability Statement: All the data used in this study are obtained from public datasets. Readers should be able to obtain those data by requesting the dataset sources described in this study.

Conflicts of Interest: The authors declare no conflict of interest.

References

1. Irigoyen, M.-C.; de Angelis, K.; Santos, F.d.; Dartora, D.R.; Rodrigues, B.; Consolim-Colombo, F.M. Hypertension, Blood Pressure Variability, and Target Organ Lesion. *Curr. Hypertens. Rep.* **2016**, *18*, 31. [CrossRef] [PubMed]
2. Schoettker, P.; Degott, J.; Hofmann, G.; Proença, M.; Bonnier, G.; Lemkaddem, A.; Lemay, M.; Schorer, R.; Christen, U.; Knebel, J.-F.; et al. Blood pressure measurements with the OptiBP smartphone app validated against reference auscultatory measurements. *Sci. Rep.* **2020**, *10*, 17827. [CrossRef] [PubMed]
3. Hypertension, World Heart Federation. (n.d.). Available online: https://world-heart-federation.org/what-we-do/hypertension/ (accessed on 23 November 2021).
4. Siu, A.L. Screening for High Blood Pressure in Adults: U.S. Preventive Services Task Force Recommendation Statement. *Ann. Intern. Med.* **2015**, *163*, 778. [CrossRef]
5. Mills, K.T.; Bundy, J.D.; Kelly, T.N.; Reed, J.E.; Kearney, P.M.; Reynolds, K.; Chen, J.; He, J. Global Disparities of Hypertension Prevalence and Control. *Circulation* **2016**, *134*, 441–450. [CrossRef]
6. NCD Risk Factor Collaboration (NCD-RisC). Long-term and recent trends in hypertension awareness, treatment, and control in 12 high-income countries: An analysis of 123 nationally representative surveys. *Lancet* **2019**, *394*, 639–651. [CrossRef]
7. Siaron, K.B.; Cortes, M.X.; Stutzman, S.E.; Venkatachalam, A.; Ahmed, K.M.; Olson, D.M. Blood Pressure measurements are site dependent in a cohort of patients with neurological illness. *Sci. Rep.* **2020**, *10*, 3382. [CrossRef]
8. Li, P.; Laleg-Kirati, T.-M. Central Blood Pressure Estimation From Distal PPG Measurement Using Semiclassical Signal Analysis Features. *IEEE Access* **2021**, *9*, 44963–44973. [CrossRef]
9. İlhan, İ.; Yıldız, İ.; Kayrak, M. Development of a wireless blood pressure measuring device with smart mobile device. *Comput. Methods Programs Biomed.* **2016**, *125*, 94–102. [CrossRef]
10. Zakrzewski, A.M.; Huang, A.Y.; Zubajlo, R.; Anthony, B.W. Real-Time Blood Pressure Estimation From Force-Measured Ultrasound. *IEEE Trans. Biomed. Eng.* **2018**, *65*, 2405–2416. [CrossRef]
11. Ding, X.-R.; Zhang, Y.-T.; Liu, J.; Dai, W.-X.; Tsang, H.K. Continuous Cuffless Blood Pressure Estimation Using Pulse Transit Time and Photoplethysmogram Intensity Ratio. *IEEE Trans. Biomed. Eng.* **2016**, *63*, 964–972. [CrossRef]
12. Ding, X.; Zhang, Y.; Tsang, H.K. Impact of heart disease and calibration interval on accuracy of pulse transit time-based blood pressure estimation. *Physiol. Meas.* **2016**, *37*, 227–237. [CrossRef] [PubMed]
13. Zheng, Y.-L.; Yan, B.P.; Zhang, Y.-T.; Poon, C.C.Y. An Armband Wearable Device for Overnight and Cuff-Less Blood Pressure Measurement. *IEEE Trans. Biomed. Eng.* **2014**, *61*, 2179–2186. [CrossRef]
14. Ding, X.-R.; Zhao, N.; Yang, G.-Z.; Pettigrew, R.I.; Lo, B.; Miao, F.; Li, Y.; Liu, J.; Zhang, Y.-T. Continuous Blood Pressure Measurement From Invasive to Unobtrusive: Celebration of 200th Birth Anniversary of Carl Ludwig. *IEEE J. Biomed. Health Inform.* **2016**, *20*, 1455–1465. [CrossRef] [PubMed]
15. Mukkamala, R.; Hahn, J.-O.; Inan, O.T.; Mestha, L.K.; Kim, C.-S.; Töreyin, H.; Kyal, S. Toward Ubiquitous Blood Pressure Monitoring via Pulse Transit Time: Theory and Practice. *IEEE Trans. Biomed. Eng.* **2015**, *62*, 1879–1901. [CrossRef]
16. He, R.; Huang, Z.-P.; Ji, L.-Y.; Wu, J.-K.; Li, H.; Zhang, Z.-Q. Beat-to-beat ambulatory blood pressure estimation based on random forest. In Proceedings of the 2016 IEEE 13th International Conference on Wearable and Implantable Body Sensor Networks (BSN), San Francisco, CA, USA, 14–17 June 2016; pp. 194–198. [CrossRef]
17. Li, Y.-H.; Harfiya, L.N.; Purwandari, K.; Lin, Y.-D. Real-Time Cuffless Continuous Blood Pressure Estimation Using Deep Learning Mode. *Sensors* **2020**, *20*, 5606. [CrossRef]
18. Miao, F.; Wen, B.; Hu, Z.; Fortino, G.; Wang, X.-P.; Liu, Z.-D.; Tang, M.; Li, Y. Continuous blood pressure measurement from one-channel electrocardiogram signal using deep-learning techniques. *Artif. Intell. Med.* **2020**, *108*, 101919. [CrossRef]
19. Miao, F.; Liu, Z.-D.; Liu, J.-K.; Wen, B.; He, Q.-Y.; Li, Y. Multi-Sensor Fusion Approach for Cuff-Less Blood Pressure Measurement. *IEEE J. Biomed. Health Inform.* **2020**, *24*, 79–91. [CrossRef]
20. Pitson, D.J.; Sandell, A.; van den Hout, R.; Stradling. Use of pulse transit time as a measure of inspiratory effort in patients with obstructive sleep apnoea. *Eur. Respir. J.* **1995**, *8*, 1669–1674. [CrossRef]
21. Mejía-Mejía, E.; May, J.M.; Elgendi, M.; Kyriacou, P.A. Classification of blood pressure in critically ill patients using photoplethysmography and machine learning. *Comput. Methods Programs Biomed.* **2021**, *208*, 106222. [CrossRef]

22. Lin, W.-H.; Wang, H.; Samuel, O.W.; Liu, G.; Huang, Z.; Li, G. New photoplethysmogram indicators for improving cuffless and continuous blood pressure estimation accuracy. *Physiol. Meas.* **2018**, *39*, 025005. [CrossRef]
23. Qin, K.; Huang, W.; Zhang, T. Deep generative model with domain adversarial training for predicting arterial blood pressure waveform from photoplethysmogram signal. *Biomed. Signal Processing Control.* **2021**, *70*, 102972. [CrossRef]
24. Huang, J.-C.; Tsai, Y.-C.; Wu, P.-Y.; Lien, Y.-H.; Chien, C.-Y.; Kuo, C.-F.; Hung, J.-F.; Chen, S.-C.; Kuo, C.-H. Predictive modeling of blood pressure during hemodialysis: A comparison of linear model, random forest, support vector regression, XGBoost, LASSO regression and ensemble method. *Comput. Methods Programs Biomed.* **2020**, *195*, 105536. [CrossRef]
25. Baker, S.; Xiang, W.; Atkinson, I. A hybrid neural network for continuous and non-invasive estimation of blood pressure from raw electrocardiogram and photoplethysmogram waveforms. *Comput. Methods Programs Biomed.* **2021**, *207*, 106191. [CrossRef]
26. Slapničar, G.; Mlakar, N.; Luštrek, M. Blood Pressure Estimation from Photoplethysmogram Using a Spectro-Temporal Deep Neural Network. *Sensors* **2019**, *19*, 3420. [CrossRef]
27. Athaya, T.; Choi, S. An Estimation Method of Continuous Non-Invasive Arterial Blood Pressure Waveform Using Photoplethysmography: A U-Net Architecture-Based Approach. *Sensors* **2021**, *21*, 1867. [CrossRef]
28. Elgendi, M.; Fletcher, R.; Liang, Y.; Howard, N.; Lovell, N.H.; Abbott, D.; Lim, K.; Ward, R. The use of photoplethysmography for assessing hypertension. *Npj Digit. Med.* **2019**, *2*, 1–11. [CrossRef]
29. Moody, G.B.; Mark, R.G. A database to support development and evaluation of intelligent intensive care monitoring. In Proceedings of the Computers in Cardiology, Indianapolis, IN, USA, 8–11 September 1996; 65, pp. 7–660. [CrossRef]
30. Johnson, A.E.W.; Pollard, T.J.; Shen, L.H.; Lehman, L.H.; Feng, M.; Ghassemi, M.; Moody, B.; Szolovits, P.; Anthony Celi, L.; Mark, R.G. MIMIC-III, a freely accessible critical care database. *Sci. Data* **2016**, *3*, 160035. [CrossRef]
31. Goldberger, A.L.; Amaral, L.A.N.; Glass, L.; Hausdorff, J.M.; Ivanov, P.C.; Mark, R.G.; Mietus, J.E.; Moody, G.B.; Peng, C.-K.; Stanley, H.E. PhysioBank, PhysioToolkit, and PhysioNet. *Circulation* **2000**, *101*, e215–e220. [CrossRef]
32. Athaya, T.; Choi, S. An Efficient Fingertip Photoplethysmographic Signal Artifact Detection Method: A Machine Learning Approach. *J. Sens.* **2021**, *2021*, e9925033. [CrossRef]
33. Fan, X.; Wang, H.; Xu, F.; Zhao, Y.; Tsui, K.-L. Homecare-Oriented Intelligent Long-Term Monitoring of Blood Pressure Using Electrocardiogram Signals. *IEEE Trans. Ind. Inform.* **2020**, *16*, 7150–7158. [CrossRef]
34. Beheshti, N.; Johnson, L. Squeeze U-Net: A Memory and Energy Efficient Image Segmentation Network. In Proceedings of the 2020 IEEE/CVF Conference on Computer Vision and Pattern Recognition Workshops (CVPRW), Seattle, WA, USA, 14–19 June 2020; pp. 1495–1504. [CrossRef]
35. Iandola, F.N.; Han, S.; Moskewicz, M.W.; Ashraf, K.; Dally, W.J.; Keutzer, K. SqueezeNet: AlexNet-level accuracy with 50× fewer parameters and <0.5 MB model size. *arXiv* **2016**, arXiv:1602.07360.
36. Saadatifard, L.; Mobiny, A.; Govyadinov, P.; Nguyen, H.; Mayerich, D. DVNet: A Memory-Efficient Three-Dimensional CNN for Large-Scale Neurovascular Reconstruction. *arXiv* **2020**, arXiv:2002.0156.
37. Elgendi, M.; Norton, I.; Brearley, M.; Abbott, D.; Schuurmans, D. Systolic Peak Detection in Acceleration Photoplethysmograms Measured from Emergency Responders in Tropical Conditions. *PLoS ONE* **2013**, *8*, e76585. [CrossRef] [PubMed]
38. Papaioannou, T.G.; Protogerou, A.D.; Vrachatis, D.; Konstantonis, G.; Aissopou, E.; Argyris, A.; Nasothimiou, E.; Gialafos, E.J.; Karamanou, M.; Tousoulis, D.; et al. Mean arterial pressure values calculated using seven different methods and their associations with target organ deterioration in a single-center study of 1878 individuals. *Hypertens. Res.* **2016**, *39*, 640–647. [CrossRef]
39. Botchkarev, A. A New Typology Design of Performance Metrics to Measure Errors in Machine Learning Regression Algorithms. *Interdiscip. J. Inf. Knowl. Manag.* **2019**, *14*, 45–76. [CrossRef]
40. Chobanian, A.V.; Bakris, G.L.; Black, H.R.; Cushman, W.C.; Green, L.A.; Joseph, J.; Izzo, L.; Jones, D.W.; Materson, B.J.; Oparil, S.; et al. The Seventh Report of the Joint National Committee on Prevention, Detection, Evaluation, and Treatment of High Blood Pressure: The JNC 7 Report. *JAMA* **2003**, *289*, 2560–2571. [CrossRef]
41. Stergiou, G.; Alpert, B.; Mieke, S.; Asmar, R.; Atkins, N.; Eckert, S.; Frick, G.; Friedman, B.; Graßl, T.; Ichikawa, T.; et al. A Universal Standard for the Validation of Blood Pressure Measuring Devices: Association for the Advancement of Medical Instrumentation/European Society of Hypertension/International Organization for Standardization (AAMI/ESH/ISO) Collaboration Statement. *J. Hypertens.* **2018**, *36*, 472–478. [CrossRef]
42. White, W.B.; Berson, A.S.; Robbins, C.; Jamieson, M.J.; Prisant, L.M.; Roccella, E.; Sheps, S.G. National standard for measurement of resting and ambulatory blood pressures with automated sphygmomanometers. *Hypertension* **1993**, *21*, 504–509. [CrossRef]
43. O'Brien, E.; Petrie, J.; Littler, W.A.; De Swiet, M.; Padfield, P.L.; Altman, D.; Bland, M.; Coats, A.; Atkins, N. The British Hypertension Society protocol for the evaluation of blood pressure measuring devices. *J. Hypertens.* **1993**, *11*, S43–S62.
44. Athaya, T.; Choi, S. A Review of Noninvasive Methodologies to Estimate the Blood Pressure Waveform. *Sensors* **2022**, *22*, 3953. [CrossRef]
45. TensorFlow Lite | ML for Mobile and Edge Devices, TensorFlow. (n.d.). Available online: https://www.tensorflow.org/lite (accessed on 26 October 2021).
46. Yuan, Y.; Zhang, C.; Wang, Y.; Liu, C.; Ji, J.; Feng, C. Linear interpolation process and its influence on the secondary equipment in substations. In Proceedings of the 2017 China International Electrical and Energy Conference (CIEEC), Beijing, China, 25–27 October 2017; pp. 205–209. [CrossRef]
47. Hossain, S.; Gupta, S.S.; Kwon, T.-H.; Kim, K.-D. Derivation and validation of gray-box models to estimate noninvasive in-vivo percentage glycated hemoglobin using digital volume pulse waveform. *Sci. Rep.* **2021**, *11*, 12169. [CrossRef] [PubMed]

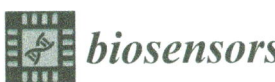

Communication

Short-Term Effect of Cigarette Smoke on Exhaled Volatile Organic Compounds Profile Analyzed by an Electronic Nose

Silvano Dragonieri [1,*], Vitaliano Nicola Quaranta [1], Enrico Buonamico [1], Claudia Battisti [1], Teresa Ranieri [1], Pierluigi Carratu [2] and Giovanna Elisiana Carpagnano [1]

1 Respiratory Diseases Unit, Department SMBNOS, University of Bari, 70121 Bari, Italy; vitalianonicola.quaranta@asl.bari.it (V.N.Q.); enrico.buonamico@policlinico.ba.it (E.B.); c.battisti1@studenti.uniba.it (C.B.); teresa.ranieri@uniba.it (T.R.); elisiana.carpagnano@uniba.it (G.E.C.)
2 Internal Medicine "A.Murri", University of Bari, 70121 Bari, Italy; pierluigi.carratu@uniba.it
* Correspondence: silvano.dragonieri@uniba.it

Abstract: Breath analysis using an electronic nose (e-nose) is an innovative tool for exhaled volatile organic compound (VOC) analysis, which has shown potential in several respiratory and systemic diseases. It is still unclear whether cigarette smoking can be considered a confounder when analyzing the VOC-profile. We aimed to assess whether an e-nose can discriminate exhaled breath before and after smoking at different time periods. We enrolled 24 healthy smokers and collected their exhaled breath as follows: (a) before smoking, (b) within 5 min after smoking, (c) within 30 min after smoking, and (d) within 60 min after smoking. Exhaled breath was collected by a previously validated method and analyzed by an e-nose (Cyranose 320). By principal component analysis, significant variations in the exhaled VOC profile were shown for principal component 1 and 2 before and after smoking. Significance was higher 30 and 60 min after smoking than 5 min after ($p < 0.01$ and <0.05, respectively). Canonical discriminant analysis confirmed the above findings (cross-validated values: baseline vs. 5 min = 64.6%, AUC = 0.833; baseline vs. 30 min = 83.6%, AUC = 0.927; baseline vs. 60 min = 89.6%, AUC = 0.933). Thus, the exhaled VOC profile is influenced by very recent smoking. Interestingly, the effect seems to be more closely linked to post-cigarette inflammation than the tobacco-related odorants.

Keywords: electronic nose; volatile organic compounds; breath analysis; smoking

1. Introduction

Breathomics is the study of exhaled breath composition, which could ease the diagnosis and phenotyping of several respiratory diseases [1]. Exhaled breath contains thousands of volatile organic compounds (VOCs), including exogenous VOCs such as environmental compounds, food, drinks, and drugs and endogenous VOCs such as metabolic derivates and microbiota. Basically, any changes occurring in the cell biochemistry, including those caused by pathologies, can change the blood composition and can be reflected in breath by the interchange of VOCs in the lungs [2]. Breath is a less complex medium compared to blood, stool, and urine, making its sampling and/or data analysis less complicated [2].

Gas chromatography–mass spectrometry (GC–MS) is the gold standard for measuring exhaled breath VOCs. However, GC–MS is a cumbersome and expensive instrument and requires well-trained personnel; thus, its application in breath analysis is limited [1].

The electronic nose (e-nose) is a quick and non-invasive tool which can detect exhaled VOC profiles. Interestingly, an increasing number of studies have shown its potential in various respiratory diseases, including asthma, COPD, lung cancer, pneumonia, interstitial lung disease [1], and even non-respiratory conditions such as breast and colon cancer, neurodegenerative diseases, diabetes mellitus, and liver failure [3].

Despite being a promising diagnostic technique, before obtaining full validation of exhaled breath profiling, there are still several methodological limitations due to different factors such as smoking, diet, race, physical exercise, pregnancy, and medication use, which may have an impact on the exhaled VOC composition [4].

Among the aforementioned factors, smoking plays a crucial role, since VOCs derive from metabolic and inflammatory processes related to physiological and/or pathophysiological changes occurring in the respiratory tract [5], and smoking may contribute to the alteration of these processes [6]. Moreover, more than 90 VOCs are known to be present in the mainstream smoke of cigarettes, including nitrogenous compounds, aldehydes, esters, alkenes, aromatic hydrocarbons, ketones, alcohols, furfurans, acids, alkanes, and ethers, which have well-known injurious and carcinogenic effects [7,8].

To date, it remains unclear how exhaled VOCs are influenced by smoking status. Based on the above, the aim of our study was to assess whether an e-nose can discriminate exhaled breath before and after smoking at different time periods in a group of healthy volunteers.

2. Materials and Methods

2.1. Patients

A total number of 24 healthy smokers (11 males, 13 females) were enrolled in our study. All participants had a negative clinical history of chest symptoms and/or systemic diseases, and none of the subjects were taking any medications. The age range was 24–47. All individuals had a normal lung function. Subjects with upper or lower respiratory tract infections in the four weeks before testing were excluded from the study. Baseline characteristics are shown in Table 1.

Table 1. Clinical characteristics of the studied population.

Parameter	Value
Subjects (n.)	24
M/F (n.)	11\13
Age (y.)	35.4 ± 11.3
FEV1%pred.	101.5 ± 11.8
BMI (kg/m^2)	25.77 ± 3.2
Current smokers (n.)	24
Comorbidities (n.)	0

FEV1 = forced expiratory volume in the 1st second.

Exhaled breath was collected from all individuals as follows: (a) before smoking (T0), (b) within 5 min after smoking (T1), (c) within 30 min after smoking (T2) and (d) within 60 min after smoking (T3).

All participants were volunteers and were enrolled from hospital staff relatives.

The current study was previously approved by the local ethics committee (protocol number 46403/15), and all individuals were required to sign an informed consent form before participating in the current study.

2.2. Study Design

A longitudinal study was performed. Two separate visits were required to complete all measurements. During visit one, all participants were judiciously screened for inclusion/exclusion criteria and, after definitive inclusion in the study, flow-volume spirometry was executed (MasterscreenPneumo, Jaeger, Würzburg, Germany).

During visit two, exhaled breath was collected before smoking (T0) and after smoking one cigarette (tar content: 10 mg, nicotine level: 0.8 mg, carbon monoxide level: 10 mg) at T1, T2, and T3 as described above and immediately analyzed by the e-nose. All participants were asked not to smoke at least 12 h prior to the test. Subjects were asked to refrain from eating and drinking, as well as from performing active physical activity, for at least 3 h before visit two. Exhaled breath was collected as previously validated [6,7]: first, a 5-min wash-in period by a 3-way non-rebreathing valve connected to an inspiratory VOC filter (A2; North Safety, Middelburg, the Netherlands) to minimize the impact of environmental VOCs and to an expiratory silica reservoir to reduce the effect of humidity on sensors (which are very sensitive to H_2O). Subsequently, participants exhaled into a Tedlar bag connected to the e-nose until approximately reaching their residual volume. A nose clip was worn during all the maneuvers. All participants were remotely monitored by text messages or phone calls for any kind of symptoms within 24 h from breath collection. None of the participants experienced hyperventilation or other related symptoms during breath collection and in the following 24 h.

2.3. Electronic Nose

A commercially available e-nose was used for the current study (Cyranose 320, Sensigent, Irwindale, CA, USA). It is based on a nano-composite array of 32 organic polymer sensors. If exposed to VOC combinations, the polymers swell, thereby modifying their electrical resistance. Raw data are registered the as increase in resistance of any single sensors in an onboard built database, resulting in a "breathprint" which labels the VOC spectrum and that can be successively used for pattern-recognition algorithms (Figure 1). According to the instruction manual, we used the following operating parameters: baseline purge: 30 s (pump speed: low); sampling time: 60 s (pump speed: medium), purging time: 200 s (pump speed: high), total run time: 300 s, temperature 42 °C. Post-run purges between samples: 5 min. Moreover, before the first sample of the day, 5 min exposure to room air followed by a "blank measurement" was performed to stabilize sensor outputs. Relative humidity for exhaled samples was around 55%.

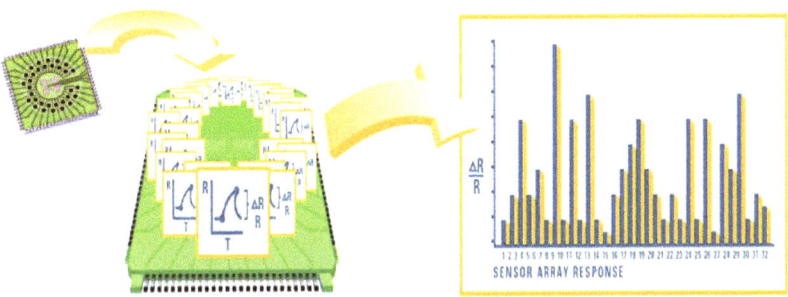

Figure 1. Working principle of Cyranose 320: it is based on a nano-composite array of 32 organic polymer sensors. If exposed to VOC combinations, the polymers swell, thereby modifying their electrical resistance. Raw data are registered as the increase in resistance of any single sensors and the combination of all signals results in a "breathprint".

2.4. Statistical Analysis

All data analyses were performed using SPSS for Windows 26.0 (SPSS, Chicago, IL, USA). The normal distribution of our data was verified by Kolmogorov–Smirnov and Shapiro–Wilk tests. We analyzed categorical values with the Fisher's exact test or χ^2 test as appropriate and reported as n (%). We compared continuous variables by ANOVA and Student's t-test for independent samples. Continuous parameters with normal distribution were reported as mean $\pm$ standard deviation (SD).

We performed data reduction of the whole set of 32 sensors by principal component analysis. All 4 principal components (PCs) were compared at different times (before smoking, 5 min after smoking, 30 min after smoking, and 60 min after smoking) by ANOVA test. When significant, the individual groups were compared 2 to 2 with Student's t-test for independent samples.

The significant principal components were analyzed by linear discriminant analysis (CDA) for categorizing VOC patterns. The "leave-one-out" validation method was used to calculate the cross-validated accuracy % (CVA%), which estimates the accuracy of a predictive model in practice. Additionally, a receiver operating characteristic curve (ROC curve) was built using predicted probabilities to determine the area under the curve (AUC). The sample size was estimated to limit the standard error to 10%. Assuming 80% accuracy, the current sample size per subgroup sufficed. We considered a p-value of <0.05 as statistically significant.

3. Results

The characteristics of the study population are described in Table 1. Males and females were almost equal, and the lung function as well as body mass index (BMI) were within ranges of normality.

We verified by the Kolmogorov test that the principal component had a normal distribution. By principal component analysis (PCA), significant variations in the exhaled VOC profile were shown for PCs 2 and 4 before and after smoking (Table 2); hence, we selected these two factors for further analysis. Interestingly, significance was higher 30 and 60 min after smoking than 5 min after (T0 vs. T2 and T0 vs. T3, $p < 0.01$ and T0 vs. T1 $p < 0.05$, see Table 3). The two-dimensional PCA plot showed the discrimination of breathprints before smoking and 5 min after smoking (Figure 2). Similarly, the 2-D PCA plot showed the distinction of breathprints before smoking and 30 min after smoking (Figure 3). Finally, the discernment of breathprints before smoking and 60 min after smoking was also shown (Figure 4). Subsequent linear discriminant analysis confirmed the above findings with the following cross-validated values: T0 vs. T1 = 64.6%, T0 vs. T2 = 83.6% and T0 vs. T3 = 89.6%. The area under the curve of the ROC curve for the discrimination between exhaled VOC profiles before and after smoking were the following: T0 vs. T1 = 0.832, T0 vs. T2 = 0.927 and T0 vs. T3 = 0.933 (Figure 5).

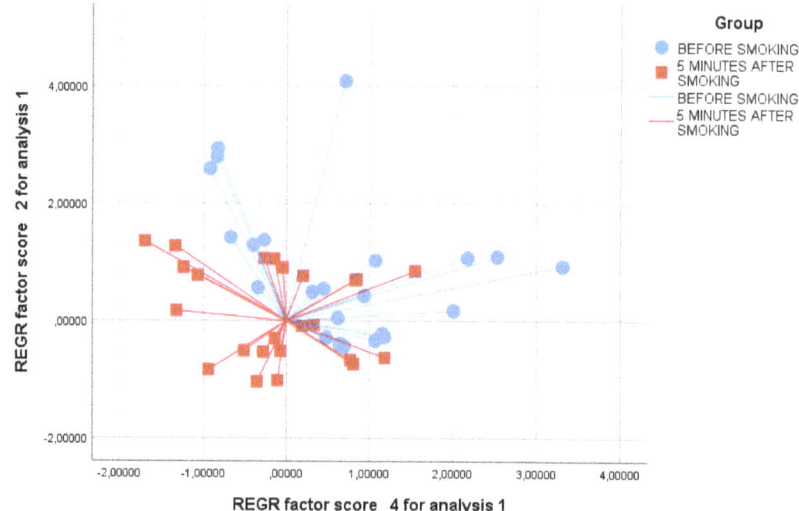

Figure 2. Two-dimensional PCA plot showing the discrimination of breathprints before smoking (blue circles) and 5 min after smoking (red squares). REGR = regression.

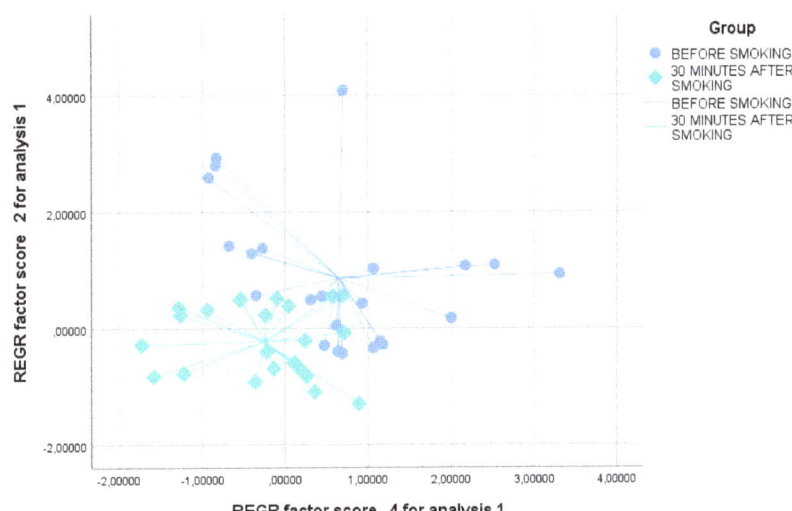

Figure 3. Two dimensional PCA plot showing the discrimination of breathprints before smoking (blue circles) and 30 min after smoking (green diamonds). REGR = regression.

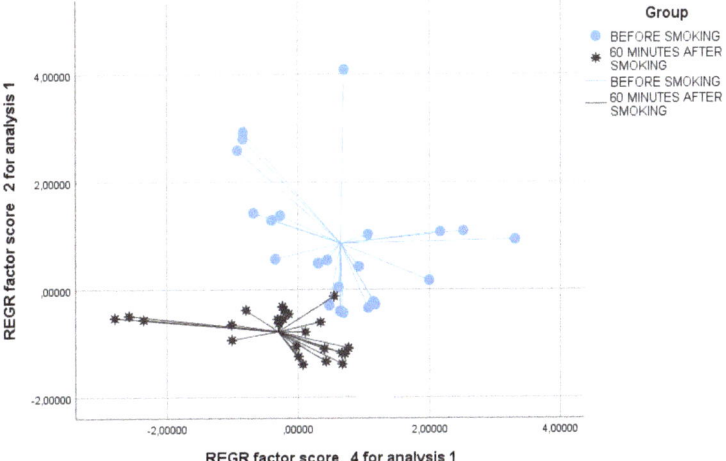

Figure 4. Two-dimensional PCA plot showing the discrimination of breathprints before smoking (blue circles) and 60 min after smoking (black stars). REGR = regression.

Table 2. ANOVA of principal components at different time periods.

	PC1	PC2	PC3	PC4	p
T0	-0.259 ± 0.499	0.858 ± 1.215	-0.210 ± 0.723	0.654 ± 1.092	0.114
T1	-0.009 ± 0.644	0.151 ± 0.800	0.023 ± 1.004	-0.114 ± 0.854	0.000
T2	0.402 ± 0.506	-0.218 ± 0.609	0.381 ± 0.947	-0.235 ± 0.753	0.140
T3	-0.133 ± 1.718	-0.790 ± 0.382	-0.193 ± 1.209	-0.305 ± 1.012	0.002

Table 3. Discriminant analysis by means of PC2 and PC4 between before smoking and after smoking time periods.

Time	Cross Validate Value (%)	AUC [CI]; p Value
T0 vs. T1	64.6	0.832 [0.715–0.948]; $p < 0.05$
T0 vs. T2	83.6	0.927 [0.853–1.000]; $p < 0.01$
T0 vs. T3	89.6	0.933 [0.977–1.000]; $p < 0.01$

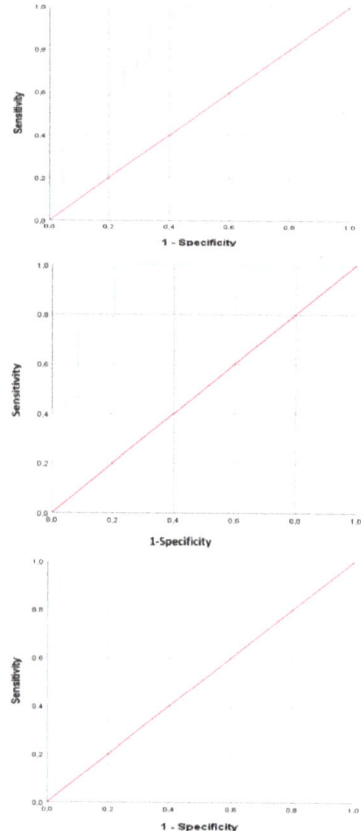

Figure 5. ROC curves between T0 and T1 (**upper**), between T0 and T2 (**center**), and between T0 and T3 (**lower**).

4. Discussion

In our study, we demonstrated that the use of an e-nose to analyze the exhaled VOC profiles is influenced by very recent smoking. Interestingly, the effect seems to be more closely linked to the post-cigarette inflammation than the tobacco-related odorants.

E-nose-based exhaled breath analysis has been increasingly used in recent years for various pathologies for screening and diagnostic purposes [1,9]. Breath analysis might be preferable compared to other biological samples such as blood, feces, and urine since breath is a totally non-invasive matrix, much easier to acquire, and has the potential to offer real-time monitoring [2].

The novelty of our study is the assessment of e-nose analyzed exhaled breath VOC composition in relation to short-term smoke exposure in a population of well-characterized, healthy subjects.

The strengths of our study are the careful selection of our population of smokers, with the exclusion of any known diseases and the use of standardized methods for e-nose analysis, with all participants smoking the same type of cigarette. On the other hand, a few limitations must be disclosed. The first is our relatively small number of enrolled subjects. However, based on previous observations, [10,11] and based on our sample size estimation, we believe that our total population of 24 individuals might warrant further investigations including larger cohorts and a validation group.

Second, we arbitrarily chose sampling periods after smoking for each group and we lack data on longer periods after smoking; therefore, we may have missed some relevant information.

Third, although being non-invasive, easy to use, and with promptly available results, e-nose analysis does not allow the identification and quantification of single VOCs. Incontestably, further investigations should integrate chemical analytical techniques such as gas chromatography–mass spectrometry (GC–MS) to identify discriminant VOCs.

How can we interpret our data?

Tobacco smoke is known to directly affect the level of several VOCs in human breath [12]. Nonetheless, previous studies on exhaled breath analyzed by an e-nose indicate that signals most likely derive from pathophysiological modifications driven by the underlying chronic airway disease and by chronic smoking exposure. In detail, a recent investigation by Principe et al. [13] showed that an e-nose could discriminate ever- from never-smokers in a population of subjects with COPD and asthma. However, their e-nose could not distinguish recent smokers as effectively, denoting that recent smoking might not be a confounding factor of the VOC spectrum [13].

Similarly to the above, previous studies with e-nose recruiting smoking or ex-smoking patients with asthma and COPD concluded that several types of e-nose can discriminate among patients with chronic smoking habits, whereas it cannot detect active smoking in patients according to the time of last cigarette consumption [14–20].

Our data are in line with the above observations; thus, we may speculate that e-nose detects the effect of cigarette smoking on airways rather than the smoke itself.

5. Conclusions

In conclusion, our data indicate that very short-term smoking may be considered as a confounder which affects e-nose measurements. Therefore, we suggest that patients should abstain from smoking for a certain period before testing their exhaled breath for e-nose-based VOC analysis. Future studies with larger cohorts and with different types of e-nose technology should be addressed to extend our findings and to explore other confounding factors.

Author Contributions: Conceptualization, S.D. and P.C.; methodology, V.N.Q.; software V.N.Q.; validation, V.N.Q.; formal analysis, C.B.; investigation, E.B.; resources, S.D. and T.R.; data curation, C.B.; writing—original draft preparation, S.D.; writing—review and editing, S.D.; visualization, G.E.C.; supervision, G.E.C.; project administration, G.E.C.; funding acquisition, G.E.C. All authors have read and agreed to the published version of the manuscript.

Funding: This research received no external funding.

Institutional Review Board Statement: The study was conducted in accordance with the Declaration of Helsinki and approved by the local ethics committee (protocol number 46403/15).

Informed Consent Statement: All participants signed an informed consent form before taking part in the study.

Data Availability Statement: Not applicable.

Conflicts of Interest: The authors declare no conflict of interest.

References

1. Dragonieri, S.; Pennazza, G.; Carratu, P.; Resta, O. Electronic Nose Technology in Respiratory Diseases. *Lung* **2017**, *195*, 157–165. [CrossRef] [PubMed]
2. Haddadi, S.; Koziel, J.A.; Engelken, T.J. Analytical approaches for detection of breath VOC biomarkers of cattle diseases—A review. *Anal. Chim. Acta* **2022**, *1206*, 339565. [CrossRef] [PubMed]
3. Bosch, S.; Lemmen, J.P.M.; Menezes, R.; Van Der Hulst, R.; Kuijvenhoven, J.; Stokkers, P.C.F.; De Meij, T.G.J.; De Boer, N.K. The influence of lifestyle factors on fecal volatile organic compound composition as measured by an electronic nose. *J. Breath Res.* **2019**, *13*, 046001. [CrossRef] [PubMed]
4. Horváth, I.; Barnes, P.J.; Loukides, S.; Sterk, P.J.; Högman, M.; Olin, A.-C.; Amann, A.; Antus, B.; Baraldi, E.; Bikov, A.; et al. A European Respiratory Society technical standard: Exhaled biomarkers in lung disease. *Eur. Respir. J.* **2017**, *49*, 1600965. [CrossRef] [PubMed]
5. Zarogoulidis, P.; Freitag, L.; Besa, V.; Teschler, H.; Kurth, I.; Khan, A.M.; Sommerwerck, U.; Baumbach, J.I.; Darwiche, K. Exhaled volatile organic compounds discriminate patients with chronic obstructive pulmonary disease from healthy subjects. *Int. J. Chronic Obstr. Pulm. Dis.* **2015**, *10*, 399–406. [CrossRef] [PubMed]
6. Tamimi, A.; Serdarevic, D.; Hanania, N.A. The effects of cigarette smoke on airway inflammation in asthma and COPD: Therapeutic implications. *Respir. Med.* **2012**, *106*, 319–328. [CrossRef] [PubMed]
7. Wang, P.; Huang, Q.; Meng, S.; Mu, T.; Liu, Z.; He, M.; Li, Q.; Zhao, S.; Wang, S.; Qiu, M. Identification of lung cancer breath biomarkers based on perioperative breathomics testing: A prospective observational study. *EClinicalMedicine* **2022**, *47*, 101384. [CrossRef] [PubMed]
8. Lu, F.; Yu, M.; Chen, C.; Liu, L.; Zhao, P.; Shen, B.; Sun, R. The Emission of VOCs and CO from Heated Tobacco Products, Electronic Cigarettes, and Conventional Cigarettes, and Their Health Risk. *Toxics* **2021**, *10*, 8. [CrossRef] [PubMed]
9. Raspagliesi, F.; Bogani, G.; Benedetti, S.; Grassi, S.; Ferla, S.; Buratti, S. Detection of Ovarian Cancer through Exhaled Breath by Electronic Nose: A Prospective Study. *Cancers* **2020**, *12*, 2408. [CrossRef] [PubMed]
10. Dragonieri, S.; Quaranta, V.N.; Carratù, P.; Ranieri, T.; Buonamico, E.; Carpagnano, G.E. Breathing Rhythm Variations during Wash-In Do Not Influence Exhaled Volatile Organic Compound Profile Analyzed by an Electronic Nose. *Molecules* **2021**, *26*, 2695. [CrossRef] [PubMed]
11. Dragonieri, S.; Scioscia, G.; Quaranta, V.N.; Carratu, P.; Venuti, M.P.; Falcone, M.; Carpagnano, G.E.; Foschino Barbaro, M.P.; Resta, O.; Lacedonia, D. Exhaled volatile organic compounds analysis by e-nose can detect idiopathic pulmonary fibrosis. *J. Breath Res.* **2020**, *14*, 047101. [CrossRef] [PubMed]
12. Gordon, M.S.; Wallace, L.A.; Brinkman, A.C. Volatile organic compounds as breath biomparkers for active and passive smoking. *Environ. Health Perspect.* **2002**, *110*, 689–698. [CrossRef] [PubMed]
13. Principe, S.; van Bragt, J.J.M.H.; Longo, C.; de Vries, R.; Sterk, P.J.; Scichilone, N.; Vijverberg, S.J.H.; Maitland-van der Zee, A.H. The Influence of Smoking Status on Exhaled Breath Profiles in Asthma and COPD Patients. *Molecules* **2021**, *26*, 1357. [CrossRef] [PubMed]
14. Gaida, A.; Holz, O.; Nell, C.; Schuchardt, S.; Lavae-Mokhtari, B.; Kruse, L.; Boas, U.; Langejuergen, J.; Allers, M.; Zimmermann, S.; et al. A dual center study to compare breath volatile organic compounds from smokers and non-smokers with and without COPD. *J. Breath Res.* **2016**, *10*, 026006. [CrossRef]
15. Papaefstathiou, E.; Stylianou, M.; Andreou, C.; Agapiou, A. Breath analysis of smokers, non-smokers, and e-cigarette users. *J. Chromatogr. B* **2020**, *1160*, 122349. [CrossRef]
16. Van Bragt, J.J.; Brinkman, P.; De Vries, R.; Vijverberg, S.J.; Weersink, E.J.; Haarman, E.G.; De Jongh, F.H.; Kester, S.; Lucas, A.; in't, Veen, J.C.C.M.; et al. Identification of recent exacerbations in COPD patients by electronic nose. *ERJ Open Res.* **2020**, *6*, 00307-2020. [CrossRef]
17. De Groot, J.C.; Amelink, M.; Storm, H.; Reitsma, B.H.; Bel, E.; Ten Brinke, A. Identification of Three Subtypes of Non-Atopic Asthma Using Exhaled Breath Analysis by Electronic Nose. *Am. Thorac. Soc.* **2014**, *189*, A2170.
18. Fens, N.; De Nijs, S.B.; Peters, S.; Dekker, T.; Knobel, H.H.; Vink, T.J.; Willard, N.P.; Zwinderman, A.H.; Krouwels, F.H.; Janssen, H.-G.; et al. Exhaled air molecular profiling in relation to inflammatory subtype and activity in COPD. *Eur. Respir. J.* **2011**, *38*, 1301–1309. [CrossRef] [PubMed]
19. Caruso, M.; Emma, R.; Brinkman, P.; Sterk, P.J.; Bansal, A.T.; De Meulder, B.; Lefaudeux, D.; Auffray, C.; Fowler, S.J.; Rattray, N.; et al. Volatile Organic Compounds Breathprinting of U-BIOPRED Severe Asthma smokers/ex-smokers cohort. *Airw. Cell Biol. Immunopathol.* **2017**, *50*, PA2018. [CrossRef]
20. Thomson, N.C. Asthma and smoking-induced airway disease without spirometric COPD. *Eur. Respir. J.* **2017**, *49*, 1602061. [CrossRef]

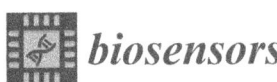

Article

Application of a Novel Biosensor for Salivary Conductivity in Detecting Chronic Kidney Disease

Chen-Wei Lin [1,2], Yuan-Hsiung Tsai [3,4], Yen-Pei Lu [5], Jen-Tsung Yang [4,6], Mei-Yen Chen [7], Tung-Jung Huang [4,8,9], Rui-Cian Weng [5,10] and Chun-Wu Tung [2,11,*]

1. School of Medicine, College of Medicine, Chang Gung University, Taoyuan 33302, Taiwan; toddgod7@cgmh.org.tw
2. Department of Medical Education, Chang Gung Memorial Hospital, Chiayi 61363, Taiwan
3. Department of Diagnostic Radiology, Chang Gung Memorial Hospital, Chiayi 61363, Taiwan; russell@cgmh.org.tw
4. College of Medicine, Chang Gung University, Taoyuan 33302, Taiwan; yljwty@cgmh.org.tw (J.-T.Y.); donaldhuang@cgmh.org.tw (T.-J.H.)
5. Taiwan Instrument Research Institute, National Applied Research Laboratories, Hsinchu 30261, Taiwan; ypl@narlabs.org.tw (Y.-P.L.); cian@tiri.narl.org.tw (R.-C.W.)
6. Department of Neurosurgery, Chang Gung Memorial Hospital, Chiayi 61363, Taiwan
7. Department of Nursing, Chang Gung University of Science and Technology, Chiayi 61363, Taiwan; meiyen@mail.cgust.edu.tw
8. Department of Internal Medicine, Chang Gung Memorial Hospital, Yunlin 63862, Taiwan
9. Department of Respiratory Care, Chang Gung University of Science and Technology, Chiayi 61363, Taiwan
10. Graduate Institute of Biomedical Electronics and Bioinformatics, National Taiwan University, Taipei 106319, Taiwan
11. Department of Nephrology, Chang Gung Memorial Hospital, Chiayi 61363, Taiwan
* Correspondence: p122219@cgmh.org.tw; Tel.: +886-(0)5-362-1000

Abstract: The prevalence of chronic kidney disease (CKD) is increasing, and it brings an enormous healthcare burden. The traditional measurement of kidney function needs invasive blood tests, which hinders the early detection and causes low awareness of CKD. We recently designed a device with miniaturized coplanar biosensing probes for measuring salivary conductivity at an extremely low volume (50 µL). Our preliminary data discovered that the salivary conductivity was significantly higher in the CKD patients. This cross-sectional study aims to validate the relationship between salivary conductivity and kidney function, represented by the estimated glomerular filtration rate (eGFR). We enrolled 214 adult participants with a mean age of 63.96 ± 13.53 years, of whom 33.2% were male. The prevalence rate of CKD, defined as eGFR < 60 mL/min/1.73 m^2, is 11.2% in our study. By multivariate linear regression analyses, we found that salivary conductivity was positively related to age and fasting glucose but negatively associated with eGFR. We further divided subjects into low, medium, and high groups according to the tertials of salivary conductivity levels. There was a significant trend for an increment of CKD patients from low to high salivary conductivity groups (4.2% vs. 12.5% vs. 16.9%, p for trend: 0.016). The receiver operating characteristic (ROC) curves disclosed an excellent performance by using salivary conductivity combined with age, gender, and body weight to diagnose CKD (AUC equal to 0.8). The adjusted odds ratio of CKD is 2.66 (95% CI, 1.10–6.46) in subjects with high salivary conductivity levels. Overall, salivary conductivity can serve as a good surrogate marker of kidney function; this real-time, non-invasive, and easy-to-use portable biosensing device may be a reliable tool for screening CKD.

Keywords: chronic kidney disease; salivary conductivity; non-invasive; portable; biosensor

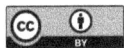

1. Introduction

Chronic kidney disease (CKD) is one of the most important public health issues and it brings an enormous socioeconomic burden [1]. The prevalence of CKD is increasing, and it affects 8–16% of the general population worldwide currently [2–4]. The progression of CKD is not only associated with end-stage renal disease but also is responsible for a wide range of morbidity and mortality. Decreased renal function is also related to longer hospitalization and poor quality of life [5–7]. CKD is estimated to become the fifth leading cause of death globally by 2040 [8]. It is well known that early identification of CKD with timely intervention plays a crucial role in preventing disease progression [9]. However, several studies have found that greater than 90% of patients with stage 3 CKD were not aware of their disorder [3,10]. The current diagnosis or staging of CKD is based on the estimated glomerular filtration rate (eGFR) which is calculated from serum creatinine [11,12]. The need for invasive procedures to collect serum creatinine is a great limitation for screening and monitoring of CKD outside the hospital. Since most patients with early-stage CKD is asymptomatic, it makes the early diagnosis difficult if a blood test is not performed [13]. In addition, blood collection may cause short-term complications such as hematomas after venipuncture, vasovagal fainting, or phlebitis [14]. Therefore, developing an easy-to-use, non-invasive, and cost-effective biodevice for the detection of CKD is essential for large-scale screening and reducing undiagnosed CKD.

Saliva is a kind of body fluid that can be obtained easily in a non-invasive manner and serves as a potential specimen for monitoring our health situation [15–18]. The saliva has complex compositions, such as electrolytes, cytokines, enzymes, antibodies, metabolites, etc. [19]. The complexity of salivary components renders it a promising diagnostic fluid to reflect the biological changes of systemic diseases. Recent literature has demonstrated the usefulness of saliva as a monitoring biological indicator in several diseases [20–22]. Moreover, the area of using salivary biomarkers for screening CKD is attracting considerable interest because it can be performed non-invasively, repeatedly without trained personnel in a low-resource setting. An increasing number of clinical studies have tried to adopt saliva as a diagnostic material for CKD [14,23–27]. Most of these studies focused on the usage of salivary urea nitrogen or salivary creatinine levels to detect CKD. In early-stage CKD, reduced permeability of salivary gland cells and reduced plasma-to-saliva gradient would lead to incorrect measurement of salivary creatinine level. Compared to salivary creatinine, salivary urea has been shown as a more sensitive marker for CKD, particularly in earlier stages [23]. Although some studies reported that salivary urea was a useful screen tool for CKD [26,27], a cohort study by Evans et al. showed suboptimal diagnostic performance of salivary urea with the area under the receiver operating characteristic (ROC) curve equal to 0.61 [23]. Therefore, our research team has been committed to exploiting a portable, miniaturized, and ready-to-use saliva detection instrument, and trying to explore more reliable diagnostic biomarkers for CKD.

The composition of saliva changes with progressive CKD [23]. Salivary concentrations of urea nitrogen, creatinine, and most electrolytes, except calcium, are significantly higher in CKD patients than in healthy controls. The change of pH, increase in electrolytes, and accumulation of uremic particles may contribute to the alteration of the electrical conductivity of saliva. We recently fabricated a novel biodevice with miniaturized sensing probes for measuring salivary conductivity [28]. The features of this portable sensing system include a disposable printed-circuit-board (PCB) electrode and the usage of highly biocompatible, stable, and reusable gold as the conductive material. Additionally, with the co-planar design of coating-free gold electrodes, the conductivity test could be achieved with a saliva specimen at an extremely low volume (50 μL). This reduces the difficulty of collecting saliva, eliminates the need for trained personnel, and increases people's willingness to the test. Our previous study has shown that the increase in salivary conductivity was associated with the increase in serum and urinary osmolality in dehydrated healthy adults [29]. Moreover, we also noticed that age and serum osmolality correlated well with salivary conductivity in hemodialysis patients [30]. Our preliminary data including 10 CKD patients and 10 healthy controls discovered that the salivary conductivity was significantly higher in the CKD population [28]. Although this result is encouraging, it still needs to be confirmed by large-scale studies. Consequently, this pilot study aims to validate the correlation between salivary conductivity and eGFR in a healthy population and to investigate whether the biodevice can act as a useful tool for screening and detecting CKD.

2. Materials and Methods

2.1. The Sensing Device and System

The portable biodevice was implemented to measure salivary conductivity. In brief, the construction steps were composed of three main steps, including biodevice design, the collection and analysis of saliva, and the test of reusability and selectivity of the electrodes.

2.1.1. Design of the Biodevice for Measuring Conductivity

The proposed system is composed of two main parts, including a PCB with coating-free gold electrodes and a conductivity meter (Figure 1). The size of the micro-fabricated electrode is 2×2 mm^2 which can be covered with testing samples with only 50 µL required. The $10 \times 5.5 \times 2.2$ cm^3 conductivity meter was fabricated as the previous study, which composes of an analog-to-digital converter (ADC) (AD5933, Analog Devices, Norwood, MA, USA), a micro control unit (MCU system) (STMicroelectronics, Geneva, Switzerland), a temperature sensor (Aosong, Guangzhou, China), and an organic light-emitting diode (OLED) (Zhongjingyuan, Henan, China). The electrode was bonded to the PCB by using nickel immersion gold wired. The conductivity meter can be implemented with 1 Vpp and 1 kHz sine waves via ADC to accomplish the measurement. The electrical conductivity parameters can be acquired through a discrete Fourier transform. The conductivity signal at 25 °C can be calculated through temperature compensation by the MCU system and be displayed on the OLED within 10 s.

2.1.2. The Collection and Analysis of Saliva

Salivary samples of all eligible subjects were collected and processed as previously described [28,29]. Briefly, the participants were asked to swallow several times for emptying their mouths before collection. The saliva was then collected by placing a mouth care cotton swab (diameter = 0.9 cm, length = 15.24 cm) under the tongue for 2 min. The collected salivary specimens were loaded into the well of the sensing probe and then analyzed for electrical conductivity through the conductivity meter which was connected to the portable device through a USB port (Figure 2). With the design of coplane, miniaturized, and coating-free gold electrodes, the conductivity test could be achieved with a saliva specimen at an extremely low volume (50 µL). A minimum measurement volume of 50 uL was determined according to the area of the electrodes, as this is the appropriate sample volume to fully cover the surface of micro-electrodes. Furthermore, stable conductivity data can be obtained when evaluating under this condition. The conductivity meter was pre-calibrated using the standard conductivity solution and examined coefficient of variation was less than 1% The detection time including sample preparation is within 5 min. The saliva solution is quite stable during the period. We had demonstrated that there was no significant change in the conductivity measurement of salivary samples at room temperature for at least 15 min (Figure S1 in Supplemental Materials).

2.1.3. Reusability of the Electrode

For testing the reusability of the electrode, salivary samples were tested 20 times with the same electrode. We used ultrapure water to clean the well until confirming the conductivity drops to the same level as the baseline before every measurement. In the clinical study, each PCB electrode was used with no more than five salivary samples to ensure the quality of the clinical data.

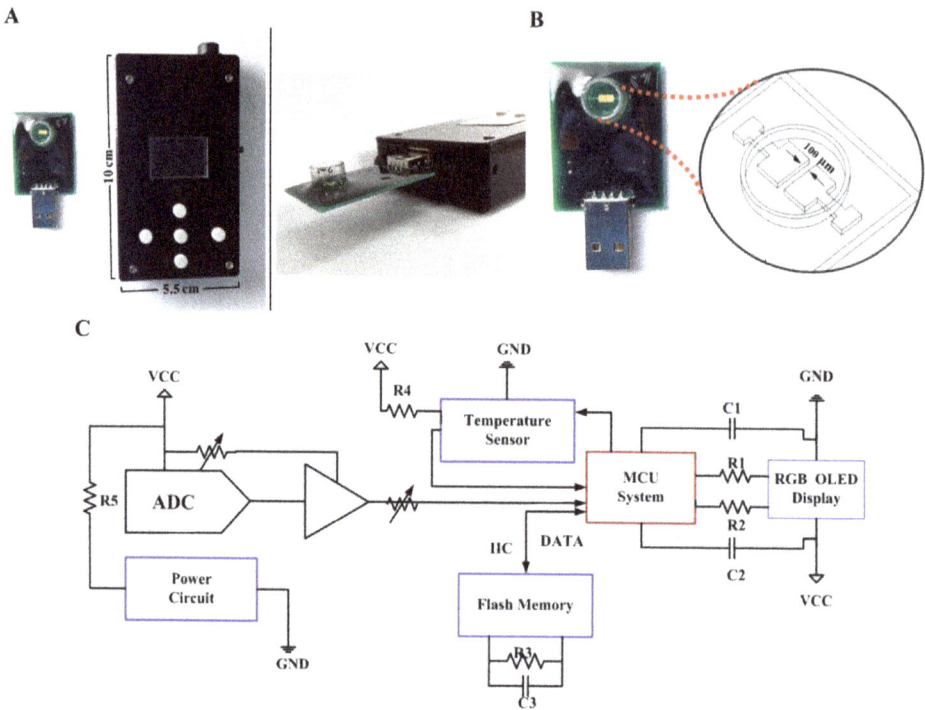

Figure 1. A tailor-made portable biodevice for measuring conductivity. (**A**) The device is composed of two parts, including a PCB with a coating-free gold microelectrode sensor in the sample well and a conductivity meter with a size of $10 \times 5.5 \times 2.2$ cm^3. (**B**) Design of the co-planar microelectrode and the sample well. The gap between two microelectrodes is only 100 μm. (**C**) Electronic schematics of the fabricated conductivity meter. Abbreviations: ADC, analog-to-digital converter; C, capacitance; GND, ground; IIC, inter-integrated circuit; MCU, micro control unit; OLED, organic light-emitting diode; R, resistance; RGB, red, green, blue color model; VCC, volt current condenser.

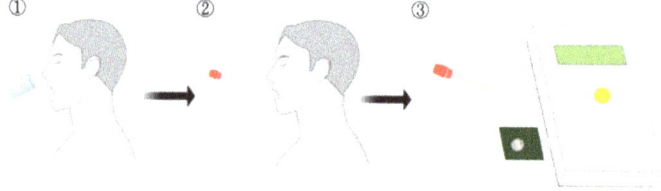

1. The participant swallowed and emptied their mouth.
2. Place a mouth care cotton swab under the tongue for 2 min.
3. Loading sample onto the printed-circuit board (PCB) electrode and analyzing the saliva conductivity through the developed portable monitor.

Figure 2. The saliva collection and salivary conductivity analysis protocol.

2.1.4. Selectivity of the Sensor

Saliva is composed of 99% water, 1% protein and salts, etc. [31]. Our sensor is used to measure the salivary conductivity which is determined by the electrical admittance between the electrodes which mostly reflects the concentration of the electrolytes. To increase the selectivity of the sensor and eliminate the interfering factors, we have adopted some special designs for our device. First, since the signal obeys the path of least impedance, the electro-path of electro-impedance spectroscopy is mainly at the edge of microelectrodes, which is approved according to the previous study [32]. Therefore, most of the interference effect caused by large particles such as food debris and nasal secretion, which fall at the top of the co-planar electrode can be minimized and have better selectivity. Second, the protein in saliva may decrease electrode sensitivity for detecting electrolytes because some proteins will adhere to the electrodes. However, with our microfabricated co-planar electrodes design, the interfering factor can be decreased compared to the commercial electrodes. This can be explained by the fact that the microelectrode edge is less vulnerable to protein adhesions than the electrode surface. To justify the hypothesis of our design, we have conducted experiments that measured the conductivity of ultrapure water, bovine serum albumin (BSA), phosphate-buffered saline (PBS) solution, different BSA concentrations mixed with PBS solution, and healthy participants' saliva. According to Lin et al., BSA can be a surrogate of the proteins secreted by the salivary glands, which is optimal for testing the selectivity of our sensor, and the mean value of human salivary protein ranged from 0.72 to 2.45 mg/mL [33]. In addition, PBS solution can be a surrogate of the electrolytes. The conductivity of each solution was measured six times repeatedly and the average was used to compare the difference between the groups. Besides, other experiments were conducted to compare our microelectrode with the commercial electrode by detection of ultrapure water spiked in with BSA to determine whether our microfabricated co-planar electrodes design has less interference with protein factors. Third, because interference particles can accumulate on the surface of the salivary solution with time, we further experimented to test the stability of the saliva sample. The conductance of six different salivary samples was repeatedly tested for 15 min with an interval of 3 min. The serial change can also reflect the stability of the saliva. Fourth, only a 50 µL saliva sample is required to perform the test. Therefore, we can assume that the sample temperature achieves equilibrium with the ambient temperature within a short period of time. It means that temperature is also not an interfering factor.

2.2. Clinical Study Design and Participants

This is a cross-sectional pilot study including adults aged ≥18 years who attended the annual health examination at Yunlin Branch of the Chang Gung Memorial Hospital, a regional teaching hospital in southern Taiwan, in August 2021. Before the investigation, we conducted a sample size calculation using PASS V.15 (NCSS, Kaysville, UT, USA). Assuming a CKD prevalence rate of 12% [2,3], with 80% power, at a two-sided statistical significance level of 5% ($\alpha = 0.05$), the sample size needed for an acceptable area under the ROC curve of 0.70 is 171. During the study period, 241 consecutive subjects completed the general health examinations. Among them, nine subjects could not cooperate with the saliva collection. Another 18 subjects were excluded owing to active illness, recent hospitalization for acute diseases, or past histories of head and neck treatments, such as surgery or radiotherapy. Therefore, a total of 214 adult subjects were included in the final analysis, exceeding the sample size required for the desired study power. The post hoc power analysis demonstrated a sample size of 214 achieved 99% power for salivary conductivity plus age and 80% power for only salivary conductivity as diagnostic tools at a 5% significance level. This study complied with the guidelines of the Declaration of Helsinki and was approved by the Medical Ethics Committee of Chang Gung Memorial Hospital (institutional review board number: 202000109B0 and 202002186B0). Before the beginning of the study, all participants agreed and signed the informed consent form.

2.3. Procedures of Clinical Study

Before health examination, all subjects received a comprehensive questionnaire survey conducted by trained nurses to provide information about previous head and neck surgery or radiotherapy and comorbid diseases, including diabetes, hypertension, chronic kidney disease, ischemic heart disease, stroke, dyslipidemia, gout, and chronic liver disease.

Anthropometric data of their body weight (kg) and height (cm) were obtained, and the corresponding body mass index (BMI) was calculated as weight in kilograms divided by height in meters squared (kg/m^2). The blood pressure was measured with a validated electronic automated sphygmomanometer on the right arm of seated participants after 15 min' rest in a quiet and comfortable environment. Two blood pressure readings were obtained at an interval of 5 min; if the readings differed by more than 20 mmHg, a third measurement was made, and the two closest blood pressure values were averaged. After an 8 to 12 h overnight fasting, venous blood and salivary samples were collected. Blood specimens were left undisturbed at room temperature for 30 min to allow the blood to clot. The clot was then removed by centrifuging at 3000 rpm for 10 min. The resulting supernatant was the serum which was analyzed for biochemical data using an automatic chemistry analyzer (Beckman DXC880i, Brea, CA, USA) following standardized laboratory procedures.

2.4. Definition of Chronic Kidney Disease

We used the revised Modification of Diet in Renal Disease (IDMS-MDRD) equation to calculate the eGFR: $175 \times Cr^{-1.154} \times Age^{-0.203} \times (0.742, \text{if female})$ [34]. The definition of chronic kidney disease is the presence of an eGFR less than 60 mL/min/1.73 m^2.

2.5. Statistical Analysis

Continuous variables are expressed as means ± standard deviations and categorical variables are displayed as numbers with their percentages. For examining the normality of numerical variables, the Kolmogorov–Smirnov method was performed. The independent two-tailed Student's t-test was used to compare the means of the continuous variables of normal distribution, while the Mann–Whitney U test was applied for continuous but not normally distributed data. For comparison between multiple groups, the Analysis of Variance (ANOVA) with post hoc analysis were used for quantitative variables. The Pearson's chi-square test was conducted for the comparison of categorical variables. The association between salivary conductivity and other quantitative variables was analyzed by univariate linear regression models. Furthermore, the multivariate linear regression analysis with backward selection was utilized to form a predictive model for salivary conductivity. Statistically significant factors identified in the univariate analysis were incorporated into the multivariate regression analysis. ROC curve analysis was used to evaluate the diagnostic accuracy of salivary conductivity on CKD. To improve the diagnostic ability, we performed the multivariable logistic regression analysis with backward selection using combined variables. The diagnostic power of different models was determined by calculating the area under the ROC curve (AUROC). Multivariate logistic regression with stepwise backward selection was utilized to estimate the odds ratios (ORs) of CKD, with salivary conductivity and other risk factors as independent variables. Subgroup analyses for heterogeneity in saliva conductivity effect were further performed, with subgroups defined according to age (<75 years or ≥75 years), gender, BMI (<25 kg/m^2 or ≥25 kg/m^2), history of diabetes (yes or no), underlying hypertension (yes or no), and coexisting dyslipidemia (yes or no). All statistical analyses were two-sided and were performed using the Statistical Program for Social Sciences (SPSS) version 22 (IBM Corporation, Armonk, NY, USA). Values of $p < 0.05$ were considered statistically significant.

3. Results

3.1. Reusability of the Sensor

After serial measurements of the salivary conductivity of the same saliva sample 20 times, the mean absolute percentage error (MAPE) is 0.88%, with a maximum error of 2.39% (Figure 3).

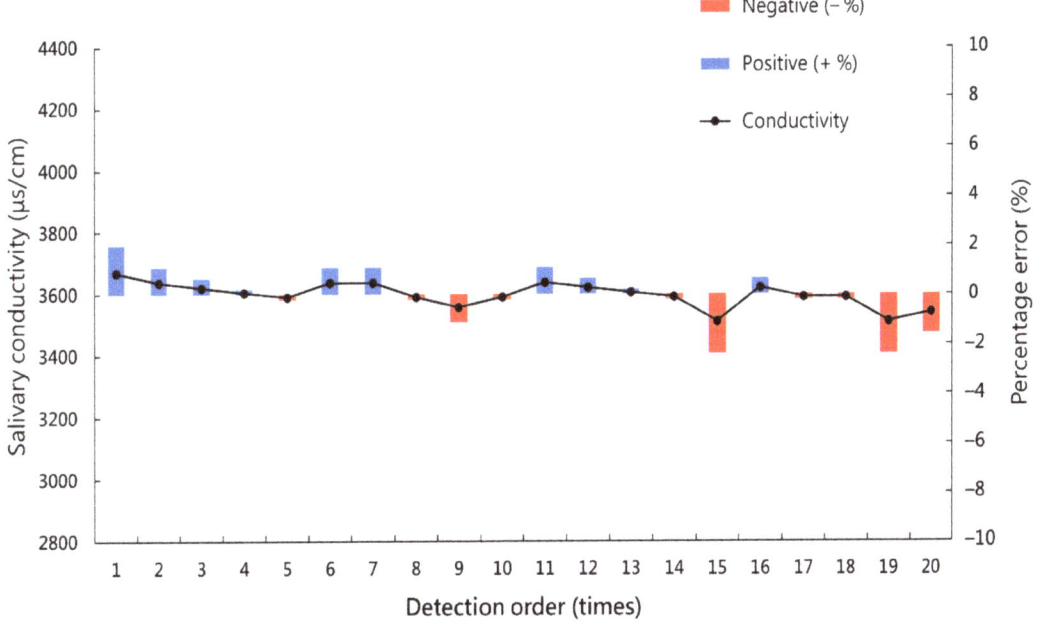

Figure 3. Serial measurements of the salivary conductivity of the same saliva sample 20 times.

3.2. Selectivity of the Sensor

For determining the selectivity of the sensor, we measured the conductivity of ultrapure water, BSA, PBS solution, different BSA concentrations mixed with PBS solution, and healthy participants' saliva. The results revealed that our co-planar microelectrodes have almost no interference from BSA and the majority of the conductivity was originated from the electrolytes in the solution (Figure 4A). By detection of ultrapure water spiked in with BSA, we noticed that the slope of the commercial electrode is three times significantly higher than our tailor-made design, which means our design is less vulnerable to BSA influence (Figure 4B). In addition, the conductivity of the saliva samples was stable for at least 15 min, which indicates that the proposed device has great resistance to interference particles accumulation (Figure 4C).

3.3. Demographic Characteristics of Study Participants

This cross-sectional study included 214 subjects with a mean age of 63.96 ± 13.53 years, of whom 33.2% were male. The mean salivary conductivity value was 5.91 ± 1.79 ms/cm. Diabetes mellitus, hypertension, chronic kidney disease, ischemic heart disease/stroke, dyslipidemia, gout, and chronic liver disease were recognized in 26 (12.1%), 62 (29.0%), 3 (1.4%), 16 (7.5%), 30 (14.0%), 9 (4.2%) and 24 (11.2%) participants, respectively. Their mean eGFR was equal to 86.33 ± 22.81 mL/min/1.73 m^2. Other biochemical parameters, anthropometric data, and blood pressure were shown in Table 1.

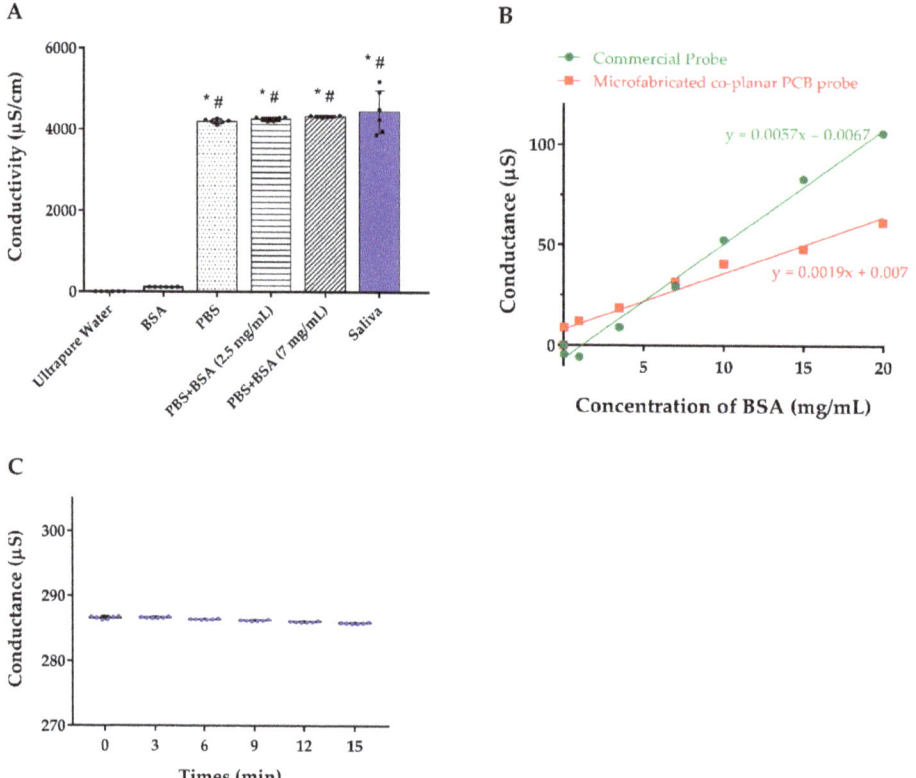

Figure 4. (**A**) Conductivity of the solution with different components. (**B**) Detection of the conductance of ultrapure water spiked in with BSA comparing our co-planar microelectrode and the commercial electrode. (**C**) Serial conductance measurements of the 6 individuals' saliva at different time points. Abbreviations: BSA, bovine serum albumin; PBS, phosphate-buffered saline. * indicates $p < 0.05$ compared to ultrapure water; # indicates $p < 0.05$ compared to the BSA.

Table 1. Characteristics of the study population and the correlation between salivary conductivity and continuous variables.

	All (N = 214)	Pearson r	p Value for r
Salivary conductivity, ms/cm	5.91 ± 1.79		
Demographics			
Age, years	63.96 ± 13.53	0.362	<0.01
Gender (male), n (%)	71 (33.2)		
Body weight, kg	63.08 ± 10.79	0.049	0.48
Body height, cm	158.97 ± 7.67	0.037	0.59
Body mass index, kg/m^2	24.90 ± 3.36	0.027	0.69
Systolic blood pressure, mmHg	131.26 ± 20.74	0.193	<0.01
Diastolic blood pressure, mmHg	75.24 ± 11.79	0.046	0.50

Table 1. Cont.

	All (N = 214)	Pearson r	p Value for r
Comorbid conditions, n (%) @			
Diabetes mellitus	26 (12.1)		
Hypertension	62 (29.0)		
Chronic kidney disease	3 (1.4)		
Ischemic heart disease/stroke	16 (7.5)		
Dyslipidemia	30 (14.0)		
Gout	9 (4.2)		
Chronic liver disease	24 (11.2)		
Laboratory parameters			
BUN, mg/dL	15.26 ± 5.28	0.178	<0.01
Creatinine, mg/dL	0.81 ± 0.26	0.251	<0.01
eGFR, mL/min/1.73 m^2	86.33 ± 22.81	−0.323	<0.01
Serum osmolality, mOsm/kgH$_2$O	287.69 ± 5.48	0.106	0.12
Fasting glucose, mg/dL	103.09 ± 25.31	0.153	0.03
Hemoglobin A1c, %	5.89 ± 0.98	0.045	0.51
ALT, U/L	22.10 ± 20.91	0.027	0.70
Triglyceride, mg/dL	113.19 ± 74.33	0.105	0.13
Total cholesterol, mg/dL	198.86 ± 39.48	−0.056	0.41
LDL-C, mg/dL	120.77 ± 33.63	−0.066	0.33
HDL-C, mg/dL	55.56 ± 13.22	−0111	0.11

Values are expressed as the mean ± standard deviation or number (percentage). @ The information of comorbid conditions was obtained by questionnaires. Abbreviations: ALT, alanine aminotransferase; BUN, blood urea nitrogen; eGFR, estimated glomerular filtration rate; HDL-C, high-density lipoprotein cholesterol; LDL-C, low-density lipoprotein cholesterol.

3.4. Association between Salivary Conductivity and Clinical Variables

The relationship between salivary conductivity and continuous variables was analyzed by Pearson's correlation coefficient. Salivary conductivity was positively associated with age, systolic blood pressure, blood urea nitrogen (BUN), creatinine, and fasting glucose, but was inversely related to the eGFR (Table 1).

We then conducted the backward multivariate linear regression analyses to determine the salivary conductivity level from clinical parameters. Only Significant factors identified in the simple regression analysis were applied to the multivariate analysis. A co-linearity analysis showed all tolerance > 0.1 and variance inflation factor (VIF) < 5, thus no co-linearity exists among independent variables (Table S1). Adjusted variables in regression model 1 consisted of age, systolic blood pressure, BUN, fasting glucose, and eGFR. Only older age (standardized β – 0.264, $p < 0.001$), higher fasting glucose (standardized β = 0.132, $p = 0.037$), and lower eGFR (standardized β = −0.186, p – 0.010) were significantly associated with higher salivary conductivity (R^2 = 0.176, model 1 in Table 2). Because eGFR is calculated from serum creatinine, we replaced eGFR with creatinine in regression model 2. It is noted that creatinine was still positively correlated with salivary conductivity (standardized β = 0.151, $p = 0.024$, model 2 in Table 2).

3.5. The Prevalence of Chronic Kidney Disease (CKD) Increases with Salivary Conductivity

To investigate the association of salivary conductivity and CKD, we divided study subjects into low, medium, and high salivary conductivity groups based on the tertial of conductivity levels (Figure 5). There was a significant trend for an increment of CKD prevalence rate from low to high salivary conductivity levels (4.2% in low vs. 12.5% in middle vs. 16.9% in high conductivity group, p for trend = 0.016).

Table 2. Multivariate linear regression analyses of determinants associated with the salivary conductivity.

Model 1	Unstandardized Coefficients β (Standard Error)	Standardized β	p Value
Constant	3.974 (1.062)		<0.001
Age	0.035 (0.010)	0.264	<0.001
Fasting glucose	0.009 (0.004)	0.132	0.037
eGFR	−0.015 (0.006)	−0.186	0.010
	$R^2 = 0.176$		
Model 2	**Unstandardized Coefficients β (Standard Error)**	**Standardized β**	**p Value**
Constant	1.452 (0.724)		0.046
Age	0.040 (0.009)	0.306	<0.001
Fasting glucose	0.010 (0.004)	0.141	0.026
Creatinine	1.043 (0.459)	0.151	0.024
	$R^2 = 0.170$		

Parameters included in model 1: age, systolic blood pressure, BUN, fasting glucose, and eGFR. Parameters included in model 2 are the same as in model 1, except that creatinine is used to replace eGFR. Abbreviations: BUN, blood urea nitrogen; eGFR, estimated glomerular filtration rate. The backward multivariate linear regression analysis method was conducted.

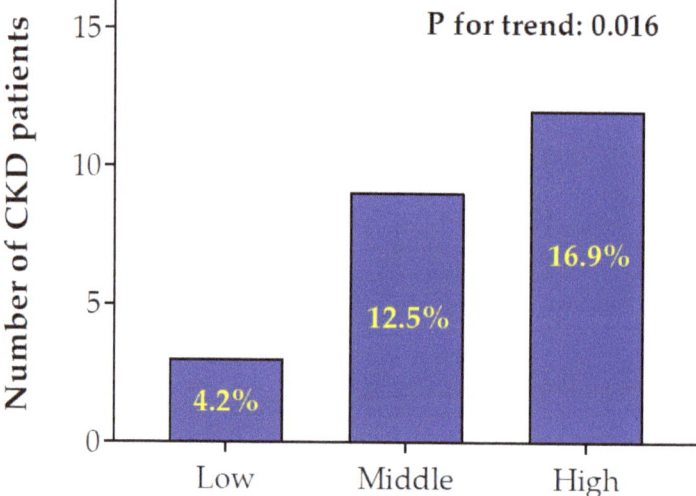

Figure 5. Bar chart of the number of CKD patients with low to high salivary conductivity levels. Participants were separated into low, middle, and high salivary conductivity levels based on the tertials of conductivity levels (low ≤ 4.84 ms/cm; 4.84 ms/cm < middle ≤ 6.60 ms/cm; high > 6.60 ms/cm). The number and percentage of patients with CKD were shown in the bar chart (p for trend: 0.016). CKD, chronic kidney disease.

3.6. The Use of Salivary Conductivity to Detect Individuals with CKD

To examine the diagnostic ability of salivary conductivity on CKD, the ROC curve analysis was conducted. The AUROC was equal to 0.648 (95% CI: 0.542–0.755) when salivary conductivity is the only predicting factor. To improve the diagnostic performance, age, gender, and body weight were further combined into the prediction model. This combination model demonstrated a significant increase in AUROC to 0.798 (95% CI: 0.726–0.871) (Figure 6A). Strikingly, the AUROC would be 0.751 (95% CI: 0.577–0.926) with salivary conductivity as the only predictor if the study group was restricted to individuals ≥75 years old (Figure 6B).

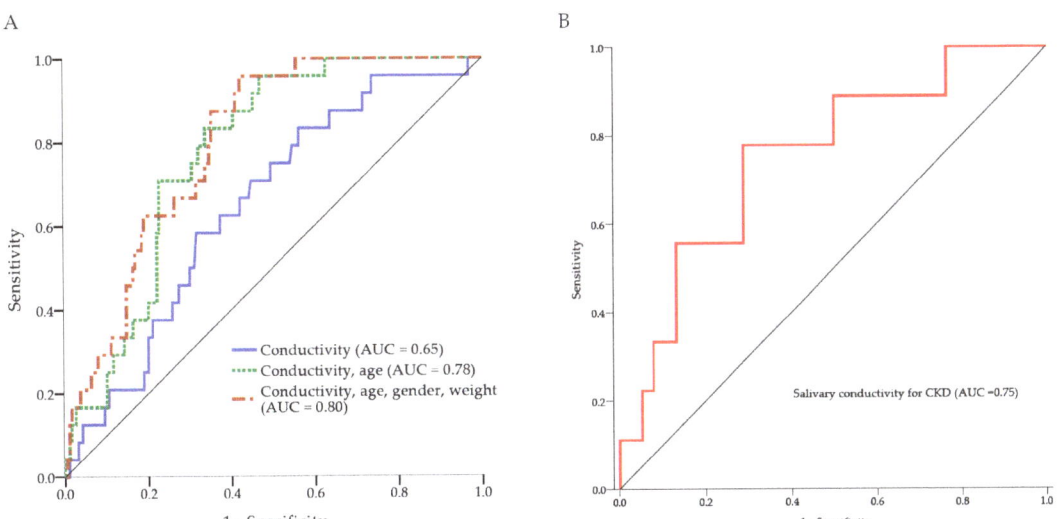

Figure 6. The receiver operating characteristic curve analysis. (**A**) Three ROC models for the diagnosis of CKD. The AUC was equal to 0.65 when salivary conductivity is the only predicting factor. The combination of salivary conductivity, age, gender, and body weight as the predicting factors showed the AUC was increased to 0.80. (**B**) The ROC curve analysis for the diagnostic accuracy of salivary conductivity on CKD among subjects older than 75 years. AUC, area under the ROC curve; CKD, chronic kidney disease; ROC, receiver operating characteristic.

3.7. Characteristics of Low Versus High Salivary Conductivity Population

To further evaluate the risk of CKD concerning salivary conductivity, the subjects were stratified into low and high salivary conductivity level groups based on the cutoff value of the ROC curve calculated by using only salivary conductivity as the predictor (6.59 ms/cm). The characteristics of low versus high salivary conductivity groups were summarized in Table 3. The mean salivary conductivity of the low and high salivary conductivity groups was 4.84 ± 1.01 and 7.94 ± 1.02 ms/cm, respectively. It was noticed that subjects with high salivary conductivity were older (69.92 ± 10.93 vs. 60.81 ± 13.75 years, $p < 0.01$). They also had higher systolic blood pressure (135.68 ± 21.91 vs. 128.93 ± 19.78 mmHg, $p = 0.02$), higher BUN (16.97 ± 5.78 vs. 14.34 ± 4.77 mg/dL, $p < 0.01$), higher creatinine (0.90 ± 0.30 vs. 0.76 ± 0.22 mg/dL, $p < 0.01$), lower eGFR (77.17 ± 21.27 vs. 91.18 ± 22.17 mL/min/1.73 m^2, $p < 0.01$), higher serum osmolality (288.69 ± 6.15 vs. 287.16 ± 5.04 mOsm/kgH$_2$O, $p = 0.05$), higher fasting glucose level (108.16 ± 20.34 vs. 100.41 ± 27.27 mg/dL, $p < 0.01$), higher hemoglobin A1c (5.97 ± 0.83 vs. $5.85 \pm 1.05\%$, $p = 0.03$), and a higher percentage of underlying diabetes mellitus (20.5 vs. 7.9%, $p < 0.01$). There were no significant differences in gender, body weight and height, body mass index, diastolic blood pressure, the prevalence of hypertension, chronic kidney disease, ischemic heart disease/stroke, dyslipidemia, gout, and chronic liver disease, ALT, triglyceride, total cholesterol, LDL-C, and HDL-C between groups.

Table 3. Population characteristics of low and high salivary conductivity groups.

	Low Salivary Conductivity Group * (N = 140)	High Salivary Conductivity Group (N = 74)	p Value
Salivary conductivity, ms/cm	4.84 ± 1.01	7.94 ± 1.02	<0.01 #
Demographics			
Age, years	60.81 ± 13.75	69.92 ± 10.93	<0.01 #
Gender (male), n (%)	42 (30.0)	29 (39.2)	0.17
Body weight, kg	62.94 ± 10.60	63.35 ± 11.21	0.94
Body height, cm	159.08 ± 7.39	158.76 ± 8.24	0.45
Body mass index, kg/m^2	24.82 ± 3.34	25.07 ± 3.40	0.61
Systolic blood pressure, mmHg	128.93 ± 19.78	135.68 ± 21.91	0.02 #
Diastolic blood pressure, mmHg	74.76 ± 11.60	76.14 ± 12.16	0.42
Comorbid conditions, n (%) @			
Diabetes mellitus	11 (7.9)	15 (20.5)	<0.01 #
Hypertension	36 (25.7)	26 (35.6)	0.13
Chronic kidney disease	1 (0.7)	2 (2.7)	0.27
Ischemic heart disease/Stroke	7 (5.0)	9 (12.3)	0.05
Dyslipidemia	20 (14.3)	10 (13.7)	0.91
Gout	4 (2.9)	5 (6.8)	0.17
Chronic liver disease	16 (11.4)	8 (11.0)	0.92
Laboratory parameters			
BUN, mg/dL	14.34 ± 4.77	16.97 ± 5.78	<0.01 #
Creatinine, mg/dL	0.76 ± 0.22	0.90 ± 0.30	<0.01 #
eGFR, mL/min/1.73 m^2	91.18 ± 22.17	77.17 ± 21.27	<0.01 #
Serum osmolality, mOsm/kgH$_2$O	287.16 ± 5.04	288.69 ± 6.15	0.05 #
Fasting glucose, mg/dL	100.41 ± 27.27	108.16 ± 20.34	<0.01 #
Hemoglobin A1c, %	5.85 ± 1.05	5.97 ± 0.83	0.03 #
ALT, U/L	22.89 ± 24.87	20.62 ± 9.74	0.69
Triglyceride, mg/dL	107.50 ± 62.19	123.95 ± 92.62	0.10
Total cholesterol, mg/dL	198.18 ± 36.15	200.15 ± 45.37	0.73
LDL-C, mg/dL	120.09 ± 30.79	122.05 ± 38.65	0.69
HDL-C, mg/dL	56.46 ± 12.81	53.84 ± 13.89	0.17

Values are expressed as mean ± standard deviation or number (percentage). * Study populations were stratified into low and high groups according to the cutoff value of salivary conductivity (6.59 ms/m). @ The information of comorbid conditions was obtained by questionnaires. # indicates p-value < 0.05. Abbreviations: ALT, alanine aminotransferase; BUN, blood urea nitrogen; eGFR, estimated glomerular filtration rate; HDL-C, high-density lipoprotein cholesterol; LDL-C, low-density lipoprotein cholesterol.

3.8. Subgroup Analysis of the Risk of CKD, Comparing High versus Low Salivary Conductivity

The subgroup analysis of the risk of CKD, comparing high versus low salivary conductivity was shown in Figure 7. Overall, the risk of CKD was higher in the high salivary conductivity group, with an adjusted odds ratio of 2.66 (95% CI, 1.10–6.46). There was no significant difference in the risk for CKD among subgroups of age and BMI. In the male population, and those without DM, without hypertension, and without dyslipidemia, the risk of CKD was significantly higher in the high salivary conductivity group, with the odds ratio of 4.60 (95% CI, 1.01–21.04), 2.99 (95% CI, 1.15–7.73), 3.71 (95% CI, 1.11–12.37), and 3.29 (95% CI, 1.27–8.55), respectively. To avoid bias introduced by unequal distribution of confounding variables, we further conducted sensitivity analyses in subjects without histories of diabetes and hypertension (Tables S2-1 and S2-2 in Supplemental Materials) and used a propensity score-matched dataset. The results were in concordance with the original analysis (Tables S3-1 and S3-2 in Supplemental Materials).

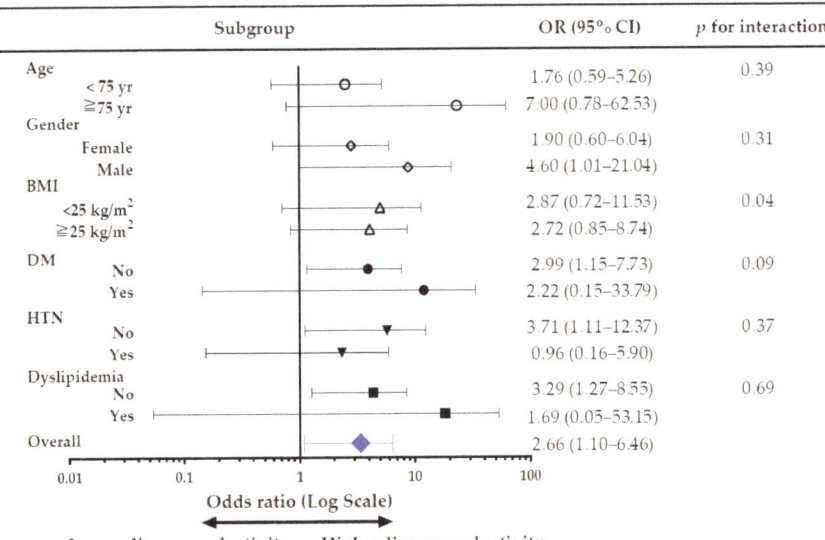

Figure 7. Forest plot for subgroup analysis of CKD risk. The adjusted odds ratio (OR) is for the high versus low salivary conductivity group. Study subjects were divided into high and low salivary conductivity groups based on the cutoff value of the ROC curve analysis (6.59 ms/cm). BMI, body mass index; CKD, chronic kidney disease; DM, diabetes mellitus; HTN, hypertension.

4. Discussion

The results reported here reveal that salivary conductivity is negatively correlated with eGFR and can serve as a potential biomarker for detecting CKD. Traditionally, the golden standard of measuring kidney function requires the collection of 24 h urine creatinine amount and the blood test of serum creatinine, which is cumbersome for patients [11,35]. Simplified estimation of renal function by MDRD equation still needs an invasive venipuncture. As mentioned in the Results section, there was a notably negative correlation between salivary conductivity and eGFR in the simple and multivariate Pearson's correlation analyses (Tables 1 and 2). In addition, there was an increasing trend of CKD prevalence from low to high salivary conductivity levels (Figure 5). Hence, the salivary conductivity may be an alternative surrogate marker for kidney function.

The prevalence rate of CKD, defined as eGFR < 60 mL/min/1.73 m^2 by the revised MDRD equation, is 11.2% in our study. A large-scale cohort study based on 462,293 adults in Taiwan showed that the national prevalence of CKD was 11.93% [3]. This indicates the representativeness of our research subjects. In addition, only three participants in our study answered that they had CKD by the questionnaire. It revealed that the awareness of CKD in our study population was very low (12.5%). In line with this observation, previous research has also pointed out the serious problem of unawareness in the management of CKD, especially in patients with early-stage CKD [3,10,36]. Since saliva collection is an easier and non-invasive method, this makes large-scale screening or continuous self-monitoring of CKD less difficult.

Furthermore, multivariate linear regression analyses also showed a significantly positive correlation between salivary conductivity with age or fasting glucose (Table 2). Subjects with high salivary conductivity were prone to be older and had higher fasting sugar, higher hemoglobin A1c, and a higher percentage of diabetic history (Table 3). Several studies have found that the secretion and properties of saliva change with age [37,38]. Similar to CKD patients, most electrolytes increase in the saliva of healthy elderly individuals [23,37], which may contribute to the increase in salivary conductivity. Recent studies have also shown a strong association between salivary conductivity and age [30,39]. Further, salivary glucose concentrations were proved to be related to serum glucose levels [40,41]. Since CKD patients are mostly the elderly and prone to develop hyperglycemia [42], this may partly explain why they have higher salivary conductivity. Besides, we also noticed a significant correlation between systolic blood pressure and salivary conductivity. Subjects in the high salivary conductivity group were shown to have higher systolic blood pressure. A recent report by Labat et al. has shown that salivary electrolytes increased with age and were associated with hypertension [39], which was compatible with our findings.

The ROC curve of our study implied that using salivary conductivity combined with age, gender, and body weight can yield an excellent prediction model with AUC equal to 0.8 [43]. The traditional concept of the elderly is defined as an age of 65 years or older. However, many of the elderly, especially those aged younger than 75 years, are still healthy and active due to the progress of modern medicine and nutritional support. Ouchi et al. had redefined aged from 65 to 74 years as pre-elderly and aged over 75 years as the new definition of elderly [44]. In addition, aging is a significant risk factor for developing CKD. Mallappallil et al. had demonstrated that the patients aged from 75 to 79 years had a 40% higher risk of having CKD than those aged from 65 to 74 years. [45]. Therefore, we further performed ROC curve and logistic regression analyses among patients greater than 75 years. Although using only salivary conductivity to predict CKD was not good enough with AUC only equal to 0.65, we found the model could perform well in the subgroup of individuals older than 75 years with AUC equal to 0.75 (Figure 6). This finding is consistent with the result in Figure 7 that older patients with higher salivary conductivity had a higher odds ratio to have CKD. A previous finding that salivary electrolytes concentration increases with age [39] provides support for these results. The morphology and function of nephrons are affected by the aging process, which causes the elderly vulnerable to acute or chronic kidney damages [46]. The prevalence of CKD is markedly higher in elder populations [47,48]. The property of better diagnostic performance in the high-risk elderly makes salivary conductivity a promising tool for CKD screening.

Figure 7 shows a strong association of salivary conductivity with the risk of CKD. Although there was a tendency for higher blood pressure and higher fasting blood glucose in subjects with high salivary conductivity (Tables 1 and 3), the subgroup analyses demonstrated that salivary conductivity distinguished CKD better among subjects without diabetes, hypertension, and dyslipidemia (Figure 7). One possible explanation for this discrepancy was that subjects with these comorbidities were little in number, 26, 72, and 30 respectively, which created a wider confidence interval. Despite that higher salivary conductivity in the patients older than 75 years did not have a significantly higher risk of CKD, there was a trend of increasing risk for CKD compared to those younger than 75 years old. However, the phenomenon of better discrimination of CKD in healthier subjects may represent salivary conductivity as a good diagnostic tool. Further analysis with a larger population is warranted to clarify these findings. In addition, patients with CKD usually had many comorbidities such as diabetes and hypertension. Salivary conductivity may merely reflect the comorbidities but not kidney function. However, we can find that those patients with higher salivary conductivity but without diabetes or hypertension still had a higher risk of having CKD. This finding can again suggest our conclusion that salivary conductivity has a positive correlation with CKD.

There are several limitations needed to be mentioned in this research. First, this is a cross-sectional study; therefore, the true relationship between salivary conductivity and eGFR or CKD could not be confirmed by a single test. Second, CKD in our study was defined by a single eGFR measurement, which may erroneously include subjects with acute kidney injury. Third, CKD was defined as an eGFR < 60 mL/min/1.73 m^2, thus individuals of higher eGFR but with kidney damage were not diagnosed. This would underestimate the occurrence or risk of CKD. In addition, current criteria for diagnosing CKD need eGFR and albuminuria or proteinuria data. A lack of urinalysis, proteinuria, or albuminuria data in study participants may underestimate the prevalence of CKD. However, the percentage of CKD is 11.2% in our study, which was comparable with the reported 12% national prevalence of CKD in Taiwan, reported by Wen et al. [3]. This suggests that our research subjects are still representative. Fourth, this study was performed only in the Asian population, thus the results may not be correctly applied to other ethnicities. Besides, serum electrolytes status was not measured during the health examination. Since salivary electrolyte concentrations may vary with serum, the lack of serum electrolyte data may affect the assessment of salivary conductivity. Finally, we did not analyze the components of saliva in CKD versus non-CKD subjects. Therefore, we could not fully explain the nature of why salivary conductivity increases in CKD subjects.

5. Conclusions

Timely screening and detection for undiagnosed CKD are decisive for delaying the disease progression and reducing its complications or mortality. The results of this study demonstrate a significant correlation between salivary conductivity and eGFR. Higher salivary conductivity is associated with an increased risk of CKD. We have also shown an acceptable diagnostic accuracy and sensitivity of salivary conductivity in distinguishing CKD, especially for the elderly. Taken together, salivary conductivity can serve as a good surrogate marker of renal function; this real-time, non-invasive, and easy-to-use portable biosensing device may be a reliable tool for screening early-stage CKD.

Supplementary Materials: The following supporting information can be downloaded at: https://www.mdpi.com/article/10.3390/bios12030178/s1, Figure S1: Conductance measurement of human saliva samples at different times; Table S1: Co-linearity analysis of covariates put into the multivariate linear regression model; Table S2-1: Characteristics of study populations without histories of diabetes and hypertension; Table S2-2: Logistic regression analyses for the risk of chronic kidney disease in study populations without histories of diabetes and hypertension; Table S3-1: Population characteristics in the propensity-score matched dataset; Table S3-2: Logistic regression analyses for the risk of chronic kidney disease in the propensity-score matched dataset.

Author Contributions: Conceptualization, C.-W.L., J.-T.Y. and C.-W.T.; methodology, C.-W.L., J.-T.Y., Y.-P.L., R.-C.W. and C.-W.T.; software, C.-W.L., Y.-P.L. and C.-W.T.; validation, C.-W.L., J.-T.Y. and C.-W.T.; formal analysis, C.-W.L., Y.-P.L. and C.-W.T.; investigation, C.-W.L. and J.-T.Y.; resources, Y.-H.T., J.-T.Y., M.-Y.C. and T.-J.H.; data curation, C.-W.L. and J.-T.Y.; writing—original draft preparation, C.-W.L.; writing—review and editing, R.-C.W. and C.-W.T.; visualization, C.-W.T.; supervision, Y.-H.T. and J.-T.Y.; project administration, J.-T.Y.; funding acquisition, J.-T.Y., M.-Y.C. and T.-J.H. All authors have read and agreed to the published version of the manuscript.

Funding: This research was supported by grants from the Chang Gung Medical Research Project to Yuan-Hsiung Tsai and Jen-Tsung Yang (CORPG6G0183, CORPG6G0211, CORPG6G0212, CORPG6G0213, and CORPG6G0233), and from the Taiwan Formosa Plastic group (FCRPF6L0011).

Institutional Review Board Statement: The study was conducted following the ethical principles of the Declaration of Helsinki, and it was approved by the Ethics Committee of Chang Gung Memorial Hospital (institutional review board number: 202000109B0 and 202002186B0).

Informed Consent Statement: Written informed consent was obtained from all subjects involved in the study.

Data Availability Statement: The data presented in this study are available on request from the corresponding author. The data are not publicly available due to privacy.

Conflicts of Interest: The authors declare no conflict of interest. The funders had no role in the design of the study; in the collection, analyses, or interpretation of data; in the writing of the manuscript, or in the decision to publish the results.

References

1. Cockwell, P.; Fisher, L.-A. The global burden of chronic kidney disease. *Lancet* **2020**, *395*, 662–664. [CrossRef]
2. Coresh, J.; Selvin, E.; Stevens, L.A.; Manzi, J.; Kusek, J.W.; Eggers, P.; Van Lente, F.; Levey, A.S. Prevalence of chronic kidney disease in the United States. *JAMA* **2007**, *298*, 2038–2047. [CrossRef] [PubMed]

3. Wen, C.P.; Cheng, T.Y.D.; Tsai, M.K.; Chang, Y.C.; Chan, H.T.; Tsai, S.P.; Chiang, P.H.; Hsu, C.C.; Sung, P.K.; Hsu, Y.H. All-cause mortality attributable to chronic kidney disease: A prospective cohort study based on 462,293 adults in Taiwan. *Lancet* **2008**, *371*, 2173–2182. [CrossRef]
4. Chen, T.K.; Knicely, D.H.; Grams, M.E. Chronic Kidney Disease Diagnosis and Management: A Review. *JAMA* **2019**, *322*, 1294–1304. [CrossRef] [PubMed]
5. Gansevoort, R.T.; Correa-Rotter, R.; Hemmelgarn, B.R.; Jafar, T.H.; Heerspink, H.J.; Mann, J.F.; Matsushita, K.; Wen, C.P. Chronic kidney disease and cardiovascular risk: Epidemiology, mechanisms, and prevention. *Lancet* **2013**, *382*, 339–352. [CrossRef]
6. Go, A.S.; Chertow, G.M.; Fan, D.; McCulloch, C.E.; Hsu, C.Y. Chronic kidney disease and the risks of death, cardiovascular events, and hospitalization. *N. Engl. J. Med.* **2004**, *351*, 1296–1305. [CrossRef] [PubMed]
7. Perlman, R.L.; Finkelstein, F.O.; Liu, L.; Roys, E.; Kiser, M.; Eisele, G.; Burrows-Hudson, S.; Messana, J.M.; Levin, N.; Rajagopalan, S.; et al. Quality of life in chronic kidney disease (CKD): A cross-sectional analysis in the Renal Research Institute-CKD study. *Am. J. Kidney Dis.* **2005**, *45*, 658–666. [CrossRef] [PubMed]
8. Foreman, K.J.; Marquez, N.; Dolgert, A.; Fukutaki, K.; Fullman, N.; McGaughey, M.; Pletcher, M.A.; Smith, A.E.; Tang, K.; Yuan, C.W.; et al. Forecasting life expectancy, years of life lost, and all-cause and cause-specific mortality for 250 causes of death: Reference and alternative scenarios for 2016-40 for 195 countries and territories. *Lancet* **2018**, *392*, 2052–2090. [CrossRef]
9. Darlington, O.; Dickerson, C.; Evans, M.; McEwan, P.; Sörstadius, E.; Sugrue, D.; van Haalen, H.; Sanchez, J.J.G. Costs and healthcare resource use associated with risk of cardiovascular morbidity in patients with chronic kidney Disease: Evidence from a systematic literature review. *Adv. Ther.* **2021**, *38*, 994–1010. [CrossRef]
10. Plantinga, L.C.; Boulware, L.E.; Coresh, J.; Stevens, L.A.; Miller, E.R., 3rd; Saran, R.; Messer, K.L.; Levey, A.S.; Powe, N.R. Patient awareness of chronic kidney disease: Trends and predictors. *Arch. Intern. Med.* **2008**, *168*, 2268–2275. [CrossRef]
11. Levin, A.; Stevens, P.E.; Bilous, R.W.; Coresh, J.; De Francisco, A.L.; De Jong, P.E.; Griffith, K.E.; Hemmelgarn, B.R.; Iseki, K.; Lamb, E.J. Kidney Disease: Improving Global Outcomes (KDIGO) CKD Work Group. KDIGO 2012 clinical practice guideline for the evaluation and management of chronic kidney disease. *Kidney Int. Suppl.* **2013**, *3*, 1–150.
12. Kilbride, H.S.; Stevens, P.E.; Eaglestone, G.; Knight, S.; Carter, J.L.; Delaney, M.P.; Farmer, C.K.; Irving, J.; O'Riordan, S.E.; Dalton, R.N.; et al. Accuracy of the MDRD (Modification of Diet in Renal Disease) study and CKD-EPI (CKD Epidemiology Collaboration) equations for estimation of GFR in the elderly. *Am. J. Kidney Dis.* **2013**, *61*, 57–66. [CrossRef] [PubMed]
13. Berns, J.S. Routine screening for CKD should be done in asymptomatic adults . . . selectively. *Clin. J. Am. Soc. Nephrol.* **2014**, *9*, 1988–1992. [CrossRef] [PubMed]
14. Celec, P.; Tothova, L.; Sebekova, K.; Podracka, L.; Boor, P. Salivary markers of kidney function—Potentials and limitations. *Clin. Chim. Acta* **2016**, *453*, 28–37. [CrossRef] [PubMed]
15. Czumbel, L.M.; Kiss, S.; Farkas, N.; Mandel, I.; Hegyi, A.; Nagy, Á.; Lohinai, Z.; Szakács, Z.; Hegyi, P.; Steward, M.C. Saliva as a candidate for COVID-19 diagnostic testing: A meta-analysis. *Front. Med.* **2020**, *7*, 465. [CrossRef]
16. Gleerup, H.S.; Hasselbalch, S.G.; Simonsen, A.H. Biomarkers for Alzheimer's disease in saliva: A systematic review. *Dis. Markers* **2019**, *2019*, 4761054. [CrossRef] [PubMed]
17. Hegde, M.N.; Attavar, S.H.; Shetty, N.; Hegde, N.D.; Hegde, N.N. Saliva as a biomarker for dental caries: A systematic review. *J. Conserv. Dent.* **2019**, *22*, 2.
18. Wang, J.; Zhao, Y.; Ren, J.; Xu, Y. Pepsin in saliva as a diagnostic biomarker in laryngopharyngeal reflux: A meta-analysis. *Eur. Arch. Oto-Rhino-Laryngol.* **2018**, *275*, 671–678. [CrossRef]
19. Chojnowska, S.; Baran, T.; Wilinska, I.; Sienicka, P.; Cabaj-Wiater, I.; Knas, M. Human saliva as a diagnostic material. *Adv. Med. Sci.* **2018**, *63*, 185–191. [CrossRef]
20. Matczuk, J.; Zalewska, A.; Lukaszuk, B.; Knas, M.; Maciejczyk, M.; Garbowska, M.; Ziembicka, D.M.; Waszkiel, D.; Chabowski, A.; Zendzian-Piotrowska, M.; et al. Insulin Resistance and Obesity Affect Lipid Profile in the Salivary Glands. *J. Diabetes Res.* **2016**, *2016*, 8163474. [CrossRef]
21. Kulak-Bejda, A.; Waszkiewicz, N.; Bejda, G.; Zalewska, A.; Maciejczyk, M. Diagnostic Value of Salivary Markers in Neuropsychiatric Disorders. *Dis. Markers* **2019**, *2019*, 4360612. [CrossRef] [PubMed]
22. Maciejczyk, M.; Bielas, M.; Zalewska, A.; Gerreth, K. Salivary Biomarkers of Oxidative Stress and Inflammation in Stroke Patients: From Basic Research to Clinical Practice. *Oxid. Med. Cell. Longev.* **2021**, *2021*, 5545330. [CrossRef]
23. Tomas, I.; Marinho, J.S.; Limeres, J.; Santos, M.J.; Araujo, L.; Diz, P. Changes in salivary composition in patients with renal failure. *Arch. Oral Biol.* **2008**, *53*, 528–532. [CrossRef] [PubMed]
24. Evans, R.D.R.; Hemmila, U.; Mzinganjira, H.; Mtekateka, M.; Banda, E.; Sibale, N.; Kawale, Z.; Phiri, C.; Dreyer, G.; Calice-Silva, V.; et al. Diagnostic performance of a point-of-care saliva urea nitrogen dipstick to screen for kidney disease in low-resource settings where serum creatinine is unavailable. *BMJ Glob. Health* **2020**, *5*, e002312. [CrossRef] [PubMed]
25. Korytowska, N.; Sankowski, B.; Wyczalkowska-Tomasik, A.; Paczek, L.; Wroczynski, P.; Giebultowicz, J. The utility of saliva testing in the estimation of uremic toxin levels in serum. *Clin. Chem. Lab. Med.* **2018**, *57*, 230–237. [CrossRef] [PubMed]
26. Rodrigues, R.; de Andrade Vieira, W.; Siqueira, W.L.; Blumenberg, C.; de Macedo Bernardino, I.; Cardoso, S.V.; Flores-Mir, C.; Paranhos, L.R. Saliva as an alternative to blood in the determination of uremic state in adult patients with chronic kidney disease: A systematic review and meta-analysis. *Clin. Oral Investig.* **2020**, *24*, 2203–2217. [CrossRef] [PubMed]
27. Rodrigues, R.; Vieira, W.A.; Siqueira, W.L.; Agostini, B.A.; Moffa, E.B.; Paranhos, L.R. Saliva as a tool for monitoring hemodialysis: A systematic review and meta-analysis. *Braz. Oral Res.* **2020**, *35*, e016. [CrossRef] [PubMed]

28. Lu, Y.P.; Huang, J.W.; Lee, I.N.; Weng, R.C.; Lin, M.Y.; Yang, J.T.; Lin, C.T. A Portable System to Monitor Saliva Conductivity for Dehydration Diagnosis and Kidney Healthcare. *Sci. Rep.* **2019**, *9*, 14771. [CrossRef]
29. Chen, C.H.; Lu, Y.P.; Lee, A.T.; Tung, C.W.; Tsai, Y.H.; Tsay, H.P.; Lin, C.T.; Yang, J.T. A Portable Biodevice to Monitor Salivary Conductivity for the Rapid Assessment of Fluid Status. *J. Pers. Med.* **2021**, *11*, 577. [CrossRef]
30. Lee, A.-T.; Lu, Y.-P.; Chen, C.-H.; Chang, C.-H.; Tsai, Y.-H.; Tung, C.-W.; Yang, J.-T. The Association of Salivary Conductivity with Cardiomegaly in Hemodialysis Patients. *Appl. Sci.* **2021**, *11*, 7405. [CrossRef]
31. Iorgulescu, G. Saliva between normal and pathological. Important factors in determining systemic and oral health. *J. Med. Life* **2009**, *2*, 303. [PubMed]
32. Kuo, Y.-C.; Lee, C.-K.; Lin, C.-T. Improving sensitivity of a miniaturized label-free electrochemical biosensor using zigzag electrodes. *Biosens. Bioelectron.* **2018**, *103*, 130–137. [CrossRef] [PubMed]
33. Lin, L.; Chang, C. Determination of protein concentration in human saliva. *Kaohsiung J. Med. Sci.* **1989**, *5*, 389–397.
34. Levey, A.S.; Coresh, J.; Greene, T.; Stevens, L.A.; Zhang, Y.L.; Hendriksen, S.; Kusek, J.W.; Van Lente, F.; Chronic Kidney Disease Epidemiology Collaboration. Using standardized serum creatinine values in the modification of diet in renal disease study equation for estimating glomerular filtration rate. *Ann. Intern. Med.* **2006**, *145*, 247–254. [CrossRef] [PubMed]
35. Manns, B.; Hemmelgarn, B.; Tonelli, M.; Au, F.; So, H.; Weaver, R.; Quinn, A.E.; Klarenbach, S.; Canadians Seeking Solutions and Innovations to Overcome Chronic Kidney Disease. The Cost of Care for People With Chronic Kidney Disease. *Can. J. Kidney Health Dis.* **2019**, *6*, 2054358119835521. [CrossRef]
36. Chu, C.D.; McCulloch, C.E.; Banerjee, T.; Pavkov, M.E.; Burrows, N.R.; Gillespie, B.W.; Saran, R.; Shlipak, M.G.; Powe, N.R.; Tuot, D.S. CKD awareness among US adults by future risk of kidney failure. *Am. J. Kidney Dis.* **2020**, *76*, 174–183. [CrossRef]
37. Xu, F.; Laguna, L.; Sarkar, A. Aging-related changes in quantity and quality of saliva: Where do we stand in our understanding? *J. Texture Stud.* **2019**, *50*, 27–35. [CrossRef]
38. Ashton, N.J.; Ide, M.; Zetterberg, H.; Blennow, K. Salivary Biomarkers for Alzheimer's Disease and Related Disorders. *Neurol. Ther.* **2019**, *8*, 83–94. [CrossRef]
39. Labat, C.; Thul, S.; Pirault, J.; Temmar, M.; Thornton, S.N.; Benetos, A.; Back, M. Differential Associations for Salivary Sodium, Potassium, Calcium, and Phosphate Levels with Carotid Intima Media Thickness, Heart Rate, and Arterial Stiffness. *Dis. Markers* **2018**, *2018*, 3152146. [CrossRef]
40. Bilancio, G.; Cavallo, P.; Lombardi, C.; Guarino, E.; Cozza, V.; Giordano, F.; Palladino, G.; Cirillo, M. Saliva for assessing creatinine, uric acid, and potassium in nephropathic patients. *BMC Nephrol.* **2019**, *20*, 242. [CrossRef]
41. Jung, D.G.; Jung, D.; Kong, S.H. A Lab-on-a-Chip-Based Non-Invasive Optical Sensor for Measuring Glucose in Saliva. *Sensors* **2017**, *17*, 2607. [CrossRef] [PubMed]
42. Buse, J.B.; Wexler, D.J.; Tsapas, A.; Rossing, P.; Mingrone, G.; Mathieu, C.; D'Alessio, D.A.; Davies, M.J. 2019 Update to: Management of Hyperglycemia in Type 2 Diabetes, 2018. A Consensus Report by the American Diabetes Association (ADA) and the European Association for the Study of Diabetes (EASD). *Diabetes Care* **2020**, *43*, 487–493. [CrossRef] [PubMed]
43. Mandrekar, J.N. Receiver operating characteristic curve in diagnostic test assessment. *J. Thorac. Oncol.* **2010**, *5*, 1315–1316. [CrossRef] [PubMed]
44. Ouchi, Y.; Rakugi, H.; Arai, H.; Akishita, M.; Ito, H.; Toba, K.; Kai, I.; Joint Committee of Japan Gerontological Society (JGLS) and Japan Geriatrics Society (JGS) on the Definition and Classification of the Elderly. Redefining the elderly as aged 75 years and older: Proposal from the Joint Committee of Japan Gerontological Society and the Japan Geriatrics Society. *Geriatr. Gerontol. Int.* **2017**, *17*, 1045–1047. [CrossRef] [PubMed]
45. Mallappallil, M.; Friedman, E.A.; Delano, B.G.; McFarlane, S.I.; Salifu, M.O. Chronic kidney disease in the elderly: Evaluation and management. *Clin. Pract.* **2014**, *11*, 525–535. [CrossRef]
46. Nitta, K.; Okada, K.; Yanai, M.; Takahashi, S. Aging and chronic kidney disease. *Kidney Blood Press. Res.* **2013**, *38*, 109–120. [CrossRef]
47. Anderson, S.; Halter, J.B.; Hazzard, W.R.; Himmelfarb, J.; Horne, F.M.; Kaysen, G.A.; Kusek, J.W.; Nayfield, S.G.; Schmader, K.; Tian, Y.; et al. Prediction, progression, and outcomes of chronic kidney disease in older adults. *J. Am. Soc. Nephrol.* **2009**, *20*, 1199–1209. [CrossRef]
48. Prakash, S.; O'Hare, A.M. Interaction of aging and chronic kidney disease. *Semin. Nephrol.* **2009**, *29*, 497–503. [CrossRef]

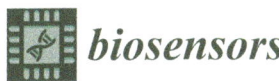

Review

Medical Devices for Tremor Suppression: Current Status and Future Directions

Jiancheng Mo and Ronny Priefer *

Massachusetts College of Pharmacy and Health Sciences University, School of Pharmacy, Boston, MA 02115, USA; jmo1@stu.mcphs.edu
* Correspondence: ronny.priefer@mcphs.edu

Abstract: Tremors are the most prevalent movement disorder that interferes with the patient's daily living, and physical activities, ultimately leading to a reduced quality of life. Due to the pathophysiology of tremor, developing effective pharmacotherapies, which are only suboptimal in the management of tremor, has many challenges. Thus, a range of therapies are necessary in managing this progressive, aging-associated disorder. Surgical interventions such as deep brain stimulation are able to provide durable tremor control. However, due to high costs, patient and practitioner preference, and perceived high risks, their utilization is minimized. Medical devices are placed in a unique position to bridge this gap between lifestyle interventions, pharmacotherapies, and surgical treatments to provide safe and effective tremor suppression. Herein, we review the mechanisms of action, safety and efficacy profiles, and clinical applications of different medical devices that are currently available or have been previously investigated for tremor suppression. These devices are primarily noninvasive, which can be a beneficial addition to the patient's existing pharmacotherapy and/or lifestyle intervention.

Keywords: tremor; medical devices; transcutaneous electrical nerve stimulation; electrical stimulation systems; wearable orthoses; assistive feeding devices

1. Introduction

Tremors, as defined by the task force of the International Parkinson and Movement Disorder Society (IPMDS), are an involuntary, rhythmic, oscillatory movement of a body part [1]. Essential tremor (ET) is recognized as the most prevalent pathological tremor among adults, affecting about 0.9% of the global population [2]. However, the true prevalence of ET may be higher, as it is believed that these patients may not seek medical attention [3]. Tremors, usually asymmetrically distributed, are frequently seen in patients with Parkinson's disease (PD), which affects more than six million individuals worldwide [4]. The presence of resting tremor supports the diagnosis of PD [5]. Different clinical subtypes and classifications of tremor disorders have also been identified [1]. The etiologies of tremor include other neurodegenerative diseases such as Wilson's disease, chromosomal aneuploidy, mitochondrial genetic disorders, infectious and inflammatory diseases, endocrine and metabolic disorders, neuropathies and spinal muscular atrophies, toxin-/drug-induced tremor pathology, and brain neoplasms and injury, as well as several environmental causes [1].

Tremors impact many aspects of the patient's daily living and interfere with many physical activities at home and in the workplace [6–10]. One clinical-epidemiological study compared the quality of life, including physical and psychosocial aspects, between patients with ET and PD using the Quality of Life in Essential Tremor (QUEST) questionnaire [11]. Patients with ET had a higher QUEST total score and QUEST physical subscore than patients with PD ($p < 0.05$). This suggests that patients with ET suffers significantly more physical and psychosocial impairment than those with PD [11]. Additionally, among patients suffering from tremor, their psychological strain may be significantly more affected than their physical disabilities [6,12]. The psychological toll of tremor may extend beyond the patients themselves. The Clinical Pathological Study of Cognitive Impairment in Essential Tremor (COGNET), a longitudinal study that evaluates cognitive function in older adults with ET, reported that both patients with ET and those close to them suffer psychological stress [13]. In addition, patients may develop feelings of social isolation [11,14] and depression [6,11,13]. Due to the incredible burden put on individuals diagnosed with ET or PD, a multitude of approaches have been investigated to improve the symptoms and quality of life of those afflicted. These range from lifestyle interventions, pharmacotherapy, and surgical treatments.

Lifestyle interventions focusing on the use of weighted utensils can reduce the amplitude of tremor and alleviate the challenges patients face in their activities of daily living (ADLs) [15,16]. With additional weights, these utensils (e.g., spoon) can assist patients to eat and drink. In 2017, the National Institute for Health and Care Excellence (NICE) produced guidelines for the management of PD in adults [5]. Patients in the early stages of PD may benefit from physio- and occupational therapy if they experience motor symptoms or have difficulties with ADLs [5]. However, lifestyle and the nonpharmacological management of ET were not discussed in the guidelines produced by the American Academy of Neurology (AAN) and the IPMDS [17–19]. A systematic review of 19 studies found that physical therapy, limb cooling, vibration therapy, use of limb weights, bright light therapy, and transcranial magnetic stimulation were all examples of investigated treatments of tremor [20]. However, these studies mainly included convenience samples, and the long-term effectiveness of these interventions was not assessed [20].

Pharmacotherapy for the treatment of ET is suboptimal and only treats the symptoms. Many patients do not respond to the existing medications indicated for ET and do not experience a significant improvement in their daily living. Currently, propranolol and primidone are the two first-line therapies [15–19,21]. Across randomized controlled trials (RCTs), propranolol and primidone monotherapy produce a mean reduction in the tremor amplitude of 54.1% and 59.9%, respectively, as measured by accelerometry [22]. Nonetheless, 56.3% of patients eventually discontinued the use of either medications [23]. Topiramate is also recommended as a first-line therapy by the guidelines of the Italian Movement Disorders Association (IMDA) [24] and is considered clinically useful at higher doses by the IPMDS task force [19]. However, it is recommended by the AAN guidelines as a second-line therapy [17,18]. Second-line medications have been reported to be less efficacious in reducing the amplitude of tremors. These include alprazolam, atenolol, gabapentin, and sotalol, as well as the aforementioned topiramate [17,18]. In contrast, there is no consensus in the management of PD tremors. The current NICE guidelines recommend levodopa as the first-line therapy for management of all motor symptoms in patients in the early stages of PD [5].

Deep brain stimulation (DBS), whose efficacy has been demonstrated through closed loop approaches [25,26] and interleaving stimulation [27], is the most common surgical treatment to date, providing durable tremor control, especially for patients with medically refractory ET or advanced PD. The effectiveness of DBS in ET and PD tremor is thought to be due to the direct electrical stimulation to the ventral intermediate nucleus (VIM) possibly disrupting the synchronous firing of thalamic neurons [28,29]. In addition to the VIM, the subthalamic nucleus, internal globus pallidus, and pedunculopontine nucleus are also effective targets for DBS in patients with PD tremors [30]. The use of DBS was approved by the Food and Drug Administration (FDA) for ET in 1997, for advanced PD in 2002, and for mid-stage PD in 2016. As of late, radiofrequency thalamotomy has become less favored. An RCT comparing DBS with thalamotomy in 68 patients with tremor due to ET, PD, or multiple sclerosis found that DBS results in fewer adverse effects ($p = 0.024$) and a greater increase in the Frenchay Activities Index score, which assess 15 ADLs. This suggests a greater improvement in the functional status when compared to thalamotomy [31]. Although surgical treatments for tremors, including DBS, stereotactic radiosurgery (SRS), and magnetic resonance-guided focused ultrasound (MRgFUS), are more efficacious than pharmacotherapy [32], the utilization of these procedures remains low. Limiting factors may include high surgical costs [33,34], access to care [35,36], and patient preference [35]. Other perceived barriers to DBS include practitioner preference [34,37], high resource and labor intensity [34,38], and perceptions of serious surgical risk [34,38,39].

Thus, a growing unmet need for safe and effective tremor control and suppression sets the stage for a range of therapies to bridge this gap between lifestyle modifications, pharmacotherapy, and surgical treatment. Using a variety of noninvasive suppression mechanisms, medical devices fit within this gap to provide effective tremor suppression at a lower risk than surgery. The increasing interest in this area has led to the birth of a new classification of external upper limb tremor stimulators. In 2018, the de novo classification request of Cala ONE (Cala Health, Burlingame, CA, USA) received FDA approval [40].

Herein, we focus on the mechanisms of action, safety and efficacy profiles, and clinical applications of different categories of medical devices that are available clinically or previously investigated for tremor suppression. Furthermore, we highlight the limitations of these devices. Such information may then be translated biomechanically and clinically for potential future advancements of medical device for tremor suppression.

2. Early Innovations

Over the past several decades, a variety of different orthotic and stimulatory approaches has been proposed to target or reverse the abnormal rhythmic activities in the neural pathways of the cerebellum and the thalamus. Beginning 1987, Rosen and colleagues proposed several devices that employed energy dissipation to suppress tremors. The damped joystick is a hand control device designed to facilitate the control of wheelchairs and other applications [41–44]. This device consists of a sealed chamber filled with viscous fluid and a spherical ball that acts as a damping element to suppress the involuntary movements of the position-sensing actuator. The controlled energy-dissipation orthosis (CEDO) is a wheelchair-mounted device that provides velocity-dependent loading with magnetic particle brakes to a limb coupling cuff [45–47]. Similarly, the modulated energy dissipation (MED) manipulator also provides damping via magnetic particle brakes with real-time digital control [48,49].

The success of these early works in showing that velocity-dependent loading can attenuate tremor and involuntary motions led to the development of wearable orthosis with mechanical loading. Other approaches, including electrical stimulation systems and assistive feeding devices, have also been proposed. Most of these are classified as Class I medical devices, meaning that they are registered with the FDA but not subjected to any premarketing review.

3. Electrical Stimulation Systems

3.1. Median and Radial Nerve Excitation

High frequency transcutaneous electrical nerve stimulation (TENS) has been widely studied and used in the treatment of nociceptive and neuropathic pain [50–53]. The use of TENS in the treatment of movement disorders, including myoclonic dystonia and ET, was first explored by Toglia and Izzo in 1985 [54]. While the exact mechanism of TENS remains unclear, putative mechanisms focus on its ability to modulate the afferent transmission of sensory information from the periphery to the central nervous system (CNS) [50]. Conventional TENS intends to selectively stimulate the large, myelinated peripheral proprioceptive A-beta (Aβ) sensory fibers [50]. The excitation of the Aβ fibers reduces the transmission of the sensory signals elicited by noxious stimulus, thereby reducing the pain perception [55–58]. These Aβ fibers carry proprioceptive sensory information into the thalamic circuits that are hypothesized to be involved in tremor generation [59]. Most [54,60–63], but not all [64], studies suggest that treatment with TENS in patients who have tremors was associated with improved muscle strength and tremor reduction. However, sham-controlled randomized trials are needed to confirm these findings due to potential confounding effects associated with the reason for use.

In 2018, Cala ONE was the first wearable transcutaneous electrical nerve stimulator to be approved by the FDA [40]. The newer version of this device, Cala Trio (Cala Health, USA; previously known as Cala TWO), is currently FDA-registered. The PROspective study for SymPtomatic relief of Essential tremor with Cala Therapy (PROSPECT) pivotal trial for Cala Trio was completed in 2019 [65], but it is still waiting for approval by the FDA. Clinically, Cala Trio is designed to replace Cala ONE for use in the transient, symptomatic relief of hand tremors in adults with ET. This device can be worn for therapy on the left or right wrist.

Cala Trio involves two working electrodes positioned over the median and radial nerves on the anterior surface of the wrist and a counter electrode placed on the posterior surface of the wrist. An accelerometer within this device measures the frequency of the patient's tremor, allowing individualized calibration of the stimulation intensity. The two working electrodes deliver electrical signals that intermittently excite the median and radial nerves in the upper limbs. Peripheral sensory nerves, including the median and radial nerves, also project to the VIM and the neural circuits that are implicated in ET. Similar to DBS, electrical stimulation of the VIM peripherally via the median [66,67] and radial [68] nerves elicits very fast oscillations, which induce thalamicneuronal oscillations and disrupt the pathological oscillations of tremors (Figure 1). A study involving five patients with tremors due to ET or PD demonstrated that electrical stimulation of the median and radial nerves leads to a 57% tremor suppression ($p < 0.01$) [69]. Over time, this stimulation with Cala Trio aims to normalize the neural firing in the pathological tremor network in the CNS to reduce tremors.

The pivotal trial for Cala ONE, a sham-controlled randomized trial of a single 40-min TENS session among 77 patients with ET, found no significant improvements in the Archimedes spiral task, as measured using the Tremor Research Group Essential Tremor Rating Assessment Scale (TETRAS) ($p = 0.26$) [70]. However, the Cala ONE stimulation did show significantly improved upper limb TETRAS tremor scores ($p = 0.017$) and subject-rated Bain and Findley ADL scores ($p = 0.001$), corresponding to a 42% (versus 28% with sham) and a 49% (versus 27% with sham) reduction in tremor amplitude, respectively [70]. The PROSPECT pivotal trial for Cala Trio, an open-label study of TENS treatment in adults with ET, compared twice-daily home therapy TENS sessions over a three-month period among 263 patients [71]. The results, based on 205 patients who completed the study, showed that TENS treatment via Cala Trio resulted in significant improvements in both the TETRAS and subject-rated Bain and Findley ADL scores ($p < 0.0001$) [71]. Among the 193 patients included in the secondary analysis, 54% experienced a $\geq 50\%$ reduction in tremor amplitude [71]. However, 14 patients did not respond to the therapy, suggesting that not all patients with ET will benefit from Cala Trio [71]. It is important to note that the open label, single-arm design of the PROSPECT trial limits the generality of Cala Trio's effect; therefore, future studies with more robust designs (e.g., RCTs) would be valuable to assess its efficacy.

Device-related adverse events were mild to moderate in severity. Nonserious adverse events were observed in 18% of patients, including skin irritations (redness, itchiness, and/or swelling); soreness or lesions; and discomfort (stinging and/or sensation of weakness) or burns [71]. These adverse events were all resolved with the use of a topical ointment, decreased stimulation intensity, or discontinued therapy [71]. Contraindications to the use of Cala Trio include having currently implanted electrical medical device (e.g., pacemaker, defibrillator, and deep brain stimulator), suspected or diagnosed epilepsy or other seizure disorders or pregnancy. This device should also not be applied on skin eruptions, open wounds, cancerous lesions, or swollen/infected/inflamed areas.

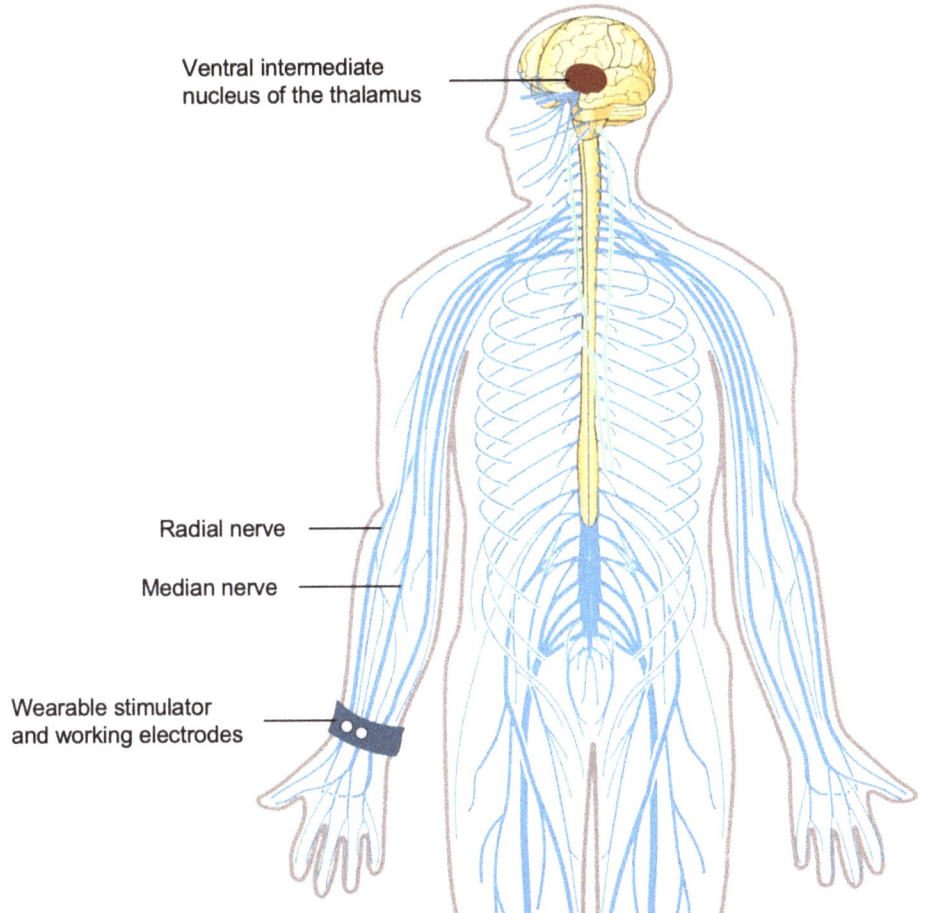

Figure 1. Cala Trio transcutaneous electrical nerve stimulation. The median and radial nerves, which project to the ventral intermediate nucleus of the thalamus, are stimulated by Cala Trio (Cala Health, Burlingame, CA, USA) through two working electrodes placed on the anterior surface of the wrist.

A 50% reduction of tremor amplitude is comparable to the first-line propranolol and primidone pharmacotherapies [17], which are considered clinically useful for the treatment of ET [19]. Cala Trio can play an important role in patients who are not eligible for surgical intervention or do not respond to pharmacotherapy. It has a similar, favorable safety profile to Cala ONE, whose risk and benefit determination met the FDA's requirements. This device is noninvasive, with 85% of patients reporting its convenience and ease of use [71]. Currently, it is uncertain whether Cala Trio could reduce or replace the need of medications in the treatment of ET. Thus, physicians need to evaluate how it will fit along with pharmacotherapy and/or lifestyle interventions for each patient with the consideration of tremor severity. Post-approval studies could address this question and provide further insights into the long-term safety and efficacy of Cala Trio.

3.2. Antagonistic Muscles Activation

In contrast to TENS, which stimulates sensory nerves, functional electrical stimulation (FES) provides stimulation to motor nerves to trigger muscle contraction. FES for tremor suppression was pioneered by Prochazka and colleagues in 1989 [72,73] and clinically assessed in 1992 [74,75]. Briefly, FES was associated with a tremor suppression of 73% in ET, 62% in PD tremors, and 38% in cerebellar tremors [75]. The recognized limitations of these early works included the potentially unreliable placement of surface electrodes, which could lead to insufficient tremor suppression [74,75]. Although the implantation of percutaneous intramuscular electrodes could solve this problem, this approach is invasive and reserved for patients with severe tremor [64]. Nonetheless, the results from these pilot works led to the first functional electrical stimulator developed specifically for tremor suppression [76,77]. Comparing the previous approach using an analog filter [72–75], the use of an optimized digital filter [76,77] in a portable functional electrical stimulator, with the enabled self-tuning and adaptation of more complex algorithms, showed improvements in suppressing tremors. In six participants who were healthy or with PD tremor, the functional electrical stimulator based on a digital filter showed an 84% tremor suppression, compared to a 65% when an analog filter was used [77]. The current approaches in utilizing FES to suppress tremors echo these early works, involving primarily two strategies: out-of-phase and co-contraction stimulations [78].

The MOTIMOVE system (3F-Fit Fabricando Faber, Belgrade, Serbia), based on an out-of-phase stimulation, obtained a CE marking for use in the European Union in 2019 but has not been approved by the FDA (Figure 2). The use of the MOTIMOVE system has been studied in patients with ET, PD tremors [79], and hemiplegia [80]. Two prototypes, the TREMOR neurorobot and the Tremor's glove, have adapted the co-contraction stimulation. Both devices have been assessed in patients with ET or PD but are currently not approved for clinical use.

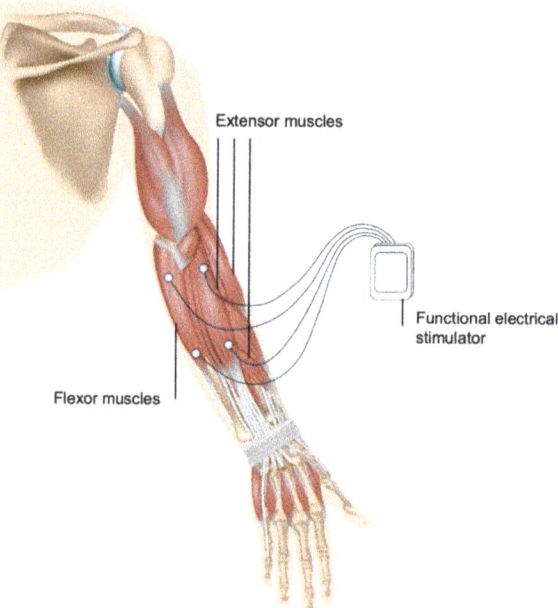

Figure 2. MOTIMOVE functional electrical stimulation system. This device (3F-Fit Fabricando Faber, Serbia) comprises a multichannel stimulator that attaches to several electrodes placed on the flexor and extensor muscles of the forearm, enabling muscle activation.

The MOTIMOVE system consists of a multichannel stimulator that provides support to activate several electrodes, placed on the forearm and upper arm above the flexor and extensor muscle points, that enable the selective muscle activation via distributed, asynchronous electrical stimulation. The inertial sensors within MOTIMOVE deliver real-time estimation of tremulous movements to a host computer, which provides control over the stimulation of muscles. This system delivers out-of-phase stimulation by sending electrical current pulses to the flexor and extensor muscles, triggering the depolarization of motor neurons that counteracts the tremorgenic activity. A pilot study of MOTIMOVE revealed a 67% tremor suppression in six of seven patients with ET or PD [79]. One patient, however, did not respond, suggesting that out-of-phase stimulation may not work for all patients with tremor [79]. Additional clinical studies evaluating the MOTIMOVE system are claimed to be currently in progress in Serbia, France, and Hungary, which will hopefully demonstrate its efficacy in tremor suppression and feasibility.

The TREMOR neurorobot and the Tremor's glove adopt a similar design as the MOTIMOVE, consisting of electrodes that provide muscle stimulation, inertial sensors that capture biomechanical characterization signals of tremor, and a controller. Both devices adapt the co-contraction stimulation strategy, which applies mechanical loading via continuous transcutaneous stimulation to a pair of antagonistic muscles, increasing the stiffness of the limb. In turn, this filters out the mechanical manifestation of tremorgenic activity, which are oscillations in the muscle tissue. Like MOTIMOVE, the TREMOR neurorobot stimulates the flexor and extensor muscles of the forearm. This device was found to have a 52% tremor suppression in six patients with ET or PD tremors ($p < 0.001$) [81]. Conversely, the Tremor's glove stimulates the abductor pollicis brevis and the first and second dorsal interossei muscles of the hand. In a sham-controlled randomized trial of 30 patients with medically refractory tremor in PD, the use of the Tremor's glove was associated with a significant reduction in the Unified Parkinson's Disease Rating Scale (UPDRS) score ($p = 0.001$), suggesting improved experiences of daily living and motor complications [82].

The A-alpha (Aα) sensory fiber, a primary afferent nerve fiber that innervates antagonistic muscle pairs, appears to have a crucial role in the complex neural pathways that are involved in tremor pathophysiology. The reciprocal inhibition of Aα fibers seems to decrease the excitability of antagonistic motor neurons and increase the excitability of agonist motor neurons [83]. While it is not entirely clear whether the reciprocal activation of Aα fibers results in tremor, intermittent stimulation of the Aα fibers innervating the flexor and extensor muscles via FES has been studied in patients with ET or PD, showing a 58% tremor suppression [78]. Another study of 14 patients with PD tremor also observed reduction in tremor amplitude and frequency [84]. This suggests that the excitability of antagonist and agonist motor neurons can be modulated, thereby supporting the mechanism by which FES attenuates tremor.

Muscle fatigue is commonly seen as a nonserious adverse event in patients who are treated with FES, owing to the fact that both out-of-phase and co-contraction stimulations lead to the activation of joints and muscle contraction [85]. The use of the Tremor's glove can also result in numbness of the hand and burning sensation [82]. Contraindications for FES include a prior implanted electrical device, cancer, osteomyelitis, thrombosis/hemorrhage, epilepsy, or pregnancy [86]. In each case, it is incumbent on physicians to evaluate the risk and benefit of a FES treatment based on the patient's medical history.

Functional electrical stimulators are minimally invasive and demonstrate sufficient efficacy in the suppression of tremor. However, muscle fatigue during repeated FES-induced contraction limits their long-term use. To address this limitation, several emerging technologies have been proposed to reduce or counter muscle fatigue during FES [85]. These functional electrical stimulators have only been studied in small cohorts of patients. Large scale, sham-controlled randomized trials are necessary to validate the efficacy and safety of these devices.

4. Wearable Orthoses

The first reported mechanical solution for the suppression of hand tremors was focused on clasping the patient's arm to prevent involuntary spasms, patented by Terry and Hoyt in 1980 [87]. However, this approach was not developed further. In 1998, the Viscous Beam orthosis [88] was developed based on previously established principles of energy dissipation [45,46,48] to suppress tremor along the wrist flexion/extension. This device showed success, demonstrating that energy dissipation could be employed in an orthosis. However, it was limited by the fixed damping rate, leading to inconsistent tremor suppression [88].

Tremor suppression orthoses for the upper limbs, wrist, and elbow joints are classified into active, semi-active, or passive. Active orthoses work by generating an active force that counteracts the involuntary motions while supporting the voluntary motions in patients with tremors. In contrast, semi-active and passive orthoses leverage energy dissipation or absorption to suppress involuntary movements. Unlike passive orthoses, the damping magnitude of semi-active orthoses can be adjusted by an active controller. Tremelo (Five Microns, Fresno, CA, USA), Steadi-One (Steadiwear, Toronto, ON, Canada), and Readi-Steadi (Readi-Steadi, Gonzales, LA, USA) are the three passive orthoses currently available for use in patients with tremor. Both Tremelo and Steadi-One are FDA-registered, while Readi-Steadi is FDA-exempted. Active and semi-active orthoses are currently being researched but are not clinically available.

4.1. Active Suppression

In 2005, the Wearable Orthosis for Tremor Assessment and Suppression (WOTAS) exoskeleton was developed as part of the Dynamically Responsive Interventions for Tremor Suppression (DRIFTS) project of the European Commission [89–92]. WOTAS consists of sensors that measure rotational motions around the joints, electrical direct current (DC) motors that act as actuators to exert force to suppress tremor by converting electrical energy into mechanical energy, and a controller. This device is placed parallel to the upper limb, suppressing tremor in the wrist flexion/extension and pronation/supination and the elbow flexion/extension. In ten patients with tremors, WOTAS demonstrated a 40% tremor suppression [92]. The major drawback of this device is that it is large and bulky, posing social exclusion concerns [91].

Subsequent active orthoses were developed with similar designs and mechatronics to WOTAS but vary in the types of actuators to reduce the weight and improve the tremor suppression efficacy. The pneumatic actuator, which has a large power-to-weight ratio, was implemented in an orthosis, along with an adaptive tremor estimation algorithm, to suppress tremors in the wrist flexion/extension and adduction/abduction [93–95]. The results at the testbench using datasets from ten patients with ET or PD tremor showed a 98.1% tremor suppression [95]. The adaptive disturbance rejection controller, utilizing a permanent magnet linear motor (PMLM), demonstrated a 97.6% tremor suppression when examined with five tremulous signals from patients with PD [96]. Compared to the pneumatic actuator, the PMLM is simpler and faster to control and requires only one sensor [96]. The voluntary-driven elbow orthosis, using an electronically communicated (EC) motor, provided a 99.8% tremor suppression in lab simulation using data from a patient with ET [97]. The wearable tremor suppression glove (WTSG), consisting of an actuation box that includes a multi-channel mechatronic splitter (MMS), aims to provide power support from a single input source to multiple output applications [98]. The MMS incorporates a power EC motor and a steering EC motor to suppress tremors in the wrists and hands [98]. The efficacy of this actuation system, however, has not been evaluated.

Other active orthoses have sought to integrate complex sensor systems to characterize voluntary motions and detect tremors. The myoelectric-controlled upper limb orthosis incorporated an algorithm that recognizes and extracts voluntary movements from surface myoelectric signals [99–102]. The results from six participants who were healthy or with ET showed a recognition rate of 82% [102]. The newer version of this orthosis adopted a different design that improved flexibility and ease of wear [103,104]. In a healthy participant with FES-induced muscle contraction, the myoelectric-controlled orthosis reduced oscillations in the elbow flexion/extension by about 50–80% [104]. Huen and colleagues implemented context aware body sensor network (BSN) sensors into an upper limb orthosis to enable the detection of six ADLs [105]. In six healthy participants with simulated tremor movements, the BSN-integrated exoskeleton exhibited a 70% accuracy rate in identifying ADLs and a 77% tremor suppression [105].

4.2. Semi-Active Suppression

Several semi-active orthoses utilize magnetorheological (MR) fluids as a strategy to provide tremor suppression. MR fluids consist of magnetizable, microscopic particles dispersed in oil or water. Upon encountering a magnetic field, these particles experience attractive force, and the viscosity of the MR fluids increases, opposing the existing flow. This rheological property has been exploited in tremor suppression orthoses by varying magnetic field intensities to tune the resistance force for tremor suppression [106].

The Double Viscous Beam (DVB) orthosis, positioned on the dorsal surface of the forearm, consists of a chamber of MR fluids and two shear plates to make up a passive actuator, applying mechanical loads for tremor suppression [107]. Compared to the previous approach [88], the DVB orthosis has an improved responsiveness to the viscous resistance as a result of the increased shear strength. This orthosis is coupled to a sensor and a controller to optimize the actuation performance.

Case and colleagues developed a wearable orthosis that incorporated four MR dampers for the wrist flexion/extension and abduction/adduction, the elbow flexion/extension, and the forearm pronation/supination [108–111]. An estimation algorithm for tremor frequency and a controller were used to measure the amount of resistance force needed to counteract tremulous movements. The resistance force generated by the MR dampers depends on a piston-coil design.

More recently, the MR damper-based soft exoskeleton for the tremor suppression (SETS) system was proposed to suppress tremor in the wrist [112]. Unlike previously designed semi-active orthoses, the SETS system equips a controllable flexible semi-active actuator that dynamically adapts to the motions of the wrist joint, providing tremor suppression in the wrist flexion/extension, abduction/adduction, rotation. This device also integrates passive suppression with two hyper-elastic blades, which suppress tremor in the wrist supination/pronation. The SETS system demonstrates potential clinical utility with its compatibility with the human wrist, real-time tunability based on tremor frequency, and lightweight design.

The carbon fiber-based, lightweight orthosis developed by Herrnstadt and Menon is magnetically activated by an electromagnetic brake (EB) [113]. When the tremor frequency and joint angular displacement are detected by a sensor and potentiometer, respectively, a pulse width modulation signal is sent from the controller to produce a magnetic field, exciting the EB. In turn, the EB actuates the orthosis to generate a resistive force for tremor suppression. In comparison to electric motors such as the DC motor, EBs are capable of producing a higher force while consuming less power. In three healthy participants with simulated tremor motions, the use of the EB-based orthosis demonstrated an 88% tremor suppression [113].

Apart from magnetically driven semi-active orthoses, Kalaiarasi and Kumar designed a pneumatically controlled hand cuff [114]. Similarly, this device is built along with an accelerometer that sends tremor frequency data to a controller. When the threshold is met, an air pump inflates the hand cuff, yielding a resistance force in a reciprocating, linear motion to suppress the tremor. Inflation and deflation of the hand cuff are enabled by two separate valves. The limited efficacy of this approach was observed in one patient with ET who experienced a 30% tremor suppression [114].

4.3. Passive Suppression

Tremelo utilized two tuned vibration absorbers (TVAs) that are positioned over the dorsal and ventral surfaces of the arm (Figure 3). Each TVA contains a mass-spring-damper system in which the vibration energy of involuntary motions of the shaking arm during tremor are transferred from the spring to the added mass. This results in reduced tremulous movements and substantial motions of the added mass within the TVA. This device is purely mechanical, eliminating the need of a power source. Preliminary results showed an 85% tremor suppression in a patient with PD tremors [115]. Recruitment for a pilot clinical study is ongoing, which should provide further data.

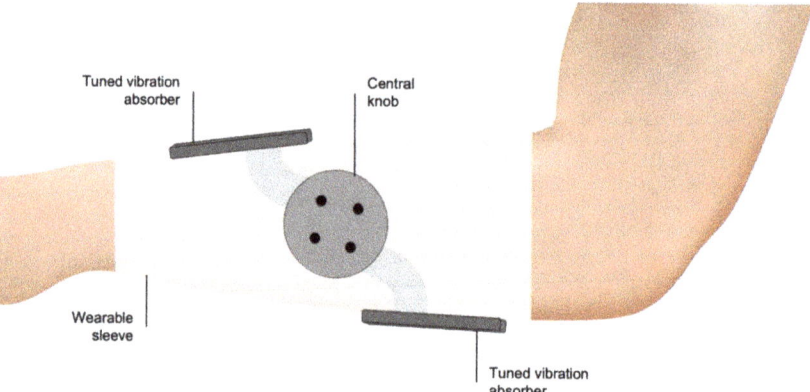

Figure 3. Tremelo passive orthosis. The vibration energy of tremor is being transferred to a mass-spring-damper system within the two tuned vibration absorbers of Tremelo (Five Microns, Fresno, CA, USA), positioned over the dorsal and ventral surfaces of the arm to counteract the involuntary motions.

Steadi-One is mechanical device that integrates a tuned mass damper (TMD), which obviates the need for a power source [116] (Figure 4). Like TVAs, the TMD embodies a mass-spring-damper system. The difference between TMDs and TVAs is the presence of a dissipating element, which, in Steadi-One, is a non-Newtonian fluid in the interior space of the TMD. When the vibration energy is transferred to the added mass, this non-Newtonian fluid becomes viscous, reducing its amplitude of motions. There are no publicly available data to support its efficacy. However, it is claimed (https://www.steadiwear.com, accessed on 26 March 2021) to have an 85–90% tremor suppression during the lab simulation.

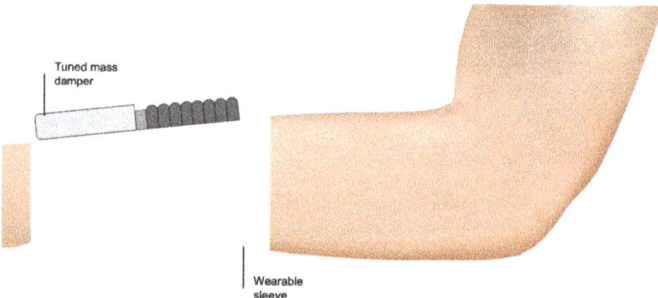

Figure 4. Steadi-One passive orthosis. The non-Newtonian fluid within the tuned mass damper of Steadi-One (Steadiwear, Toronto, ON, Canada) becomes viscous when the vibration energy of tremor is transferred to a mass-spring-damper system, acting as a dissipating element that reduces the amplitude of motions.

The Readi-Steadi glove embeds a multitude of metal disks that aims to add inertia to the tremulous hand. A preliminary study involving 40 participants who were healthy or with ET observed a 50% tremor suppression [117]. The metal disks function as sensory tricks that influence the aberrant sensorimotor integration to suppress tremor. While there is no study that examines the effectiveness of the sensory trick phenomenon in patients with ET or PD tremor, it has been studied in 30 patients with musician's dystonia [118].

By wearing a glove, patients with more severe symptoms of dystonia showed better improvements in fine motor control (Pearson's r = −0.45; p = 0.01) [118].

The Task-Adjustable Passive Orthosis (TAPO) has a textile glove design to enhance wearability and comfort for daily activities. An air-filled structure, inflated on-demand by hand or electrical pump, is fitted within the glove on the dorsal surface of the hand. The inflated TAPO applies pressure to the back of the hand and the forearm, suppressing the involuntary motions in the wrist flexion/extension, ulnar/radial deviation, and pronation/supination. The proof of concept of TAPO has been examined in a patient with PD tremors performing six ADLs. The use of TAPO was associated with a significant tremor suppression in three specific tasks, including 82% while drinking ($p = 0.03$), 79% while pouring ($p = 0.03$), and 74% while drawing a spiral ($p = 0.03$) [119].

More recently, Lu and Huang examined and established a mechanical model for particle damping for passive vibration suppression in tremors [120]. Particle dampers involve the potential of energy absorption and dissipation through momentum exchange between moving particles and vibrating walls. There are several advantages of using particle dampers, including simple construction, low cost, robustness and reliability, wide damping frequency band, and insensitivity to extreme temperature [120]. At a high tremor frequency, the provided damping of the particle damper became nearly independent to the frequency and amplitude of tremor, indicating that it is suitable for tremor suppression [120].

Two other passive orthoses have also been previously investigated for their use in tremor suppression. The Vib-Bracelet, also designed with an incorporated TMD, suppresses tremors in the wrist pronation/supination [121,122]. The result at the testbench using tremor data from one patient with PD showed an 85% tremor suppression [122]. Another approach, proposed by Takanokura and colleagues [123], involved implementing air dashpots into an orthosis to suppress tremors in the wrist flexion/extension and ulnar/radial deviation, as well as the elbow flexion/extension. In a healthy participant with electrical stimulation-induced muscle contraction, this orthosis demonstrated an involuntary movement suppression of 62% in the wrist when two air dashpots were used and 82% in the elbow [123].

4.4. Mechanism Underpinning the Efficacy of Wearable Orthoses in Tremor Suppression

Although some of the underlying causes of tremors remain unknown, several putative interactive factors contributing to the motor expression of tremor have been hypothesized. These include the oscillating tendencies of the joint and muscular mechanical systems, short- and long-loop reflexes of the spinal cord and the brainstem, and the closed-loop feedback systems of higher motor centers such as the cerebellum [124]. Unlike electrical stimulation systems, wearable orthoses target the clinical manifestations of tremors. By generating an opposite force of equal magnitude, these devices attempt to mechanically counteract the involuntary movements.

4.5. Comparing Active, Semi-Active, and Passive Orthoses for Tremor Suppression

Unlike semi-active and passive orthoses, active orthoses often rely on actuators coupled to a signal transmission system, resulting in their heavy and unwieldy nature. A reduction in the overall weights to improve their wearability is an important research priority. For example, Kelley and Kauffman recently proposed substituting the traditional actuators with the soft and compliant dielectric elastomer stack actuators to enable an orthosis conforming to the human joints [125,126]. In lieu of the metallic structure of previous orthoses, the BSN-integrated exoskeleton leveraged plastic materials to reduce the weight [105]. By using an MMS to support multiple output applications with one drive motor, the WTSG has a reduced size and weight [98].

Wearable orthoses are primarily noninvasive in suppressing tremors. However, their safety profile has not been established, because most wearable orthoses were only assessed in small cohorts of patients or at the testbench with data simulation. Furthermore, the small sample size of these studies may undermine the reliability of the data. It is likely that wearable orthoses will become the most widely used medical devices for tremor suppression, given their promising efficacy. Major challenges include developing orthoses that are lightweight and soft in texture, studying the orthotic placement that will result in maximized tremor suppression, and improving the ergonomic design based on the anatomy of the upper limbs. Addressing these questions with further studies should enhance our understanding of the feasibility and practicality of clinically implementing wearable orthoses to suppress tremor.

5. Assistive Feeding Devices

The Neater Eater (Neater Solutions, Derbyshire, UK) was introduced by Michaelis in 1988 [127]. However, it was not available for use in the US until its registration with the FDA in 1993. This is a table-mounted device that involves internal spring-assisted lifting to support a clip-on utensil to enable eating. It relies on viscous damping to absorb tremors and fast movements via the flowing of a viscous fluid that dissipates the kinetic energy. A brief report interviewing 39 participants with various neuromuscular conditions found that the Neater Eater is associated with positive impacts in independence, self-confidence, and quality of life [128]. Follow-up and monitoring may be necessary to prevent fatigue and muscle build-up from using this device on a regular basis.

Liftware Steady (Verily Life Sciences, South San Francisco, CA, USA), registered with the FDA in 2013, is a handheld device designed to help patients with ET or PD tremors eat. It consists of a motion-generating platform, capable of directing two DC motors to move the utensil opposite to the direction of the tremor. The patient's involuntary movements are detected by an accelerometer, which are then transmitted to a controller, providing control over the motion-generating platform. A pilot study involving 15 patients with ET demonstrated an improvement in tremor with the device, as measured by Fahn-Tolosa-Marin Tremor Rating Scale (TRS), while holding ($p = 0.016$), eating ($p = 0.001$), and transferring objects ($p = 0.001$) [129]. When using the device, patients expressed improved symptoms of ET while eating ($p < 0.001$) and transferring objects ($p = 0.013$) but not holding them ($p = 0.14$), as measured by the subject-rated Clinical Global Impression Scale (CGI-S) [129]. Data demonstrated a 73% tremor suppression across the three tasks [129]. Compared to other adaptive utensils in 22 patients with ET or PD tremor, Liftware Steady was preferred [130].

The Gyenno Spoon (GYENNO Technologies, Shenzhen, China), another handheld assistive feeding device, consists of a longitudinal motor and a transverse motor that are able to generate movements in two different directions opposite to the tremor direction [131]. Both motors are linked to a control module, which receives vibration data from multiple movement sensors within the device. Its ergonomic design and proposed efficacy led to its registration with the FDA in 2016 for use for patients with ET or PD tremors. While it claims (https://www.gyenno.com/spoon-en, accessed on 26 March 2021) to have an 85% tremor suppression, no clinical data has been published.

Contrary to Liftware Steady and the Gyenno Spoon, the Neater Eater requires no power supply and has the ability to automatically bring the spoon forward to the patient's mouth with an internal spring. However, both Liftware Steady and the Gyenno Spoon enable data collection of the patient's tremor. This can be beneficial in allowing physicians to monitor their patients' tremor improvement or progression when Liftware Steady or the Gyenno Spoon is supplemented with pharmacotherapy. Nonetheless, it is important to note that the functionality of these devices is limited to provide support in feeding only.

6. Other Devices

6.1. Gyroscopic Stabilization

The GyroGlove (GyroGear, London, UK) is developed with a plurality of gyroscopes, mounted to a fabric glove on the dorsal surface of the hand, that function to counteract tremors [132]. Each gyroscope includes a rotatable disc that is capable of rotating about an axis to resist involuntary motions. This allows its angular momentum to be conserved when a rotational displacement is encountered, with opposing force inputs from any direction. Unlike previous gyroscopic devices using a single gyroscope [133,134], the use of multiple gyroscopes in the GyroGlove allows it to suppress involuntary movements in multiple planar directions. This device is currently in the advanced stage of development, and data is needed to inform its efficacy.

6.2. Haptic Stimulation Systems

The Emma Watch (Microsoft, Redmond, WA, USA) is a wrist-worn device consisting of several vibration-generating actuators aimed at providing haptic stimulation to the wrist. Mechanosensitive receptors, such as the Pacinian and Meissner corpuscles in the upper limbs, deliver afferent signals to the cuneate nucleus in response to vibratory stimuli [135,136]. Proprioceptive inputs from the cuneate nucleus are projected to the thalamus [136–138], implicating its possible role in the neural pathway associated with tremors [139]. However, a study involving 18 patients with ET reported that a mechanical vibration to the hand and forearm via piezoelectric actuators resulted in no homogenous effect in the tremor amplitude [139]. Across different frequencies of vibratory stimuli, 50–72% of patients experienced an increase in tremor amplitude, while 5–22% of patients showed a decrease [139]. The Emma Watch will require clinical validations, since the use of haptic stimulation for tremor suppression has, to date, only led to questionable efficacy.

7. Tremor Suppression Devices: Place in Therapy

The onset of ET can occur early in childhood due to familial factors, but the majority of cases of ET appeared after the age of 40 [140]. One study investigated the correlation between the age of onset and the progression of ET in 115 patients [141]. Patients with an age of onset later than 60 years experienced a more rapid progression when compared to patients with a younger age of onset ($p < 0.001$) [141]. Since the onset of ET and PD tremors typically occurs in middle to late adulthood, aging-associated diseases such as dementia [142,143] and mild cognitive impairment [144–146] intersect with both of these conditions. These neurological disorders may further preclude patients from adhering to pharmacotherapies.

The medical devices described above offer alternative options for the suppression of tremors (Table 1), especially in patients who are not eligible for surgical interventions (i.e., DBS, SRS, and MRgFUS). However, the use of these devices is patient specific. For example, although Cala Trio has an aesthetic design that will likely not pose any social concerns, wearable orthoses may be a better option if the patient has any contraindication to the use of electrical stimulation systems. Depending on the patient's needs, assistive feeding devices may be a useful addition to the patient's daily living. Most of the devices that are available for use are subjected to the FDA's Class I general control for safety and efficacy assurance. In addition to the general control, Cala ONE requires Class II special control for its performance standards and special prescriber labeling.

Table 1. Summary of the tremor suppression devices and study results.

Type of Device	Study Participants (n)	Efficacy	Risks	Refs
Electrical Stimulation Systems: Transcutaneous Electrical Nerve Stimulators				
Cala ONE [‡]	ET (77)	• Improved upper limb TETRAS tremor scores ($p = 0.017$) • Improved subject-rated BF-ADL scores ($p = 0.001$)	• Skin irritations (redness, itchiness, and swelling) • Soreness or lesions • Discomfort (stinging and sensation of weakness) or burns	[70]
Cala Trio *	ET (205)	• Improved upper limb TETRAS tremor scores ($p < 0.0001$) • Improved subject-rated BF-ADL scores ($p < 0.0001$)		[71]
Electrical Stimulation Systems: Functional Electrical Stimulators				
MOTIMOVE	ET (3); PD tremor (4)	67% tremor suppression		[79]
TREMOR neurorobot	ET (4); PD tremor (2)	52% tremor suppression	Muscle fatigue	[81]
Tremor's glove	PD tremor (30)	Reduced UPDRS score ($p = 0.001$)		[82]
Wearable Orthoses: Active Orthoses				
WOTAS exoskeleton	ET (7); MS tremor (1); Posttraumatic tremor (1); Mixed tremor (1)	40% tremor suppression [92]		[89–92]
Pneumatic actuator-based orthosis	ET (5) [§]; PD tremor (5) [§]	98.1% tremor suppression [95]		[93–95]
PMLM-based orthosis	PD tremor (5) [§]	97.6% tremor suppression		[96]
Voluntary-driven elbow orthosis	ET (1) [§]	99.8% tremor suppression	Not reported	[97]
MMS-based WTSG	Not reported	Not reported		[98]
Myoelectric-controlled orthosis	ET (2); Healthy (4)	Not reported		[99–102]
Myoelectric-controlled orthosis (ver. 2)	Healthy (1)	50–80% tremor suppression [104]		[103,104]
BSN-based orthosis	Healthy (6) [§]	77% tremor suppression		[105]
Wearable Orthoses: Semi-Active Orthoses				
Double viscous beam orthosis	Not reported	Not reported		[107]
MR damper-based orthosis	Not reported	Not reported	Not reported	[108–111]
SETS system	Not reported	Not reported		[112]
Electromagnetic brake-based orthosis	Healthy (3) [§]	88% tremor suppression		[113]
Pneumatic hand cuff	ET (1)	30% tremor suppression		[114]

Table 1. Cont.

Type of Device	Study Participants (n)	Efficacy	Risks	Refs
Wearable Orthoses: Passive Orthoses				
Tremelo *	PD tremor (1)	85% tremor suppression		[115]
Steadi-One *	Lab simulation	85–90% tremor suppression		[116]
Readi-Steadi *	ET (20); Healthy (40)	50% tremor suppression		[117]
Task-Adjustable Passive Orthosis	PD tremor (1)	• 82% tremor suppression while drinking ($p = 0.03$) • 79% tremor suppression while pouring ($p = 0.03$) • 74% tremor suppression while drawing a spiral ($p = 0.03$)	Not reported	[119]
Particle Damper	Not reported	Not reported		[120]
Vib-Bracelet	PD tremor (1) §	85% tremor suppression		[121,122]
Air-dashpot-based orthosis	Healthy (1) ¶	• 20–62% tremor suppression in the wrist • 82% tremor suppression in the elbow		[123]
Assistive Feeding Devices				
Neater Eater *	Not reported	Not reported		[127]
Liftware Steady *	ET (15)	• Improved FTM-TRS while holding, eating, and transferring objects ($p = 0.001$) • 73% tremor suppression	Not reported	[129]
Gyenno Spoon *	Not reported	85% tremor suppression (claimed)		[131]
Gyroscopic Stabilizers				
GyroGlove *	Not reported	Not reported	Not reported	[132]
Haptic Stimulation Systems				
Emme Watch	Not reported	Not reported	Not reported	

BF-ADL, Bain and Findley Activities of Daily Living; BSN, body senor network; ET, essential tremor; FTM-TRS, Fahn-Tolosa-Marin Tremor Rating Scale; MMS, multi-channel mechatronic splitter; MS, multiple sclerosis; PMLM, permanent magnet linear motor; SETS, soft exoskeleton for tremor suppression; TETRAS, Tremor Research Group Essential Tremor Rating Assessment Scale; PD, Parkinson's disease; UPDRS, Unified Parkinson's Disease Rating Scale; WOTAS, Wearable Orthosis for Tremor Assessment and Suppression; and WTSG, wearable tremor suppression gloves. * FDA-registered; Class I medical device. ‡ FDA-approved; Class II medical device. § Test bench simulation. ¶ Induced muscle contraction.

ET is associated with a staggering cost of direct medical expenses, indirect productivity and income losses, nonmedical expenses, and disability benefits. The unemployment rate increases to about 88% in patients whose ET progresses from mild to severe [147], leading to forced early retirements. Collectively, patients with mild ET have a 1.83-year average loss of employment, corresponding to a $280 billion in income loss [147]. In patients with moderate to severe tremors, the average loss of employment is 6.5 years [147]. ET and PD tremors likely increase the economic burden more than currently estimated due to their progressive natures and the underreported cases. The development of a medical device for tremor suppression is an under-researched area. Most of the investigational devices discussed were abandoned before entering the market. However, it is imperative that the search for safe and effective tremor suppression devices continues, given the overall economic burden of tremors. Given that most of the currently available devices are based on preliminary data, more investigation is needed to understand the safety and efficacy of these devices before their use in clinical practice can be supported. Cost-effectiveness data are necessary and important to convince insurance programs to provide coverage, alleviating the financial constraints on patients and caregivers.

8. Future Perspectives

The devices currently studied have employed distinctive mechanistic approaches. The weight of evidence supporting their efficacy challenges the notion that tremors originate from a single, dominant pathway. Additional pathological insights, such as the loss of Purkinje cells in ET [148,149] and increased central oscillator synchronization in the basal ganglia in PD tremors [150], along with several mechanistic targets of tremor suppression devices, highlight the advances in our understanding of how tremors may be generated. Perhaps the most pertinent pathway implicated in tremors is the cortico-ponto-cerebello-thalamo-cortical loop, which serves as the basis for successful surgical interventions [21]. These findings suggest an integrative multi-pathway model for tremor pathogenesis. The relevance of these pathways necessitates a further clarification of the complexities and inter-related causes of tremors, which is central to spur the future development of safer and more effective devices for tremor suppression.

The lack of consensus on the characterization and electrophysiology of tremor previously represented two major diagnostic pitfalls [151]. However, in 2018, the IPMDS task force reviewed the vast uncertainties to update its consensus classification criteria for tremor disorders [1]. Besides ET and PD tremors, it is important to recognize that a wide range of other tremor conditions also affect the upper limbs with varying clinical features and etiologies [1]. Future studies could investigate whether the efficacy of these devices is generalizable to other tremor conditions. As seen in the pivotal Cala ONE trial [70], tremor suppression can, in part, be attributed to the surgical placebo effect. Since the studies of most of these devices were descriptive in design, sham-controlled randomized trials are warranted to confirm their efficacy. Lastly, evaluating the concurrent use of one or more devices, along with pharmacotherapy/lifestyle interventions, may derive insightful data to explain the benefits and overall impact of a multimodal strategy in the management of tremors.

9. Conclusions

Although tremors are not a life-threatening movement disorder, they can be disabling and negatively impact the patient's quality of life. Our limited knowledge of the pathophysiology of tremors has given rise to the challenge of developing effective or curative pharmacotherapies. In the past several decades, many medical devices, with a broad range of mechanisms, have been developed to suppress tremors in different aspects of daily living. Based on the current evidence, some of these devices appear to have promise as potentially safe and effective options in the medical armamentarium for tremor suppression. Most of these devices are noninvasive and placed externally around the wrists or the upper limbs. It is important to note that externally wearing a device could pose a cosmetic and social concern, so understanding the acceptability of tremor medical devices among patients with tremors is warranted. Nonetheless, it is likely that the future of tremor management will benefit from the addition of medical devices into the patient's existing pharmacotherapy and/or lifestyle intervention. However, given the high variability in the quality of the current studies, future research is needed to better understand the long-term efficacy, safety, and cost-effectiveness of the tremor suppression devices to fulfill this promise.

Author Contributions: Conceptualization: R.P.; Writing—original draft: J.M.; Writing—reviewing and editing—All authors. All authors have read and agreed to the published version of the manuscript.

Funding: This research received no external funding.

Institutional Review Board Statement: Not applicable.

Informed Consent Statement: Not applicable.

Data Availability Statement: Data sharing not applicable.

Acknowledgments: The authors wish to thank the School of Pharmacy at the Massachusetts College of Pharmacy and Health Sciences University for their financial support of this project.

Conflicts of Interest: The authors declare no conflict of interest.

References

1. Bhatia, K.P.; Bain, P.; Bajaj, N.; Elble, R.J.; Hallett, M.; Louis, E.D.; Raethjen, J.; Stamelou, M.; Testa, C.M.; Deuschl, G.; et al. Consensus Statement on the classification of tremors. From the task force on tremor of the International Parkinson and Movement Disorder Society. *Mov. Disord.* **2018**, *33*, 75–87. [CrossRef]
2. Louis, E.D.; Ferreira, J.J. How common is the most common adult movement disorder? Update on the worldwide prevalence of essential tremor. *Mov. Disord.* **2010**, *25*, 534–541. [CrossRef]
3. Louis, E.D.; Ottman, R.; Hauser, W.A. How common is the most common adult movement disorder? Estimates of the prevalence of essential tremor throughout the world. *Mov. Disord.* **1998**, *13*, 5–10. [CrossRef] [PubMed]
4. Dorsey, E.R.; Elbaz, A.; Nichols, E.; Abd-Allah, F.; Abdelalim, A.; Adsuar, J.C.; Ansha, M.G.; Brayne, C.; Choi, J.-Y.J.; Collado-Mateo, D.; et al. Global, regional, and national burden of Parkinson's disease, 1990–2016: A systematic analysis for the Global Burden of Disease Study 2016. *Lancet Neurol.* **2018**, *17*, 939–953. [CrossRef]
5. National Institute for Health and Care Excellence (UK). *Parkinson's Disease in Adults: Diagnosis and Management*; National Institute for Health and Care Excellence (UK): London, UK, 2017.
6. Louis, E.D.; Barnes, L.; Albert, S.M.; Cote, L.; Schneier, F.R.; Pullman, S.L.; Yu, Q. Correlates of functional disability in essential tremor. *Mov. Disord.* **2001**, *16*, 914–920. [CrossRef]
7. Elble, R.J.; Brilliant, M.; Leffler, K.; Higgins, C. Quantification of essential tremor in writing and drawing. *Mov. Disord.* **1996**, *11*, 70–78. [CrossRef]
8. Héroux, M.E.; Parisi, S.L.; Larocerie-Salgado, J.; Norman, K.E. Upper-Extremity Disability in Essential Tremor. *Arch. Phys. Med. Rehabil.* **2006**, *87*, 661–670. [CrossRef] [PubMed]
9. Norman, K.E.; D'Amboise, S.N.; Pari, G.; Héroux, M.E. Tremor during movement correlates well with disability in people with essential tremor. *Mov. Disord.* **2011**, *26*, 2088–2094. [CrossRef] [PubMed]
10. Rajput, A.H.; Robinson, C.A. Essential tremor course and disability: A clinicopathologic study of 20 cases. *Neurology* **2004**, *62*, 932–936. [CrossRef]
11. Louis, E.D.; Machado, D.G. Tremor-related quality of life: A comparison of essential tremor vs. Parkinson's disease patients. *Park. Relat. Disord.* **2015**, *21*, 729–735. [CrossRef] [PubMed]
12. Lorenz, D.; Schwieger, D.; Moises, H.; Deuschl, G. Quality of life and personality in essential tremor patients. *Mov. Disord.* **2006**, *21*, 1114–1118. [CrossRef]
13. Monin, J.K.; Gutierrez, J.; Kellner, S.; Morgan, S.; Collins, K.; Rohl, B.; Migliore, F.; Cosentino, S.; Huey, E.; Louis, E.D. Psychological Suffering in Essential Tremor: A Study of Patients and Those Who Are Close to Them. *Tremor Other Hyperkinetic Mov.* **2017**, *7*, 526. [CrossRef]
14. Schneier, F.R.; Barnes, L.F.; Albert, S.M.; Louis, E.D. Characteristics of Social Phobia among Persons with Essential Tremor. *J. Clin. Psychiatry* **2001**, *62*, 367–372. [CrossRef]
15. Damen, J.A.A.G. Author's reply to Woodward. *BMJ* **2016**, *354*, i4485. [CrossRef]
16. Elias, W.J.; Shah, B.B. Tremor. *JAMA* **2014**, *311*, 948–954. [CrossRef] [PubMed]
17. Zesiewicz, T.A.; Elble, R.; Louis, E.D.; Hauser, R.A.; Sullivan, K.L.; Dewey, R.B.; Ondo, W.G.; Gronseth, G.S.; Weiner, W.J. Practice Parameter: Therapies for essential tremor: Report of the Quality Standards Subcommittee of the American Academy of Neurology. *Neurology* **2005**, *64*, 2008–2020. [CrossRef]
18. Zesiewicz, T.A.; Elble, R.J.; Louis, E.D.; Gronseth, G.S.; Ondo, W.G.; Dewey, R.B.; Okun, M.S.; Sullivan, K.L.; Weiner, W.J. Evidence-based guideline update: Treatment of essential tremor: Report of the Quality Standards Subcommittee of the American Academy of Neurology. *Neurology* **2011**, *77*, 1752–1755. [CrossRef] [PubMed]
19. Ferreira, J.J.; Mestre, T.A.; Lyons, K.E.; Benito-León, J.; Tan, E.; Abbruzzese, G.; Hallett, M.; Haubenberger, D.; Elble, R.; Deuschl, G.; et al. MDS evidence-based review of treatments for essential tremor. *Mov. Disord.* **2019**, *34*, 950–958. [CrossRef]
20. O'Connor, R.J.; Kini, M.U. Non-pharmacological and non-surgical interventions for tremor: A systematic review. *Park. Relat. Disord.* **2011**, *17*, 509–515. [CrossRef]
21. Haubenberger, D.; Hallett, M. Essential Tremor. *N. Engl. J. Med.* **2018**, *378*, 1802–1810. [CrossRef]
22. Deuschl, G.; Raethjen, J.; Hellriegel, H.; Elble, R. Treatment of patients with essential tremor. *Lancet Neurol.* **2011**, *10*, 148–161. [CrossRef]
23. Diaz, N.L.; Louis, E.D. Survey of medication usage patterns among essential tremor patients: Movement disorder specialists vs. general neurologists. *Park. Relat. Disord.* **2010**, *16*, 604–607. [CrossRef] [PubMed]
24. Zappia, M.; Italian Movement Disorders Association (DISMOV-SIN) Essential Tremor Committee; Albanese, A.; Bruno, E.; Colosimo, C.; Filippini, G.; Martinelli, P.; Nicoletti, A.; Quattrocchi, G. Treatment of essential tremor: A systematic review of evidence and recommendations from the Italian Movement Disorders Association. *J. Neurol.* **2012**, *260*, 714–740. [CrossRef] [PubMed]

25. Velisar, A.; Syrkin-Nikolau, J.; Blumenfeld, Z.; Trager, M.; Afzal, M.; Prabhakar, V.; Bronte-Stewart, H. Dual threshold neural closed loop deep brain stimulation in Parkinson disease patients. *Brain Stimul.* **2019**, *12*, 868–876. [CrossRef]
26. Weerasinghe, G.; Duchet, B.; Cagnan, H.; Brown, P.; Bick, C.; Bogacz, R. Predicting the effects of deep brain stimulation using a reduced coupled oscillator model. *PLoS Comput. Biol.* **2019**, *15*, e1006575. [CrossRef] [PubMed]
27. Kern, D.S.; Picillo, M.; Thompson, J.A.; Sammartino, F.; Di Biase, L.; Munhoz, R.P.; Fasano, A. Interleaving Stimulation in Parkinson's Disease, Tremor, and Dystonia. *Ster. Funct. Neurosurg.* **2018**, *96*, 379–391. [CrossRef] [PubMed]
28. Chen, K.S.; Chen, R. Invasive and Noninvasive Brain Stimulation in Parkinson's Disease: Clinical Effects and Future Perspectives. *Clin. Pharmacol. Ther.* **2019**, *106*, 763–775. [CrossRef]
29. Farokhniaee, A.; McIntyre, C.C. Theoretical principles of deep brain stimulation induced synaptic suppression. *Brain Stimul.* **2019**, *12*, 1402–1409. [CrossRef]
30. Mao, Z.; Ling, Z.; Pan, L.; Xu, X.; Cui, Z.; Liang, S.; Yu, X. Comparison of Efficacy of Deep Brain Stimulation of Different Targets in Parkinson's Disease: A Network Meta-Analysis. *Front. Aging Neurosci.* **2019**, *11*, 23. [CrossRef] [PubMed]
31. Schuurman, P.R.; Bosch, D.A.; Bossuyt, P.M.; Bonsel, G.J.; Van Someren, E.J.; De Bie, R.M.; Merkus, M.P.; Speelman, J.D. A Comparison of Continuous Thalamic Stimulation and Thalamotomy for Suppression of Severe Tremor. *N. Engl. J. Med.* **2000**, *342*, 461–468. [CrossRef]
32. Elble, R.J.; Shih, L.; Cozzens, J.W. Surgical treatments for essential tremor. *Expert Rev. Neurother.* **2018**, *18*, 303–321. [CrossRef]
33. Ravikumar, V.K.; Parker, J.J.; Hornbeck, T.S.; Santini, V.E.; Pauly, K.B.; Wintermark, M.; Ghanouni, P.; Stein, S.C.; Halpern, C.H. Cost-effectiveness of focused ultrasound, radiosurgery, and DBS for essential tremor. *Mov. Disord.* **2017**, *32*, 1165–1173. [CrossRef]
34. Lozano, A.M.; Lipsman, N.; Bergman, H.; Brown, P.; Chabardes, S.; Chang, J.W.; Matthews, K.; McIntyre, C.C.; Schlaepfer, T.E.; Schulder, M.; et al. Deep brain stimulation: Current challenges and future directions. *Nat. Rev. Neurol.* **2019**, *15*, 148–160. [CrossRef] [PubMed]
35. Walters, H.; Shah, B.B. Focused Ultrasound and Other Lesioning Therapies in Movement Disorders. *Curr. Neurol. Neurosci. Rep.* **2019**, *19*, 66. [CrossRef] [PubMed]
36. Chan, A.K.; McGovern, R.A.; Brown, L.T.; Sheehy, J.P.; Zacharia, B.E.; Mikell, C.B.; Bruce, S.S.; Ford, B.; McKhann, G.M. Disparities in Access to Deep Brain Stimulation Surgery for Parkinson Disease. *JAMA Neurol.* **2014**, *71*, 291–299. [CrossRef]
37. Lange, M.; Mauerer, J.; Schlaier, J.; Janzen, A.; Zeman, F.; Bogdahn, U.; Brawanski, A.; Hochreiter, A. Underutilization of deep brain stimulation for Parkinson's disease? A survey on possible clinical reasons. *Acta Neurochir.* **2017**, *159*, 771–778. [CrossRef] [PubMed]
38. Shukla, A.W.; Deeb, W.; Patel, B.; Ramirez-Zamora, A. Is deep brain stimulation therapy underutilized for movement disorders? *Expert Rev. Neurother.* **2018**, *18*, 899–901. [CrossRef]
39. Kim, M.-R.; Yun, J.Y.; Jeon, B.; Lim, Y.H.; Kim, K.R.; Yang, H.-J.; Paek, S.H. Patients' reluctance to undergo deep brain stimulation for Parkinson's disease. *Park. Relat. Disord.* **2016**, *23*, 91–94. [CrossRef]
40. Food and Drug Administration. Medical Devices; Neurological Devices; Classification of the External Upper Limb Tremor Stimulator. Final order. *Fed. Regist.* **2018**, *83*, 52315–52316.
41. Beringhause, S.; Rosen, M.; Huang, S. Evaluation of a damped joystick for people disabled by intention tremor. In Proceedings of the 12th Annual Conference on Rehabilitation Technology, New Orleans, LA, USA, 25–30 June 1989; pp. 41–42.
42. Hendriks, J.; Rosen, M.; Berube, N.; Aisen, M. A second-generation joystick for people disabled by tremor. In Proceedings of the 14th Annual RESNA Conference, Kansas City, MO, USA, 21–26 June 1991; pp. 248–251.
43. Rosen, M.J. Tremor Suppressing Hand Controls. U.S. Patent 4,689,449, 25 August 1987.
44. Rosen, M.J. Multiple Degree of Freedom Damped Hand Controls. U.S. Patent 5,107,080, 21 April 1992.
45. Arnold, A.S.; Rosen, M.J.; Aisen, M.L. Evaluation of a controlled-energy-dissipation orthosis for tremor suppression. *J. Electromyogr. Kinesiol.* **1993**, *3*, 131–148. [CrossRef]
46. Rosen, M.J.; Arnold, A.S.; Baiges, I.J.; Aisen, M.L.; Eglowstein, S.R. Design of a controlled-energy-dissipation orthosis (CEDO) for functional suppression of intention tremors. *J. Rehabil. Res. Dev.* **1995**, *32*, 1–16. [PubMed]
47. Rosen, M.J.; Baiges, I.J. Whole-Arm Orthosis for Steadying Limb Motion. U.S. Patent 5,231,998, 3 August 1993.
48. Maxwell, S.M. A Modulated-Energy-Dissipation Manipulator and Application to Suppressing Human Arm Tremor. Ph.D. Thesis, Massachusetts Institute of Technology, Cambridge, MA, USA, 1990.
49. Maxwell, S.M. A System for Resisting Limb Movement. EP Patent 0,569,489 B1, 10 May 1995.
50. Johnson, M. Transcutaneous Electrical Nerve Stimulation: Mechanisms, Clinical Application and Evidence. *Rev. Pain* **2007**, *1*, 7–11. [CrossRef] [PubMed]
51. Gibson, W.; Wand, B.M.; Meads, C.; Catley, M.J.; E O'Connell, N. Transcutaneous electrical nerve stimulation (TENS) for chronic pain—An overview of Cochrane Reviews. *Cochrane Database Syst. Rev.* **2019**, *4*, CD011890. [CrossRef] [PubMed]
52. Johnson, M.I.; Paley, C.A.; Howe, T.E.; Sluka, K.A. Transcutaneous electrical nerve stimulation for acute pain. *Cochrane Database Syst. Rev.* **2015**, *6*, CD006142. [CrossRef]
53. Gibson, W.; Wand, B.M.; E O'Connell, N. Transcutaneous electrical nerve stimulation (TENS) for neuropathic pain in adults. *Cochrane Database Syst. Rev.* **2017**, *2017*, 011976. [CrossRef]
54. Toglia, J.U.; Izzo, K. Treatment of myoclonic dystonia with transcutaneous electrical nerve stimulation. *Neurol. Sci.* **1985**, *6*, 75–78. [CrossRef]

55. Campbell, J.N.; Raja, S.N.; Meyer, R.A.; MacKinnon, S.E. Myelinated afferents signal the hyperalgesia associated with nerve injury. *Pain* **1988**, *32*, 89–94. [CrossRef]
56. Truini, A.; Padua, L.; Biasiotta, A.; Caliandro, P.; Pazzaglia, C.; Galeotti, F.; Inghilleri, M.; Cruccu, G. Differential involvement of A-delta and A-beta fibres in neuropathic pain related to carpal tunnel syndrome. *Pain* **2009**, *145*, 105–109. [CrossRef]
57. Xu, Z.-Z.; Kim, Y.H.; Bang, S.; Zhang, Y.; Berta, T.; Wang, F.; Oh, S.B.; Ji, R.-R. Inhibition of mechanical allodynia in neuropathic pain by TLR5-mediated A-fiber blockade. *Nat. Med.* **2015**, *21*, 1326–1331. [CrossRef]
58. Nagi, S.S.; Marshall, A.G.; Makdani, A.; Jarocka, E.; Liljencrantz, J.; Ridderström, M.; Shaikh, S.; O'Neill, F.; Saade, D.; Donkervoort, S.; et al. An ultrafast system for signaling mechanical pain in human skin. *Sci. Adv.* **2019**, *5*, eaaw1297. [CrossRef]
59. Garcia, K.; Wray, J.K.; Kumar, S. *Spinal Cord Stimulation, StatPearls*; StatPearls Publishing: Treasure Island, FL, USA, 2020.
60. Ferrara, J.; Stamey, W.; Strutt, A.M.; Adam, O.R.; Jankovic, J. Transcutaneous Electrical Stimulation (TENS) for Psychogenic Movement Disorders. *J. Neuropsychiatry Clin. Neurosci.* **2011**, *23*, 141–148. [CrossRef]
61. Serrano-Muñoz, D.; Avendaño-Coy, J.; Simón-Martínez, C.; Taylor, J.; Gómez-Soriano, J. Effect of high-frequency alternating current transcutaneous stimulation over muscle strength: A controlled pilot study. *J. Neuroeng. Rehabil.* **2018**, *15*, 1–4. [CrossRef]
62. Hao, M.-Z.; Xu, S.-Q.; Hu, Z.-X.; Xu, F.-L.; Niu, C.-X.M.; Xiao, Q.; Lan, N. Inhibition of Parkinsonian tremor with cutaneous afferent evoked by transcutaneous electrical nerve stimulation. *J. Neuroeng. Rehabil.* **2017**, *14*, 75. [CrossRef] [PubMed]
63. Hao, M.-Z.; He, X.; Kipke, D.R.; Lan, N. Effects of electrical stimulation of cutaneous afferents on corticospinal transmission of tremor signals in patients with Parkinson's disease. In Proceedings of the 2013 6th International IEEE/EMBS Conference on Neural Engineering (NER), San Diego, CA, USA, 6–8 November 2013.
64. Munhoz, R.P.; Hanajima, R.; Ashby, P.; Lang, A.E. Acute effect of transcutaneous electrical nerve stimulation on tremor. *Mov. Disord.* **2002**, *18*, 191–194. [CrossRef] [PubMed]
65. U.S. National Library of Medicine. Prospective Study for Symptomatic Relief of ET with Cala Therapy (PROSPECT). 2018. Available online: https://clinicaltrials.gov/ct2/show/NCT03597100 (accessed on 20 July 2020).
66. Hanajima, R. Somatosensory evoked potentials (SEPs) recorded from deep brain stimulation (DBS) electrodes in the thalamus and subthalamic nucleus (STN). *Clin. Neurophysiol.* **2004**, *115*, 424–434. [CrossRef] [PubMed]
67. Hanajima, R.; Chen, R.; Ashby, P.; Lozano, A.M.; Hutchison, W.D.; Davis, K.D.; Dostrovsky, J.O. Very Fast Oscillations Evoked by Median Nerve Stimulation in the Human Thalamus and Subthalamic Nucleus. *J. Neurophysiol.* **2004**, *92*, 3171–3182. [CrossRef] [PubMed]
68. Bathien, N.; Rondot, P.; Toma, S. Inhibition and synchronisation of tremor induced by a muscle twitch. *J. Neurol. Neurosurg. Psychiatry* **1980**, *43*, 713–718. [CrossRef] [PubMed]
69. Dosen, S.; Muceli, S.; Dideriksen, J.L.; Romero, J.P.; Rocon, E.; Pons, J.; Farina, D. Online Tremor Suppression Using Electromyography and Low-Level Electrical Stimulation. *IEEE Trans. Neural Syst. Rehabil. Eng.* **2014**, *23*, 385–395. [CrossRef] [PubMed]
70. Pahwa, R.; Dhall, R.; Ostrem, J.; Gwinn, R.; Lyons, K.; Ro, S.; Dietiker, C.; Luthra, N.; Ms, P.C.; Hamner, S.; et al. An Acute Randomized Controlled Trial of Noninvasive Peripheral Nerve Stimulation in Essential Tremor. *Neuromodulation* **2018**, *22*, 537–545. [CrossRef] [PubMed]
71. Isaacson, S.H.; Peckham, E.; Tse, W.; Waln, O.; Way, C.; Petrossian, M.T.; Dahodwala, N.; Soileau, M.J.; Lew, M.; Dietiker, C.; et al. Prospective Home-use Study on Non-invasive Neuromodulation Therapy for Essential Tremor. *Tremor Other Hyperkinetic Mov.* **2020**, *10*, 29. [CrossRef]
72. Elek, J.; Prochazka, A. Attenuation of wrist tremor with closed-loop electrical stimulation of muscles. *J. Physiol.* **1989**, *414*, 17P.
73. Javidan, M.; Elek, J.; Prochazka, A. Tremor reduction by functional electrical stimulation. *Neurology* **1990**, *40*, 369.
74. Prochazka, A.; Elek, J.; Javidan, M. Attenuation of pathological tremors by functional electrical stimulation I: Method. *Ann. Biomed. Eng.* **1992**, *20*, 205–224. [CrossRef]
75. Javidan, M.; Elek, J.; Prochazka, A. Attenuation of pathological tremors by functional electrical stimulation II: Clinical evaluation. *Ann. Biomed. Eng.* **1992**, *20*, 225–236. [CrossRef] [PubMed]
76. Law, J.J. Reduction of Pathological Tremor by Functional Electrical Stimulation Using Digital Feedback Control. Master's Thesis, University of Alberta, Edmonton, AB, Canada, 1995.
77. Gillard, D.; Cameron, T.; Prochazka, A.; Gauthier, M. Tremor suppression using functional electrical stimulation: A comparison between digital and analog controllers. *IEEE Trans. Rehabil. Eng.* **1999**, *7*, 385–388. [CrossRef]
78. Dideriksen, J.L.; Laine, C.M.; Dosen, S.; Muceli, S.; Rocon, E.; Pons, J.L.; Benito-Leon, J.; Farina, D. Electrical Stimulation of Afferent Pathways for the Suppression of Pathological Tremor. *Front. Neurosci.* **2017**, *11*, 178. [CrossRef]
79. Maneski, L.P.; Jorgovanović, N.; Ilić, V.; Došen, S.; Keller, T.; Popović, M.B.; Popović, D.B. Electrical stimulation for the suppression of pathological tremor. *Med. Biol. Eng. Comput.* **2011**, *49*, 1187–1193. [CrossRef]
80. Popović, D.; Popović-Maneski, L. The Instrumented Shoe Insole for Rule-Based Control of Gait in Persons with Hemiplegia. *EasyChair Prepr.* 2019, p. 1345. Available online: https://easychair.org/publications/preprint/ZF3Z (accessed on 26 March 2021).
81. Gallego, J.Á.; Rocon, E.; Belda-Lois, J.M.; Pons, J.L. A neuroprosthesis for tremor management through the control of muscle co-contraction. *J. Neuroeng. Rehabil.* **2013**, *10*, 36. [CrossRef]
82. Jitkritsadakul, O.; Thanawattano, C.; Anan, C.; Bhidayasiri, R. Tremor's glove-an innovative electrical muscle stimulation therapy for intractable tremor in Parkinson's disease: A randomized sham-controlled trial. *J. Neurol. Sci.* **2017**, *381*, 331–340. [CrossRef] [PubMed]

83. Meunier, S.; Pol, S.; Houeto, J.L.; Vidailhet, M. Abnormal reciprocal inhibition between antagonist muscles in Parkinson's disease. *Brain* **2000**, *123*, 1017–1026. [CrossRef]
84. Heo, J.-H.; Jeon, H.-M.; Choi, E.-B.; Kwon, D.-Y.; Eom, G.-M. Effect of Sensory Electrical Stimulation on Resting Tremors in Patients with Parkinson's Disease and SWEDDS. *J. Mech. Med. Biol.* **2019**, *19*, 1940033. [CrossRef]
85. Bickel, C.S.; Gregory, C.M.; Dean, J.C. Motor unit recruitment during neuromuscular electrical stimulation: A critical appraisal. *Graefe's Arch. Clin. Exp. Ophthalmol.* **2011**, *111*, 2399–2407. [CrossRef] [PubMed]
86. Martin, R.; Sadowsky, C.; Obst, K.; Meyer, B.; McDonald, J. Functional Electrical Stimulation in Spinal Cord Injury: From Theory to Practice. *Top. Spinal Cord Inj. Rehabil.* **2012**, *18*, 28–33. [CrossRef]
87. Terry, T.E.; Hoyt, L.J., Sr. Cerebral Palsy Arm and Hand Brace. U.S. Patent 4,237,873, 9 December 1980.
88. Kotovsky, J.; Rosen, M.J. A wearable tremor-suppression orthosis. *J. Rehabil. Res. Dev.* **1998**, *35*, 373–387. [PubMed]
89. Rocon, E.; Ruiz, A.; Pons, J.L.; Belda-Lois, J.; Sánchez-Lacuesta, J. Rehabilitation Robotics: A Wearable Exo-Skeleton for Tremor Assessment and Suppression. In Proceedings of the Proceedings of the 2005 IEEE International Conference on Robotics and Automation, Barcelona, Spain, 18–22 April 2005.
90. Rocon, E.; Ruiz, A.; Brunetti, F.; Pons, J.L.; Belda-Lois, J.; Sánchez-Lacuesta, J. On the use of an active wearable exoskeleton for tremor suppression via biomechanical loading. In Proceedings of the 2006 IEEE International Conference on Robotics and Automation, Orlando, FL, USA, 15–19 May 2006.
91. Manto, M.; Rocon, E.; Pons, J.L.; Belda, J.M.; Camut, S. Evaluation of a wearable orthosis and an associated algorithm for tremor suppression. *Physiol. Meas.* **2007**, *28*, 415–425. [CrossRef]
92. Rocón, E.; Belda-Lois, J.M.; Ruiz, A.; Manto, M.; Moreno, J.C.; Pons, J.L. Design and Validation of a Rehabilitation Robotic Exoskeleton for Tremor Assessment and Suppression. *IEEE Trans. Neural Syst. Rehabil. Eng.* **2007**, *15*, 367–378. [CrossRef]
93. Taheri, B.; Case, D.; Richer, E. Active Tremor Estimation and Suppression in Human Elbow Joint. In Proceedings of the ASME 2011 Dynamic Systems and Control Conference, Arlington, VI, USA, 31 October–2 November 2011.
94. Taheri, B.; Case, D.; Richer, E. Robust Controller for Tremor Suppression at Musculoskeletal Level in Human Wrist. *IEEE Trans. Neural Syst. Rehabil. Eng.* **2013**, *22*, 379–388. [CrossRef]
95. Taheri, B.; Case, D.; Richer, E. Adaptive Suppression of Severe Pathological Tremor by Torque Estimation Method. *IEEE/ASME Trans. Mechatron.* **2014**, *20*, 717–727. [CrossRef]
96. Zamanian, A.H.; Richer, E. Adaptive disturbance rejection controller for pathological tremor suppression with permanent magnet linear motor. In Proceedings of the ASME 2017 Dynamic Systems and Control Conference, Tysons, VI, USA, 11–13 October 2017.
97. Herrnstadt, G.; Menon, C. Voluntary-Driven Elbow Orthosis with Speed-Controlled Tremor Suppression. *Front. Bioeng. Biotechnol.* **2016**, *4*, 29. [CrossRef]
98. Zhou, Y.; Naish, M.D.; Jenkins, M.E.; Trejos, A.L. Design and validation of a novel mechatronic transmission system for a wearable tremor suppression device. *Robot. Auton. Syst.* **2017**, *91*, 38–48. [CrossRef]
99. Ando, T.; Watanabe, M.; Fujie, M.G. Extraction of voluntary movement for an EMG controlled exoskeltal robot of tremor patients. In Proceedings of the 2009 4th International IEEE/EMBS Conference on Neural Engineering, Antalya, Turkey, 29 April–2 May 2009.
100. Seki, M.; Matsumoto, Y.; Ando, T.; Kobayashi, Y.; Fujie, M.G.; Iijima, H.; Nagaoka, M. Development of robotic upper limb orthosis with tremor suppressiblity and elbow joint movability. In Proceedings of the 2011 IEEE International Conference on Systems, Man, and Cybernetics, Anchorage, AK, USA, 9–12 October 2011.
101. Seki, M.; Matsumoto, Y.; Ando, T.; Kobayashi, Y.; Iijima, H.; Nagaoka, M.; Fujie, M.G. The weight load inconsistency effect on voluntary movement recognition of essential tremor patient. In Proceedings of the 2011 IEEE International Conference on Robotics and Biomimetics, Karon Beach, Thailand, 7–11 December 2011.
102. Ando, T.; Watanabe, M.; Nishimoto, K.; Matsumoto, Y.; Seki, M.; Fujie, M.G. Myoelectric-Controlled Exoskeletal Elbow Robot to Suppress Essential Tremor: Extraction of Elbow Flexion Movement Using STFTs and TDNN. *J. Robot. Mechatron.* **2012**, *24*, 141–149. [CrossRef]
103. Matsumoto, Y.; Amemiya, M.; Kaneishi, D.; Nakashima, Y.; Seki, M.; Ando, T.; Kobayashi, Y.; Iijima, H.; Nagaoka, M.; Fujie, M.G. Development of an elbow-forearm interlock joint mechanism toward an exoskeleton for patients with essential tremor. In Proceedings of the 2014 IEEE/RSJ International Conference on Intelligent Robots and Systems, Chicago, IL, USA, 14–18 September 2014.
104. Matsumoto, Y.; Seki, M.; Ando, T.; Kobayashi, Y.; Nakashima, Y.; Iijima, H.; Nagaoka, M.; Fujie, M.G. Development of an Exoskeleton to Support Eating Movements in Patients with Essential Tremor. *J. Robot. Mechatron.* **2013**, *25*, 949–958. [CrossRef]
105. Huen, D.; Liu, J.; Lo, B. An integrated wearable robot for tremor suppression with context aware sensing. In Proceedings of the 2016 IEEE 13th International Conference on Wearable and Implantable Body Sensor Networks (BSN), San Francisco, CA, USA, 14–17 June 2016.
106. Fromme, N.P.; Camenzind, M.; Riener, R.; Rossi, R.M. Need for mechanically and ergonomically enhanced tremor-suppression orthoses for the upper limb: A systematic review. *J. Neuroeng. Rehabil.* **2019**, *16*, 1–15. [CrossRef]
107. Loureiro, R.; Belda-Lois, J.M.; Lima, E.; Pons, J.; Sanchez-Lacuesta, J.; Harwin, W.S. Upper Limb Tremor Suppression in ADL Via an Orthosis Incorporating a Controllable Double Viscous Beam Actuator. In Proceedings of the 9th International Conference on Rehabilitation Robotics, Chicago, IL, USA, 28 June–1 July 2005.
108. Case, D.; Taheri, B.; Richer, E. Dynamic Magnetorheological Damper for Othotic Tremor Suppression. In Proceedings of the 2011 Hawaii University International Conference on Mathematics and Engineering, Honolulu, HI, USA, 13–15 June 2011.

109. Case, D.; Taheri, B.; Richer, E. Multiphysics modeling of magnetorheological dampers. *Int. J. Multiphysics* **2013**, *7*, 61–76. [CrossRef]
110. Case, D.; Taheri, B.; Richer, E. A Lumped-Parameter Model for Adaptive Dynamic MR Damper Control. *IEEE ASME Trans. Mechatron.* **2014**, *20*, 1–8. [CrossRef]
111. Case, D.; Taheri, B.; Richer, E. Active control of MR wearable robotic orthosis for pathological tremor suppression. In Proceedings of the ASME 2015 Dynamic Systems and Control Conference, Columbus, OH, USA, 28–30 October 2015.
112. Zahedi, A.; Zhang, B.; Yi, A.; Zhang, D. A Soft Exoskeleton for Tremor Suppression Equipped with Flexible Semiactive Actuator. *Soft Robot.* **2020**. [CrossRef] [PubMed]
113. Herrnstadt, G.; Menon, C. On-Off Tremor Suppression Orthosis with Electromagnetic Brake. *Int. J. Mech. Eng. Mechatron.* **2013**, *1*, 7–14. [CrossRef]
114. Kalaiarasi, A.; Kumar, L.A. Sensor Based Portable Tremor Suppression Device for Stroke Patients. *Electrother. Res.* **2018**, *43*, 29–37. [CrossRef]
115. Rudraraju, S.; Nguyen, T. Wearable Tremor Reduction Device (TRD) for Human Hands and Arms. In Proceedings of the 2018 Design of Medical Devices Conference, Minneapolis, MI, USA, 9–12 April 2018.
116. Elias, M.; Patel, S.; Maamary, E.; Araneta, L.; Obaid, N. Apparatus for Damping Involuntary Hand Motions. U.S. Patent 0,216,628 A1, 18 July 2019.
117. Hunter, R.; Pivach, L.; Madere, K.; Van Gemmert, A.W.A. Potential benefits of the Readi-Steadi on essential tremor. In Proceedings of the 5th Annual LSU Discover Day, Baton Rouge, LA, USA, 10 April 2018.
118. Paulig, J.; Jabusch, H.-C.; Groäÿbach, M.; Boullet, L.; Altenmüller, E. Sensory trick phenomenon improves motor control in pianists with dystonia: Prognostic value of glove-effect. *Front. Psychol.* **2014**, *5*, 1012. [CrossRef]
119. Fromme, N.P.; Camenzind, M.; Riener, R.; Rossi, R.M. Design of a lightweight passive orthosis for tremor suppression. *J. Neuroeng. Rehabil.* **2020**, *17*, 1–15. [CrossRef]
120. Lu, Z.; Huang, Z. Analytical and experimental studies on particle damper used for tremor suppression. *J. Vib. Control* **2020**, 1–11. [CrossRef]
121. Katz, R.; Buki, E.; Zacksenhouse, M. Attenuating Tremor Using Passive Devices. *Stud. Health Technol. Inform.* **2017**, *242*, 741–747.
122. Buki, E.; Katz, R.; Zacksenhouse, M.; Schlesinger, I. Vib-bracelet: A passive absorber for attenuating forearm tremor. *Med Biol. Eng. Comput.* **2017**, *56*, 923–930. [CrossRef] [PubMed]
123. Takanokura, M.; Sugahara, R.; Miyake, N.; Ishiguro, K.; Muto, T.; Sakamoto, K. Upper-limb orthoses implemented with air dashpots for suppression of pathological tremor in daily activities. In Proceedings of the 23rd Congress of International Society of Biomechanics, Brussels, Belgium, 2–3 July 2011.
124. Lusardi, M.M. Tremor, chorea and other involuntary movement. In *Geriatric Rehabilitation Manual*, 2nd ed.; Kauffman, T., Barr, J., Moran, M., Eds.; Elsevier: New York, NY, USA, 2007; pp. 215–225.
125. Kelley, C.R.; Kauffman, J.L. Tremor-Active Controller for Dielectric Elastomer-Based Pathological Tremor Suppression. *IEEE/ASME Trans. Mechatron.* **2020**, *25*, 1143–1148. [CrossRef]
126. Kelley, C.R.; Kauffman, J.L. Scaled Tremor Suppression with Folded Dielectric Elastomer Stack Actuators. In *Electroactive Polymer Actuators and Devices (EAPAD) XXII*; International Society for Optics and Photonics: Bellingham, WA, USA, 2020. [CrossRef]
127. Michaelis, J. Introducing the neater eater. *Action Res.* **1988**, *6*, 2–3.
128. Mandy, A.; Sims, T.; Stew, G.; Onions, D. Manual Feeding Device Experiences of People with a Neurodisability. *Am. J. Occup. Ther.* **2018**, *72*, 7203345010p1–7203345010p5. [CrossRef]
129. Pathak, A.; Redmond, J.A.; Allen, M.; Chou, K.L. A noninvasive handheld assistive device to accommodate essential tremor: A pilot study. *Mov. Disord.* **2013**, *29*, 838–842. [CrossRef]
130. Sabari, J.; Stefanov, D.G.; Chan, J.; Goed, L.; Starr, J. Adapted Feeding Utensils for People With Parkinson's-Related or Essential Tremor. *Am. J. Occup. Ther.* **2019**, *73*, 7302205120p1–7302205120p9. [CrossRef] [PubMed]
131. Zhu, Y.; Ren, K. Arm Vibration Damping Device. U.S. Patent 0,327,023 A1, 16 November 2017.
132. De Panisse, P.; Ibrahim, Y.; Medeisis, J.; Tiarvando, L.; Vaklev, N.L.; Ong, J.F.; Gan, B.; Koh, B.; Soler, X.L.; Choong Ngan Lou, W. Tremor Stabilization Apparatus and Methods. U.S. Patent 0266820 A1, 20 September 2018.
133. Hall, W.D. Hand-Held Gyroscopic Device. U.S. Patent 5,058,571 A, 22 October 1991.
134. Kalvert, M.A. Adjustable and Tunable Hand Tremor Stabilizer. U.S. Patent 6,730,049 B2, 4 May 2004.
135. Ferrington, D.G.; Nail, B.S.; Rowe, M. Human tactile detection thresholds: Modification by inputs from specific tactile receptor classes. *J. Physiol.* **1977**, *272*, 415–433. [CrossRef]
136. Douglas, P.R.; Ferrington, D.G.; Rowe, M. Coding of information about tactile stimuli by neurones of the cuneate nucleus. *J. Physiol.* **1978**, *285*, 493–513. [CrossRef] [PubMed]
137. Uemura, Y.; Haque, T.; Sato, F.; Tsutsumi, Y.; Ohara, H.; Oka, A.; Furuta, T.; Bae, Y.C.; Yamashiro, T.; Tachibana, Y.; et al. Proprioceptive thalamus receiving forelimb and neck muscle spindle inputs via the external cuneate nucleus in the rat. *Brain Struct. Funct.* **2020**, *225*, 2177–2192. [CrossRef]
138. Tracey, D.J. The projection of joint receptors to the cuneate nucleus in the cat. *J. Physiol.* **1980**, *305*, 433–449. [CrossRef] [PubMed]
139. Lora-Millán, J.S.; López-Blanco, R.; Gallego, J.Á.; Méndez-Guerrero, A.; de La Aleja, J.G.; Rocon, E. Mechanical vibration does not systematically reduce the tremor in essential tremor patients. *Sci. Rep.* **2019**, *9*, 1–11. [CrossRef]

140. Louis, E.D. The Roles of Age and Aging in Essential Tremor: An Epidemiological Perspective. *Neuroepidemiology* **2019**, *52*, 111–118. [CrossRef]
141. Louis, E.D.; Ford, B.; Barnes, L.F. Clinical subtypes of essential tremor. *Arch. Neurol.* **2000**, *57*, 1194–1198. [CrossRef]
142. Benito-León, J.; Louis, E.D.; Bermejo-Pareja, F. Elderly-onset essential tremor is associated with dementia. *Neurology* **2006**, *66*, 1500–1505. [CrossRef] [PubMed]
143. Hanagasi, H.A.; Tufekcioglu, Z.; Emre, M. Dementia in Parkinson's disease. *J. Neurol. Sci.* **2017**, *374*, 26–31. [CrossRef]
144. Park, I.-S.; Oh, Y.-S.; Lee, K.-S.; Yang, D.-W.; Song, I.-U.; Park, J.-W.; Kim, J.-S. Subtype of Mild Cognitive Impairment in Elderly Patients with Essential Tremor. *Alzheimer Dis. Assoc. Disord.* **2015**, *29*, 141–145. [CrossRef] [PubMed]
145. Benito-León, J.; Louis, E.D.; Mitchell, A.J.; Bermejo-Pareja, F. Elderly-Onset Essential Tremor and Mild Cognitive Impairment: A Population-Based Study (NEDICES). *J. Alzheimer's Dis.* **2011**, *23*, 727–735. [CrossRef]
146. Monastero, R.; Cicero, C.E.; Baschi, R.; Davì, M.; Luca, A.; Restivo, V.; Zangara, C.; Fierro, B.; Zappia, M.; Nicoletti, A. Mild cognitive impairment in Parkinson's disease: The Parkinson's disease cognitive study (PACOS). *J. Neurol.* **2018**, *265*, 1050–1058. [CrossRef] [PubMed]
147. Frost & Sullivan. Assessing the Full Impact of Essential Tremor on Patient Quality of Life and Finances in the United States. 2018. Available online: https://www.insightec.com/media/1550/fs_wp_insightec-et_010819.pdf (accessed on 20 September 2020).
148. Axelrad, J.E.; Louis, E.D.; Honig, L.S.; Flores, I.; Ross, G.W.; Pahwa, R.; Lyons, K.E.; Faust, P.L.; Vonsattel, J.P.G. Reduced Purkinje Cell Number in Essential Tremor. *Arch. Neurol.* **2008**, *65*, 101–107. [CrossRef] [PubMed]
149. Louis, E.D.; Lee, M.; Babij, R.; Ma, K.; Cortés, E.; Vonsattel, J.-P.G.; Faust, P.L. Reduced Purkinje cell dendritic arborization and loss of dendritic spines in essential tremor. *Brain* **2014**, *137*, 3142–3148. [CrossRef]
150. Helmich, R.C.; Janssen, M.J.R.; Oyen, W.J.G.; Bloem, B.R.; Toni, I. Pallidal dysfunction drives a cerebellothalamic circuit into Parkinson tremor. *Ann. Neurol.* **2011**, *69*, 269–281. [CrossRef] [PubMed]
151. Espay, A.J.; Lang, A.E.; Erro, R.; Merola, A.; Fasano, A.; Berardelli, A.; Bhatia, K.P. Essential pitfalls in "essential" tremor. *Mov. Disord.* **2017**, *32*, 325–331. [CrossRef] [PubMed]

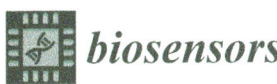

Article

Arteriovenous Fistula Flow Dysfunction Surveillance: Early Detection Using Pulse Radar Sensor and Machine Learning Classification

Cheng-Hsu Chen [1,2,3,4], Teh-Ho Tao [5,*], Yi-Hua Chou [6], Ya-Wen Chuang [1,3] and Tai-Been Chen [7,8,*]

1. Division of Nephrology, Department of Internal Medicine, Taichung Veterans General Hospital, Taichung City 40705, Taiwan; cschen@vghtc.gov.tw (C.-H.C.); coladr@yahoo.com.tw (Y.-W.C.)
2. Department of Life Sciences, Tunghai University, Taichung City 40724, Taiwan
3. School of Medicine, China Medical University, Taichung City 40640, Taiwan
4. College of Medicine, National Chung Hsing University, Taichung City 40227, Taiwan
5. Finedar Biomedical Technology Co., Ltd., Hsinchu City 30069, Taiwan
6. Center of Hemodialysis, Department of Nursing, Taichung Veterans General Hospital, Taichung City 40705, Taiwan; cihua544@gmail.com
7. Department of Medical Imaging and Radiological Science, I-Shou University, Kaohsiung City 82445, Taiwan
8. Institute of Statistics, National Yang Ming Chiao Tung University, Hsinchu 30010, Taiwan
* Correspondence: tht@finedarbtc.com (T.-H.T.); ctb@isu.edu.tw (T.-B.C.); Tel.: +886-7-6151100 (ext. 7516) (T.-B.C.); Fax: +886-7-6151100 (ext. 7802) (T.-B.C.)

Abstract: Vascular Access (VA) is often referred to as the "Achilles heel" for a Hemodialysis (HD)-dependent patient. Both the patent and sufficient VA provide adequacy for performing dialysis and reducing dialysis-related complications, while on the contrary, insufficient VA is the main reason for recurrent hospitalizations, high morbidity, and high mortality in HD patients. A non-invasive Vascular Wall Motion (VWM) monitoring system, made up of a pulse radar sensor and Support Vector Machine (SVM) classification algorithm, has been developed to detect access flow dysfunction in Arteriovenous Fistula (AVF). The harmonic ratios derived from the Fast Fourier Transform (FFT) spectrum-based signal processing technique were employed as the input features for the SVM classifier. The result of a pilot clinical trial showed that a more accurate prediction of AVF flow dysfunction could be achieved by the VWM monitor as compared with the Ultrasound Dilution (UD) flow monitor. Receiver Operating Characteristic (ROC) curve analysis showed that the SVM classification algorithm achieved a detection specificity of 100% at detection thresholds in the range from 500 to 750 mL/min and a maximum sensitivity of 95.2% at a detection threshold of 750 mL/min.

Keywords: arteriovenous fistula; SVM; harmonic ratio; vascular wall motion monitor

1. Introduction

The National Kidney Foundation Kidney Disease Outcomes Quality Initiative (NKF-K/DOQI) guidelines suggest two monitoring methods for VA flow surveillance, physical examination, and the measuring of arteriovenous VA flow through special equipment [1]. Guideline 13 of the NKF-K/DOQI specifically states that the underlying cause of AV access flow dysfunction is either stenosis or thrombosis. Hence, the purpose of flow dysfunction surveillance is to detect stenosis early on before the development of thrombosis, which then requires surgical intervention to replace the AV access.

Amongst the current monitoring instruments available, the Ultrasound Dilution (UD) flow monitoring instrument has been extensively studied. For example, the benefits of AV Fistula (AVF) flow surveillance using the UD measurement was studied [2], where the effectiveness of UD measurement in detecting stenosis and predicting thrombosis was investigated [3–5]. Our clinical experience regarding the application of the UD measurement technique shows that it is limited due to its cost, the disposable consumables used, and its dependence on the operator's experience with the instruments. However, through the use of skillful operation techniques, it has been accepted as a reference standard for AV access flow surveillance.

Studies have been performed surrounding the use of optical sensor and machine learning algorithms for the detection of stenosis or flow dysfunction. However, either two finger Photoplethysmography (PPG) sensors were used, which may cause measurement uncertainties [6] or additional physiological measurements other than the PPG signal were required as input features for classification of the algorithm [7,8]. Phono-angiography employs a digital stethoscope to record bruit sounds in the AVF. However, four locations are required in order to search for the most probable stenosis site [9,10]. Therefore, for the most part, detection sensitivity and specificity of the aforementioned methods do not meet the requirements for them to be reliable monitoring instruments. A qualified monitoring technique should possess standardized diagnostic thresholds, as well as sufficient sensitivity and specificity for the detection of flow dysfunction.

The physical examination techniques for VA flow surveillance include inspection, palpation (pulse, thrill), and auscultation (bruit) [1]. One of the clinical indicators for VA flow dysfunction is alterations in the pulse characteristics such as weak and persistent pulses which are difficult to compress in the area of stenosis. Although recommended by the NKF-K/DOQI guidelines, the technique of pulse palpation relies upon the subjective experiences of the examiner. Studies performed on the hemodynamics of stenosis in arteries were reviewed [11]. In a stenotic blood vessel, turbulent blood flow is generated approximately 1.5 to 6.0 diameters downstream from the site of stenosis. Finite element numerical simulation was employed to investigate pulsatile and turbulent blood flow in an elastic artery with single as well as double stenosis, with the results showing that the displacement of the arterial walls in the pre-stenotic regions was higher than that in the post-stenotic regions [12]. Raminari et al. investigated the potential clinical application of ultrasound Tissue Doppler Imaging (TDI) of arterial wall motion in order to quantify simple wall motion indices in normal and diseased carotid arteries. Their results showed a wide variation in arterial wall motion indices across the stenotic region. However, their experimental data showed noticeable changes in the morphology of the diseased arterial wall motion waveforms when compared to those of normal arteries [13]. The aforementioned studies demonstrate that stenosis of the arterial blood vessel, which is the underlying cause of flow dysfunction, can be detected by analyzing the characteristic changes in the waveform of arterial wall motion.

In the present work, the spectral analysis technique was adopted by analyzing the variations in the spectrum of the distorted VWM waveform due to the AVF flow dysfunction. A machine learning algorithm based on Support Vector Machines (SVM) was chosen to classify the spectrum data of VWM monitoring data. Through a comparison with the corresponding UD flow measurements, the performance of the SVM classifier was evaluated in terms of its detecting sensitivity, specificity, and accuracy.

2. Materials and Methods

2.1. The Sensing Device and System

The VWM monitor consists of a pulse radar sensor, a Microcontroller Unit (MCU), as well as a data analysis and classification unit, as shown in Figure 1A. The pulse radar sensor serves the purpose of sensing the motion of the A-V fistula vessel wall [14,15]. The operation principle of the pulse radar sensor is described as follows. Damped sinusoidal pulses with a pulse duration of 4 ns and repetition frequency of 250 K Hz are generated in the pulse generator, with its input connected to the square wave generator. As shown in Figure 1B, a sequence of damped sinusoidal pulses is emitted by the transmit antenna towards the patient's arm where the AVF is located. The damped sinusoidal pulses can be expressed by Equation (1), where A is the pulse envelope of $\widetilde{X}(t)$ and f_p is the carrier frequency of $\widetilde{X}(t)$.

$$\widetilde{X}(t) = A sin(2\pi f_p t) \quad (1)$$

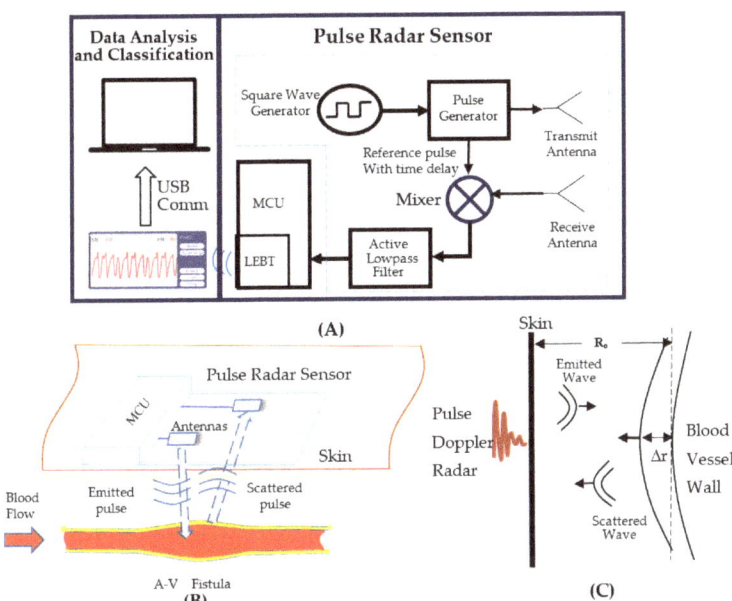

Figure 1. The system diagram of the VWM monitor and the principle of measuring the AVF vessel wall movement (**A**). The diagram of pulse radar sensor detect blood flow (**B**). The diagram of pulse Doppler radar emit and receive the signals of wave (**C**).

The scattered pulses from the AVF wall to the receiving antenna is then expressed by Equation (2), where $R(t)$ is the distance between the antenna and the AVF wall, c (meter/sec) is the speed of light, and $\in$ is the effective permittivity of the skin and subcutaneous tissue.

$$\widetilde{Y}(t) = \widetilde{X}\left(t - \frac{2R(t)}{c/\sqrt{\in}}\right) \quad (2)$$

Due to variations in blood pressure, the AVF wall is displaced towards the radar (Figure 1C), with the distance expressed by Equation (3), where R_o is the initial distance between the antenna and the AVF wall and $\Delta r(t)$ is the displacement of the AVF wall. Substitute Equation (3) into Equation (2) and the scattered pulses are expressed by Equation (4).

$$R(t) = R_o - \Delta r(t) \quad (3)$$

$$\widetilde{Y}(t) = A\sin\left(2\pi f_p\left(t - \frac{2(R_o - \Delta r(t))}{\frac{c}{\sqrt{\in}}}\right)\right) \quad (4)$$

The reference pulse (shown in Figure 1A) with a time delay of $\widetilde{X}(t)$ can be expressed.

$$\widetilde{X}(t - \tau) = A\sin(2\pi f_p(t - \tau)) \quad (5)$$

The received signal $\widetilde{Y}$ and the delayed reference pulse $\widetilde{X}(t - \tau)$ is then mixed and the carrier frequency component is filtered out to leave the baseband signal $B(t)$ expressed by Equation (6), where $\lambda_p = \frac{c}{\sqrt{\in}} \cdot \frac{1}{f_p}$ is the wavelength of the emitted and scattered pulses in the subcutaneous tissue.

$$B(t) = B\sin\left(\frac{4\pi(R_o - \Delta r(t))}{\lambda_p}\right) \quad (6)$$

For hemodialysis patients, the distance R_o between the AVF wall and skin is less than 6 mm and the diameter of the AVF is larger than 6 mm [16], with the periodical variation of the radius of the AVF, Δr estimated to be 0.028 mm [17]. Since $\Delta r(t) \ll R_o$, the motion of the AVF wall can be linearized to the following Equations (7) and (8), where $C_1 = B\left(\sin\left(\frac{4\pi}{\lambda_p}R_o\right)\right)$ and $C_2 = B\frac{4\pi}{\lambda_p}\cos\left(\frac{4\pi}{\lambda_p}R_o\right)$ are constants.

$$B(t) = B\left[\left(\sin\left(\frac{4\pi}{\lambda_p}R_o\right) - \frac{4\pi}{\lambda_p}\cos\left(\frac{4\pi}{\lambda_p}R_o\right)(\Delta r(t))\right)\right] \tag{7}$$

$$B(t) = C_1 - C_2 * (\Delta r(t)) \tag{8}$$

Therefore, as derived in Equation (8), the baseband signal $B(t)$ is linearly related to the displacement of the AVF wall $\Delta r(t)$.

The pulse radar sensor is fabricated on a flexible substrate (polyimide, size 8.0 × 3.5 cm, thickness 0.25 mm). Both antennas are planar microstrip monopoles. The input to each antenna is connected to a 50-ohm coplanar transmission microstrip line. The antenna input impedance matching was measured using a Vector Network Analyzer (Rohde & Schwartz, Muehldorfstrasse 15, 81671 Munich, Germany). The return loss was -20 dB at a resonant frequency of 1.38 GHz and the -10 dB bandwidth was 120 MHz. This lower antenna resonant frequency was chosen so that emitted pulses could penetrate the subcutaneous tissue surrounding the AVF vessel [18]. Since the antenna is working in the near field region, the medium between the sensor and skin surface is critical for coupling signal power through the skin barrier and subcutaneous tissues. Merli et al. [19] showed that the radiation efficiency of implanted antennas depended upon the dielectric properties of an insulating layer which separated the antenna from the surrounding muscle tissues. In the present work, it was found that a thin layer (0.25 to 1.0 mm) of textile material such as cotton or polyester cotton blended fiber is suitable for providing the desired properties. In addition to the insulating properties, the material's biocompatibility and adherence to the skin are also important factors when selecting coupling materials.

The active low-pass filter smooths the mixed pulsatile signal into the baseband signal $B(t)$ (Figure 1A). The cutoff frequency of the active low pass filter is 25 Hz. The baseband signal is then amplified and fed into the MCU (Nordic Semiconductor, Trondheim, Norway), in which the A to D converter's sampling frequency is set to 64 Hz. The digitized data are then transferred to a mobile phone using the built-in Low Energy Bluetooth Transceiver (LEBT) of the MCU. An App has been designed to display the signal waveform on the mobile phone during testing of the patient. To preserve the essential frequency contents of the baseband signal, a Hamming window-based bandpass, linear phase FIR filter has been designed using MATLAB 2020a (MathWorks, 1 Apple Hill Drive Natick, MA 01760, USA) in the frequency range of 0.2 to 10 Hz. The filtered data is then stored in the mobile phone and sent to a PC via a USB communication link for data analysis and classification.

Figure 2A shows baseband signals of three patients having normal AVF flows (1410, 1380, and 790 mL/min, respectively), in which stable and consistent VWM waveforms are evident. Figure 2B shows baseband signals of three patients having abnormal AVF flows (350, 430, and 360 mL/min, respectively), in which unstable and superimposed oscillations were observed on the VWM waveforms.

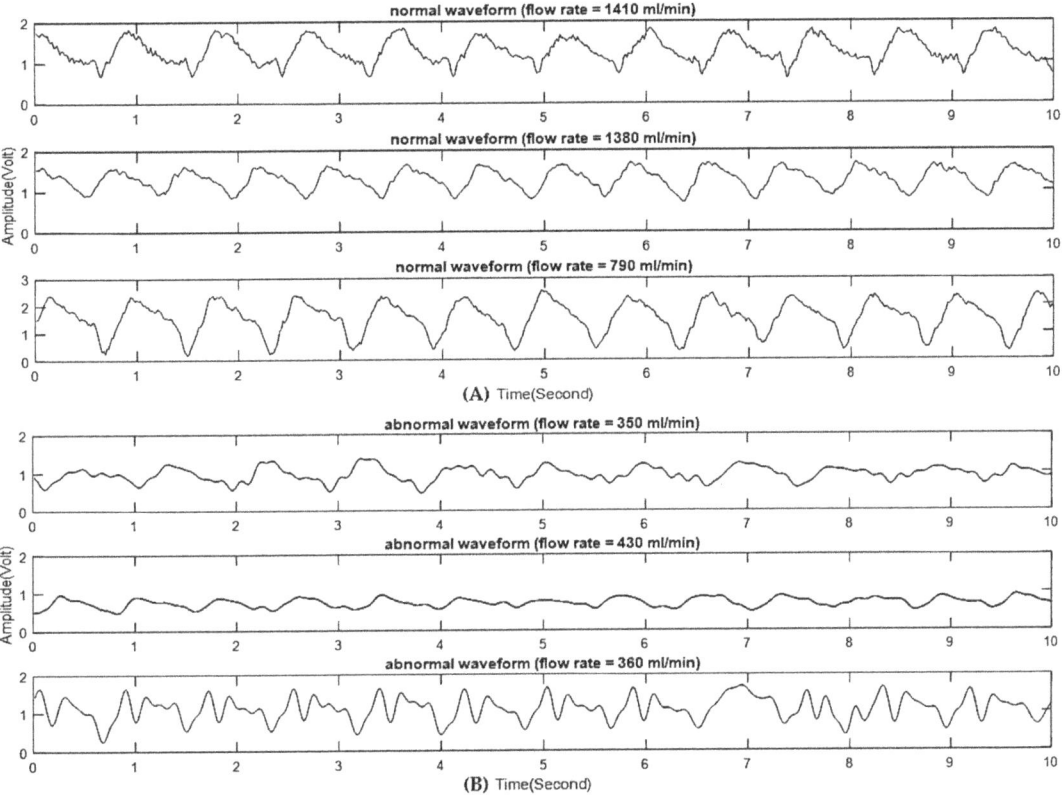

Figure 2. (**A**) Baseband signals of normal AVF with stable and consistent VWM waveforms. (**B**) Baseband signals of abnormal AVF with unstable and superimposed oscillations on VWM waveforms.

2.2. A Clinical Testing Protocol

The clinical trial was approved by the Institutional Review Board of Taichung Veterans General Hospital (TCVGH). A total of 46 patients regularly treated at the hemodialysis center in TCVGH were chosen for the clinical trial according to the inclusion criteria. There were 18 females with 67.9 ± 11.4 years old and 28 males with 61.9 ± 12.5 years old. One patient was excluded from the trial as his blood flow was not measurable due to difficulty in finding suitable sites for needle puncture. Informed consent was obtained from each patient prior to the start of the test session. The AVF locations on the tested patients were in various positions, from the wrist to the upper arm. The pulse radar sensor was attached according to each patient's AVF location, and positioned near the venous outflow side distal to the AVF, as shown in Figure 3. The patient was instructed to remain still for 1 min with their arm supported on the table top. The acquired VWM data were wirelessly transferred using a Bluetooth transceiver in real time from the pulse radar sensor to the mobile phone, where the signal waveform was displayed and data stored. The stored data were then transferred from the mobile phone through the USB communication link to a laptop PC. The hemodialysis treatment was then applied to the same patient, with AVF flow measured by the UD flow instrument (HD03, Transonic Systems Inc., Ithaca, NY, USA) within the first 30 min of the hemodialysis treatment session. The measured flow data was recorded and stored in a laptop PC for later analysis.

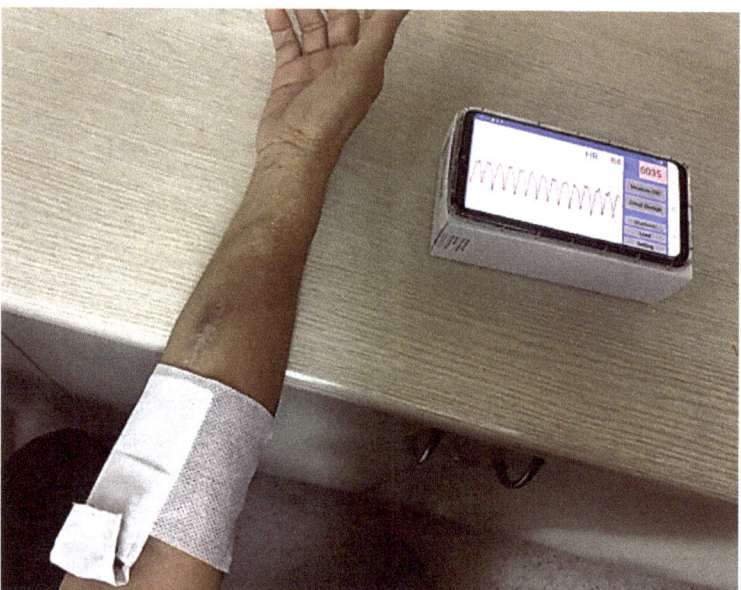

Figure 3. The hemodialysis patient during testing using a pulse radar sensor. Note that the App displays the signal waveform on a mobile phone. The detailed strategy of immobilizing as developed by the VWM monitoring system on patients, shown in Appendix A.

2.3. Data Processing and SVM Classification

The VWM data were converted to spectrum data using the Fast Fourier Transform algorithm in MATLAB 2020a. Due to its advantage in classifying small-sized complex datasets, the SVM machine learning classification algorithm was developed to predict the patient's AVF status using the features derived from the FFT spectrum data. The Radial Basis Function (RBF) kernel was chosen to train the SVM algorithm for classification of the non-linear datasets. The cutoff value between the abnormal and normal data sets was chosen according to the suggestions of the NKF-K/DOQI guidelines with a threshold of 600 mL/min and followed up in the hemodialysis center in TVGH for the detection of flow dysfunction. In addition to this regularly used cutoff value, the ROC analysis was used to verify the performance of the SVM classifier and to search for an optimal threshold in the detection of flow dysfunction.

The spectral (frequency-domain) analysis of physiological variables, using the fast Fourier transformation (FFT), has been reported [20]. A total of five features was used in this study, which are the ratios of FFT spectral peaks of the higher harmonics to those of the nearest lower harmonics, defined as the Harmonic Ratio (HR), i.e., P2/P1, P3/P2, P4/P3, P5/P4, and P6/P5. For example, Figure 4 compares the FFT spectrum of a normal VWM signal (left panel) with that of an abnormal VWM signal (right panel), in which a distinct difference exists in the ratio of P3 to P2. To validate the HRs as being features for VSM classification, the mean differences between the HRs of abnormal FFT spectrums and those of normal FFT spectrums were tested using the independent T-test ($\alpha = 0.05$). Table 1 shows that P5/P4 is a sensitive feature for a detection threshold of 600 mL/min ($p = 0.008$), and that P3/P2 is a sensitive feature for a detection threshold of 750 mL/min ($p = 0.041$). Based on this sensitivity analysis, the HRs for each patient were chosen to be the input features for the SVM classification algorithm.

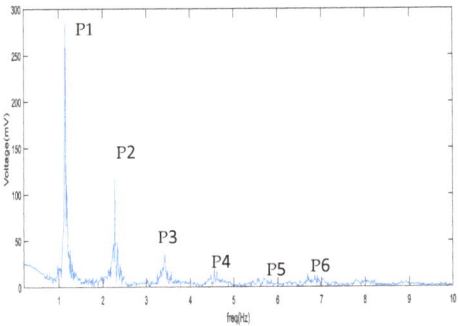 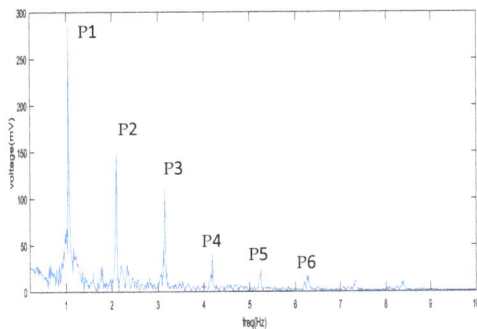

Figure 4. FFT spectrum of normal AVF wall motion signal (left), FFT spectrum of abnormal AVF wall motion signal (right).

Table 1. Independent T-test of the mean difference in harmonic ratios between low flow cases and high flow cases relative to cutoff values at 600 and 750 mL/min (referenced in Figure 4). Notice symbol * represents the p-value < 0.05.

Harmonic Ratio	≤600 (n = 11) Mean (SD)	>600 (n = 34) Mean (SD)	Difference	p-Value	≤750 (n = 21) Mean (SD)	>750 (n = 24) Mean (SD)	Difference	p-Value
P2/P1	0.357 (0.203)	0.380 (0.178)	−0.023	0.722	0.347 (0.168)	0.398 (0.195)	−0.051	0.356
P3/P2	0.665 (0.313)	0.491 (0.285)	0.174	0.093	0.630 (0.277)	0.449 (0.296)	0.181	0.041 *
P4/P3	0.591 (0.289)	0.785 (0.456)	−0.193	0.195	0.774 (0.475)	0.705 (0.387)	0.069	0.591
P5/P4	1.075 (0.601)	0.711 (0.273)	0.365	0.008 *	0.818 (0.510)	0.784 (0.293)	0.035	0.777
P6/P5	0.659 (0.235)	0.751 (0.347)	−0.092	0.417	0.696 (0.352)	0.758 (0.300)	−0.062	0.529

3. Results

Figure 5 displays the results of training the SVM classifier with detection thresholds of 600 mL/min. Each data point in the figure represents a set of two values in which the correponding value on the x axis is the value of the decision function, while that on the y axis is the measured flow data by UD. The value of the decision function shows whether an output by the SVM classifier lies to the right or left side of the hyperplane (y axis), as well as how far it is from the hyperplane. The hyperplane is an optimal plane separating the two classes with maximum margin. When the output value of the decision function is close to zero on the hyperplane, it represents a low-confidence decision, whereas when the output values of the decision function are a larger magnitude of positive or negative values, the more confident the decisions are. The locations of the data points relative to both the detection threshold (horizontal red line) and hyperplane determine whether the classification results are true or false. As defined by the hyperplane and detection threshold, when a data point is located either in the lower left or upper right region, it is being classified correctly as true positive or true negative, respectively. Alternatively, when a data point is located either in the upper left or lower right region, it is being classified incorrectly as fase positive or false negative, respectively. For a detection threshold of 600 mL/min, the outputs of the SVM classifier were mostly located in the true positive and true negative regions, with no false positive predictions and only one false negative being classified (shown in Figure 5).

The trained SVM classifier was validated using the method of 10-fold cross validation. Table 2 summarizes the validated results of the VSM classifier with a detection threshold of 600 and 750 mL/min. The performance of the SVM classifier shows a sensitivity of 90.9% (95.2%), specificity of 100.0% (100.0%), and an accuracy of 97.8% (97.8%) for 600 (750) mL/min. Notice that the prediction accuracy is 100.0% if measured by the positive prediction value.

As mentioned in the NKF-K/DOQI guidelines, there exists a need for standardized diagnostic thresholds with sufficient sensitivity as well as specificity. In the present work, the ROC curve analysis was performed with the results showing that the Area Under the Curve (AUC) was 0.994. The specificity and positive prediction value for the detection thresholds of 750, 650, 600, and 500 mL/min were all 100%, with the maximum sensitivity being 95.2% at a detection threshold of 750 mL/min (shown in Figure 6). This result indicates that the VWM monitor-based AVF flow dysfunction detector provides an excellent correlation with the UD flow monitor within a large range of AVF flow. However, a single optimal detection threshold could not be determined solely on the value of sensitivity. Instead, two levels of detection thresholds, e.g., firth level at 750 mL/min and second level at 600 mL/min, may be more reliable for the early detection of flow dysfunction before proceeding to pre-emptive angioplasty.

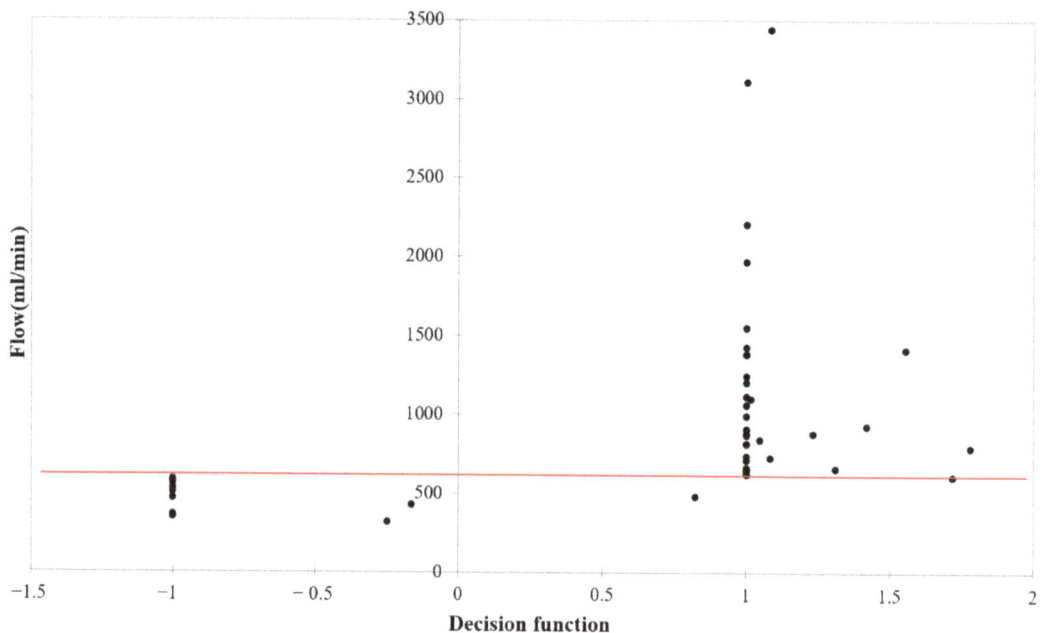

Figure 5. Results of SVM classifier training with a detection threshold of 600 mL/min.

Table 2. The 10-fold cross validation results for SVM classifier at a detection threshold of 600 and 750 mL/min, respectively.

Threshold	Prediction	Ground Truth		Total	%Correct	Index
		Flow ≤ 600	Flow > 600			
600	Flow ≤ 600	10	0	10	90.9	Sensitivity
	Flow > 600	1	34	35	100.0	Specificity
	Total	11	34	45	97.8	Accuracy
Threshold	Prediction	Flow ≤ 750	Flow > 750	Total	%Correct	Index
750	Flow ≤ 750	20	1	21	95.2	Sensitivity
	Flow > 750	0	24	24	100.0	Specificity
	Total	20	25	45	97.8	Accuracy

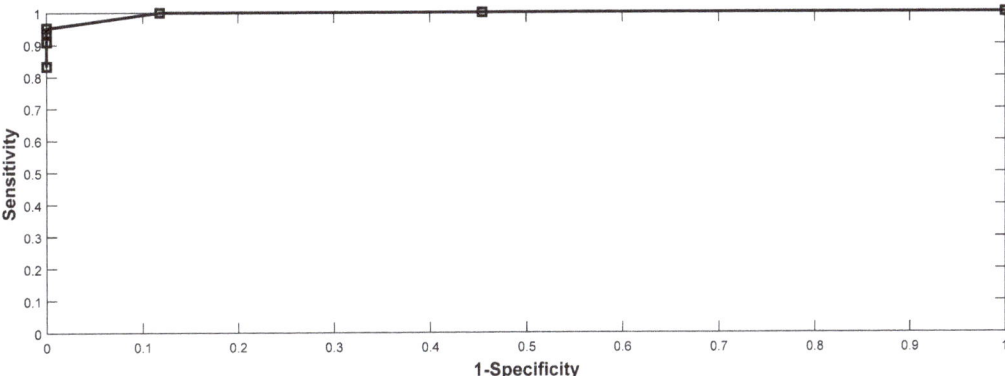

Figure 6. The results of ROC analysis on the performance of the SVM classifier.

4. Discussion

The wall motion in a stenotic carotid artery was investigated by Kanber et al. [21]. Due to the difficulty to measure stable signals in the stenotic region, the proximal shoulder of the atherosclerotic region was chosen as the measurement site, with ultrasound image sequences being acquired over several cardiac cycles. Results showed that both absolute and percentage diameter changes did not have any statistically significant relationship to the degree of stenosis. In the present work, measurement sites on patients' arms were all located at the venous outflow side of AVFs distal to where the periodical generation of flow turbulence took place. The signals acquired by the VWM monitor showed differences in waveform morphology between the abnormal flow cases and those of the normal flow cases. Figure 7A shows an example of a distorted AVF VWM signal (low flow, flow = 360 mL/min) whose waveform morphology displayed oscillations superimposed on one cycle of the original AVF VWM waveform. This is believed to be the result of the modulation of two signals, i.e., the original VWM signal and the signal with oscillations due to flow turbulence. Consequently, as shown in Figure 7B, new harmonics P3 and P5 appear with higher strengths in the FFT spectrum than those of the original VWM signal. Since the oscillating frequency is three to five times the fundamental frequency, the modulation effect would increase the strength of the higher frequency harmonics. This observation could be the basis for future work on detection of flow dysfunction by combining time domain and frequency domain analytical techniques.

Tessitore et al. [5] investigated the optimal thresholds for stenosis detection using the UD flow measurement. Their results showed that a detection threshold of 750 mL/min was optimal for AVFs at the wrist and 1000 mL/min for AVFs at the mid-forearm. In the present work, 50% of AVFs were located on patients' mid-forearms, 40% on patients' wrists, and the remaining 10% on patients' elbows. The ROC analysis results of the SVM classifier found that maximum sensitivity was achieved at a detection threshold of 750 mL/min, which was identical to that reported in [5] on stenosis detection. In the future, through the use of fistulography as the gold standard, an expanded clinical study will be needed in order to validate the SVM classifier in predicting stenosis.

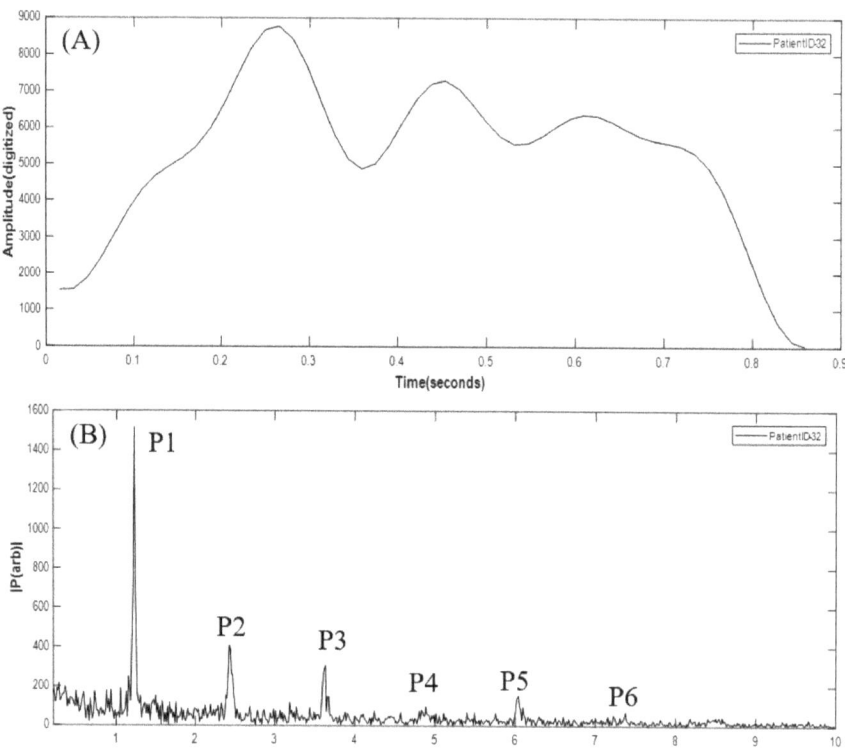

Figure 7. (**A**) Abnormal oscillations superimposed on one cycle of the VWM waveform. (**B**) The abnormal FFT spectrum with more pronounced spectral peaks at P3 and P5.

5. Conclusions

In conclusion, this study is based on previous studies which demonstrated that stenosis of the arterial blood vessel could be detected by analyzing the characteristic changes in the waveform of VWM. In this work, the operating principle of the pulse radar sensor for detection of VWM was derived theoretically and the performance of the VWM monitoring system was verified clinically. The VWM monitoring system was applied to detect the flow dysfunction in AVFs on patients who were receiving the hemodialysis treatment. Harmonic ratios derived from the FFT spectrum of the VWM monitoring signals were used as the input features to a SVM classification algorithm. Ten-fold cross validation results revealed an excellent correlation between the VWM monitor and UD flow monitor. To ensure the operation reliability of the VWM monitoring system, the long-term reproducibility of the as developed VWM monitoring system will be evaluated in the near future.

By adapting the two-level detection threshold method for early detection, the VWM monitoring technique for self-tests at home, or regular screening in hemodialysis centers, can provide the benefits of both reducing the present workload in testing AVF flow dysfunction in the hospital, as well as assuring the quality of care needed to preserve AVF patency. Meanwhile, the long-term reproducibility of the as developed VWM monitoring system should be evaluated in the near future.

Author Contributions: Initial conception, C.-H.C., T.-H.T. and T.-B.C.; design, C.-H.C., T.-H.T., Y.-H.C. and Y.-W.C.; provision of resources, C.-H.C. and T.-H.T.; collection of data, C.-H.C., Y.-H.C. and Y.-W.C.; analysis and interpretation of data, T.-H.T. and T.-B.C.; writing and revision of the paper, C.-H.C., T.-H.T and T.-B.C. All authors have read and agreed to the published version of the manuscript.

Funding: This work was supported by grant TCVGH-VHCY1098602 from Taichung Veterans General Hospital and Taichung Veterans General Hospital, Chiayi Branch.

Institutional Review Board Statement: The work was approved by the Institutional Review Board (I) 108-A-08 Board Meeting of TCVGH through Certificate of Approval TCVGH-IRB no. CF19258A.

Informed Consent Statement: The version of the Informed Consent Form was "Protocol Title: Ultra-wideband radar patch for non-invasive vascular movement detection in early vascular access stenosis of hemodialysis patients", version 1.3 on 28 August 2019.

Data Availability Statement: From 11 September 2019 to 10 September 2020.

Acknowledgments: All the authors thank Evelyn Tseng for her contribution on the VWM measurements and Yi-Ping Tsai for her partial contribution on data collection, as well as all the hemodialysis patients who participated in this study.

Conflicts of Interest: The authors C.-H.C., Y.-H.C., Y.-W.C., and T.-B.C. declare no conflict of interest. The pulse radar sensor was supplied free by Finedar Biomedical Technology Co., Ltd.

Appendix A

A detailed strategy of immobilizing the as developed VWM monitoring system on patients, as illustrated below.

1. Place the arm on the table top. Make sure that the side of the arm with AVF is in parallel with the table top and the weight of the arm should be fully supported by the table, as shown in Figure A1.
2. Position the pulse radar sensor in Figure A2 near the venous outflow junction of the AVF, as shown in Figure A3.
3. Attach the pulse radar sensor to the skin using the soft cloth tape.
4. Start the measurement while keeping the body still for 1 min.

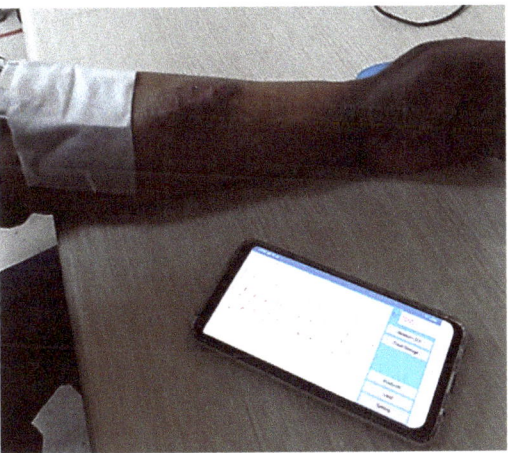

Figure A1. Placement of the arm with the AVF to be tested.

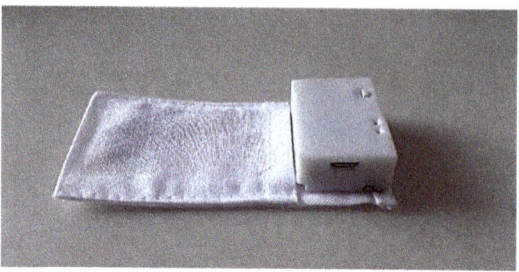

Figure A2. The pulse radar sensor.

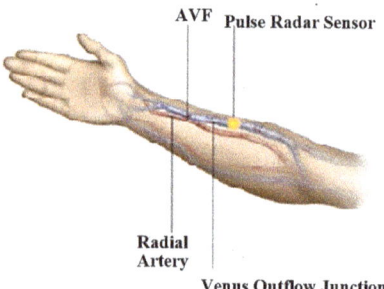

Figure A3. Attachment of the pulse radar sensor.

References

1. National Kidney Foundation. K/DOQI Clinical Practice Guidelines for Vascular Access, update 2019. *Am. J. Kidney Dis.* **2019**, *75* (Suppl. 2), 80–88.
2. Salman, L.; Rizvi, A.; Contreras, G.; Manning, C.; Feustel, P.J.; Machado, I.; Briones, P.L.; Jamal, A.; Bateman, N.; Martinez, L.; et al. A Multicenter Randomized Clinical Trial of Hemodialysis Access Blood Flow Surveillance Compared to Standard of Care: The Hemodialysis Access Surveillance Evaluation (HASE) Study. *Kidney Int. Rep.* **2020**, *5*, 1937–1944. [CrossRef] [PubMed]
3. Mccarley, P.; Wingard, R.L.; Shyr, Y.; Pettus, W.; Hakim, R.M.; Ikizler, T.A. Vascular access blood flow monitoring reduces access morbidity and costs. *Kidney Int.* **2001**, *60*, 1164–1172. [CrossRef] [PubMed]
4. Schwarz, C.; Mitterbauer, C.; Boczula, M.; Maca, T.; Funovics, M.; Heinze, G.; Matthias, M.; Kovarik, J.; Oberbauer, R. Flow Monitoring: Performance Characteristics of Ultrasound Dilution Versus Color Doppler Ultrasound Compared with Fistulography. *Am. J. Kidney Dis.* **2003**, *42*, 539–545. [CrossRef]
5. Tessitore, N.; Bedogna, V.; Gammaro, L.; Lipari, G.; Poli, A.; Baggio, E.; Firpo, M.; Morana, G.; Mansueto, G.; Maschio, G. Diagnostic Accuracy of Ultrasound Dilution Access Blood Flow Measurement in Detecting Stenosis and Predicting Thrombosis in Native Forearm Arteriovenous Fistulae for Hemodialysis. *Am. J. Kidney Dis.* **2003**, *42*, 331–341. [CrossRef]
6. Du, Y.-C.; Stephanus, A. A Novel Classification Technique of Arteriovenous Fistula Stenosis Evaluation Using Bilateral PPG Analysis. *Micromachines* **2016**, *7*, 147. [CrossRef] [PubMed]
7. Chiang, P.Y.; Chao, P.C.P.; Tarng, D.C.; Yang, C.Y. A Novel Wireless Photoplethysmography Blood-Flow Volume Sensor for Assessing Arteriovenous Fistula of Hemodialysis Patients. *IEEE Trans. Ind. Electron.* **2017**, *64*, 9626–9635. [CrossRef]
8. Chiang, P.Y.; Chao, P.C.P.; Tu, T.Y.; Kao, Y.H.; Yang, C.Y.; Tarng, D.C.; Wey, C.L. Machine Learning Classification for Assessing the Degree of Stenosis and Blood Flow Volume at Arteriovenous Fistulas of Hemodialysis Patients Using a New Photoplethysmography Sensor Device. *Sensors* **2019**, *19*, 3422. [CrossRef] [PubMed]
9. Chen, W.L.; Lin, C.H.; Chen, T.; Chen, P.J.; Kan, C.D. Stenosis Detection using Burg Method with Autoregressive Model for Hemodialysis Patients. *J. Med. Biol. Eng.* **2013**, *33*, 356–362. [CrossRef]
10. Ota, K.; Nishiura, Y.; Ishihara, S.; Adachi, H.; Yamamoto, T.; Hamano, T. Evaluation of Hemodialysis Arteriovenous Bruit by Deep Learning. *Sensors* **2020**, *20*, 4852. [CrossRef] [PubMed]
11. Ku, D.N. Blood Flow in Arteries. *Annu. Rev. Fluid Mech.* **1997**, *29*, 399–434. [CrossRef]
12. Jahangiri, M.; Saghafia, M.; Sadeghi, M.R. Numerical Simulation of Hemodynamic Parameters of Turbulent and Pulsatile Blood Flow in Flexible Artery with Single and Double Stenoses. *J. Mech. Sci. Technol.* **2015**, *29*, 3549–3560. [CrossRef]

13. Ramnarine, K.V.; Hartshorne, T.; Sensier, Y.; Naylor, M.; Walker, J.; Naylor, A.R.; Panerai, R.B.; Evans, D.H. Tissue Doppler imaging of carotid plaque wall motion: A pilot study. *Cardiovasc. Ultrasound* **2003**, *1*, 17. [CrossRef] [PubMed]
14. Tao, T.H.; Hu, S.J.; Peng, J.H.; Kuo, S.C. An Ultrawideband Radar Based Pulse Sensor for Arterial Stiffness Measurement. In Proceedings of the 29th Annual International Conference of the IEEE EMBS 2007, Lyon, France, 22–26 August 2007; pp. 1679–1682.
15. Hellbrück, H.; Ardelt, G.; Wegerich, P.; Gehring, H. Brachialis Pulse Wave Measurements with Ultra-Wide Band and Continuous Wave Radar, Photoplethysmography and Ultrasonic Doppler Sensors. *Sensors* **2021**, *21*, 165. [CrossRef] [PubMed]
16. National Kidney Foundation. KDOQI clinical practice guidelines and clinical practice recommendations for 2006 updates: Hemodialysis adequacy, peritoneal dialysis adequacy and vascular access. *Am. J. Kidney Dis.* **2006**, *48* (Suppl. 1), S1–S322.
17. Giannattasio, C.; Vincenti, A.; Failla, M.; Capra, A.; Cirò, A.; Ceglia, S.D.; Gentile, G.; Brambilla, R.; Mancia, G. Effects of Heart Rate Changes on Arterial Distensibility in Humans. *Hypertension* **2003**, *42*, 253–256. [CrossRef] [PubMed]
18. Brovoll, S.; Aardal, Ø.; Paichard, Y.; Berger, T.; Lande, T.S.; Hamran, S.-E. Optimal frequency range for medical radar Measurements of human heartbeats using body-contact radar. In Proceedings of the 35th Annual International Conference of the IEEE EMBS 2013, Osaka, Japan, 3–7 July 2013; pp. 1752–1755.
19. Merli, F.; Fuchs, B.; Mosig, J.R.; Skrivervik, A.K. The Effect of Insulating Layers on the Performance of Implanted Antennas. *IEEE Trans. Antennas Propag.* **2011**, *59*, 21–31.
20. Pybus, D.A. Real-time, spectral analysis of the arterial pressure waveform using a wirelessly-connected, tablet computer: A pilot study. *J. Clin. Monit. Comput.* **2019**, *33*, 53–63. [CrossRef] [PubMed]
21. Kanber, B.; Hartshorne, T.C.; Horsfield, M.A.; Naylor, A.R.; Robinson, T.G. and Ramnarine, K.V. Wall Motion in the Stenotic Carotid Artery: Association with Greyscale Plaque Characteristics, the Degree of Stenosis and Cerebrovascular Symptoms. *Cardiovasc. Ultrasound* **2013**, *11*, 37. [CrossRef] [PubMed]

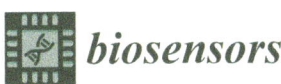

Article

Paper-Based Substrate for a Surface-Enhanced Raman Spectroscopy Biosensing Platform—A Silver/Chitosan Nanocomposite Approach

Yuri Kang [1], Hyeok Jung Kim [1], Sung Hoon Lee [2,*] and Hyeran Noh [1,3,*]

[1] Department of Optometry, Seoul National University of Science and Technology, 232 Gongneung-ro, Nowon-gu, Seoul 01811, Korea; eurikang@seoultech.ac.kr (Y.K.); hjkim@seoultech.ac.kr (H.J.K.)
[2] Corning Technology Center Korea, Corning Precision Materials Co., Ltd., 212 Tangjeong-ro, Asan 31454, Korea
[3] Convergence Institute of Biomedical Engineering and Biomaterials, Seoul National University of Science and Technology, 232 Gongneung-ro, Nowon-gu, Seoul 01811, Korea
* Correspondence: sunghoonlee@corning.com (S.H.L.); hrnoh@seoultech.ac.kr (H.N.); Tel.: +82-02-970-6231 (H.N.)

Abstract: Paper is a popular platform material in all areas of sensor research due to its porosity, large surface area, and biodegradability, to name but a few. Many paper-based nanocomposites have been reported in the last decade as novel substrates for surface-enhanced Raman spectroscopy (SERS). However, there are still limiting factors, like the low density of hot spots or loss of wettability. Herein, we designed a process to fabricate a silver–chitosan nanocomposite layer on paper celluloses by a layer-by-layer method and pH-triggered chitosan assembly. Under microscopic observation, the resulting material showed a nanoporous structure, and silver nanoparticles were anchored evenly over the nanocomposite layer. In SERS measurement, the detection limit of 4-aminothiophenol was 5.13 ppb. Furthermore, its mechanical property and a strategy toward further biosensing approaches were investigated.

Keywords: cellulose paper; chitosan; layer-by-layer; self-assembly; nanocomposite; SERS spectroscopy

Citation: Kang, Y.; Kim, H.J.; Lee, S.H.; Noh, H. Paper-Based Substrate for a Surface-Enhanced Raman Spectroscopy Biosensing Platform—A Silver/Chitosan Nanocomposite Approach. *Biosensors* **2022**, *12*, 266. https://doi.org/10.3390/bios12050266

Received: 17 March 2022
Accepted: 20 April 2022
Published: 22 April 2022

Publisher's Note: MDPI stays neutral with regard to jurisdictional claims in published maps and institutional affiliations.

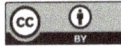

Copyright: © 2022 by the authors. Licensee MDPI, Basel, Switzerland. This article is an open access article distributed under the terms and conditions of the Creative Commons Attribution (CC BY) license (https://creativecommons.org/licenses/by/4.0/).

1. Introduction

Surface-enhanced Raman spectroscopy (SERS) is a sensitive analytical tool for the detection of chemical and biological analytes [1,2]. It reveals the intrinsic vibrational mode of chemicals in the manner of label-free detection with high sensitivity [3–5]. In recent years, diverse nanoscale structures, including those of noble metal nanocomposites, have led to the development of new substrates for label-free detection via Raman spectroscopy. Resonance-enhancing spaces known as "hot spots" can be generated between nanoparticles or at the sharp edges of individual nanoparticles, which locally enhances electromagnetic fields; thus, high density is regarded as the key to obtaining better Raman signals.

Since the first SERS effect was utilized in molecular detection by Richard P. Van Duyne and other peers, there have been attempts to connect it to the biosensing approach using biosensing molecules like enzymes and antibodies [6,7]. SERS benefits from multiplex detection and spectrometric approaches in biosensing. Also, the feasible formation of coordinate bonds between those sensing molecules and noble nanoparticles makes SERS highly applicable to biosensor research, i.e., thiol–gold, thiol–silver, amine–gold, and so on. Combined with established biosensing strategies such as ELISA [8], it can expand the analytical performance of biosensing to ultrasensitive levels. There have been several reports showing how SERS can be applied to biosensing [9–11].

SERS-active substrates are generally categorized as colloidal liquids or solid materials. Colloidal SERS substrates are relatively simpler in their preparation, and they can derive various shapes of nanoparticles to target a specific analyte. However, colloidal stability is more important due to the risk of particle aggregation, precipitation, and loss of colloidality. Thus, solid materials binding to individual nanoparticles, such as paper, glass, silicone, polydimethylsiloxane (PDMS), graphene nanosheets, and polymer films, may be preferred in some applications [12–16]. In particular, porosity is widely sought as it effectively improves the density, dispersion, and consistency of hot spots over a whole dimension [5,17–19]. Moreover, the following features of these materials are thought to be beneficial in SERS analysis: (1) effective adsorption of analytes, (2) ease of multiple adjacent nanostructure formation to increase hot spots, (3) support fixtures for nanoparticle growth, and (4) filtering for selective detection. Some recent studies in the literature elucidated how such nanoporous materials improve analytical performance. A network of carbon wires and pores showed high absorptivity and high-density hot spots, enhancing signals [20]. A porous silicon material resulted in signal enhancement around 5 times stronger than that of SERS using a flat silicon surface [21]. A nanoparticle-embedded polymer hydrogel showed high sensitivity and filtration functions excluding small matrix molecules [22].

Recently, paper as a porous base material has received attention due to its reformability, low cost, and biocompatibility, to name but a few [23–26]. There are some notable reports exploiting its filtrating and microfluidic characteristics for renovative SERS sensing [23,27–29]. These paper-based substrates can be fabricated by well-established technologies, including core–shell nanoparticles/hybridization of metals [30], chemical vaporizing deposition [31,32], and hydrophobization with wax or siloxane [24], all of which enhance sensitivity in SERS analysis.

In this study, we maximize the porosity of paper using nanoporous silver/chitosan nanocomposites on the cellulose surface, which increase the number of hot spots and provide a filtration function for small molecules. Chitosan was chosen due to its chemical similarity to cellulose. That is, the whole structure can be stabilized in a paper matrix, enhancing its mechanical and thermal stability to a level suitable for SERS-active paper substrates [33,34]. Layer-by-layer (LbL) processing was employed for a better firm structure of this soft material. This low-cost silver/chitosan nanocomposite substrate was used to detect a low concentration of a model small chemical, 4-aminothiophenol (4-ATP). Lastly, we suggest a way to enhance the analytical performance of this substrate by simply cutting it.

2. Materials and Methods

2.1. Materials and Reagents

Chitosan oligosaccharide lactate (($C_{12}H_{24}N_2O_9$)$_n$, >90% deacetylated, average M_n = 5000, oligosaccharide 60%), acetic acid (CH_3COOH, 99%), and 4-aminothiophenol (C_6H_7NO, >97%) were purchased from Sigma Aldrich. Silver nitrate ($AgNO_3$, >99%), sodium citrate dihydrate ($Na_3C_6H_5O_7 \cdot 2H_2O$, >99%), and anhydrous absolute ethanol (C_2H_5OH, 99.5%) were purchased from Daejung Chemical, Inc. (Siheung-si, Gyeonggi-do, Korea), and sodium hydroxide (NaOH, >93%) and sodium borohydride ($NaBH_4$, >98%) were purchased from Duksan Chemical, Inc. (Ansan-si, Gyeonggi-do, Korea). Whatman standard chromatography paper (Whatman 1 CHR, Cytiva, Marlborough, MA, USA) and a dialysis tubing cellulose membrane (flat width 25 mm, Sigma Aldrich, Burlington, MA, USA) were used as the base materials in SERS measurement and SEM imaging, respectively.

2.2. Fabrication of the Paper SERS Substrate

Whatman standard chromatography papers 2.5 × 7.0 cm² in size were employed. A slide rack was used to fabricate multiple sheets at once, prepared with slide glasses as dividers between the papers. To fabricate the silver/chitosan nanocomposite, a 0.1 $w/v\%$ chitosan solution (in 1% of acetic acid), a 50 mM sodium hydroxide solution, a 20 mM silver nitrate solution, and reductant solutions (20 mM sodium borohydride, 20 mM sodium citrate dihydrate) were prepared. The silver/chitosan nanocomposite was formed after the paper cellulose was dipped into the chitosan solution for 1 hour, the sodium hydroxide solution for 15 min, the silver nitrate solution for 30 min, and the reductant solution for

30 min, sequentially. After each immersion step, except for that in the chitosan solution, the paper was rinsed in water under magnetic stirring for 20 min. We then dried the paper in an oven at 60 degrees for 30 min, making this the LbL 1 cycle. This was repeatedly performed on the single-cycled paper via the same method described above to obtain 2 cycles, 3 cycles, and so on (Figure 1a).

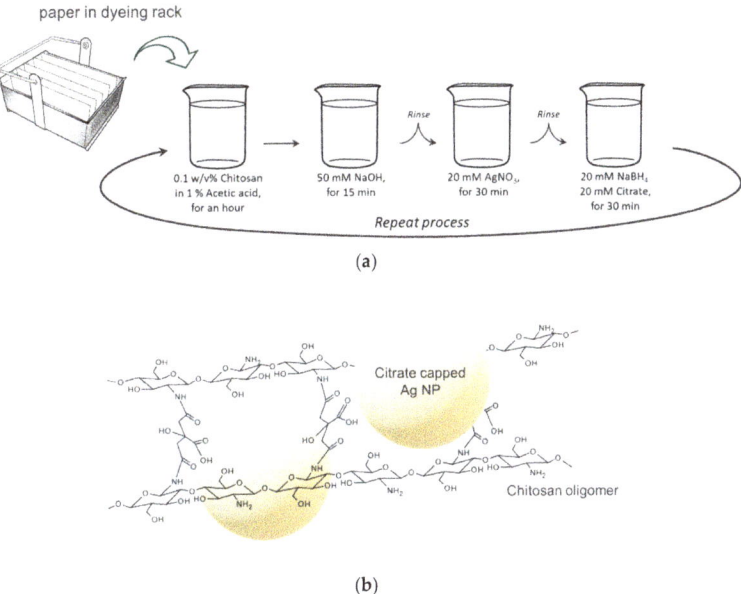

Figure 1. (a) Schematic illustration of the layer-by-layer process used to coat cellulose paper with silver/chitosan nanocomposite, where the paper substrate was submerged in each reagent solution, stepwise; (b) Configured silver/chitosan nanocomposite by coordinate bonds between citrate-capped silver nanoparticles and self-assembled chitosan.

To explain the synthesis process in detail, an acetic acid solution was used to dissolve the chitosan. This makes the chitosan molecules electrically positive through the protonation of amino groups at low pH, and this property increases the water solubility. The dissolved chitosan has an electrostatic attraction with cellulose, which is a polyanion, in aqueous solution. When the paper is placed in the next sodium hydroxide solution, the amine groups of chitosan become insoluble at high pH and may become harder on the paper. Rinsing off unwanted ions that are not used for binding and immersing the paper in a silver nitrate solution and a reductant solution results in negatively charged silver nanoparticles capped with a citrate capping agent. By repeating the cycle, citrate-capped silver nanoparticles can be coordinated with chitosan to obtain a three-dimensional nanocomposite (Figure 1b).

The synthesis method for the non-LbL model was identical to the first cycle step, but from the second cycle onwards, it consisted only of the silver nitrate solution and the reductant solution without the chitosan solution or the sodium hydroxide solution. The volume of solution used in the experiment was adjusted according to the size of the paper to be produced. For the ten sheets of paper mentioned above, amounts of 0.5 L of the solutions were used. After completion of production, the dried paper samples were wrapped in aluminum foil and stored under refrigeration at about 4 °C.

2.3. Sampling for the Detection of 4-ATP

Paper samples for the SERS measurements were cut into 4 mm diameter circles using a perforated punch. These were immersed in a 1.5 mL tube with 0.5 mL 4-ATP (12.5 ppm in ethanol) for 18 h at 45 degrees and then dried at room temperature for use with the SERS measurements. The other paper sample used here with capillary action was 4 mm wide and 20 mm long, and the tip was prepared as an isosceles triangle with a height of 4 mm. These samples were immersed in the same manner as the circle sample above, except that the volume of 4-ATP used was 1.5 mL. After immersion for 18 h, the dried sample was placed vertically in a 60 mm diameter Petri dish covered with ethanol to approximately 1 mm high. One minute after the ethanol reached the tip of the paper, it was taken out and dried at room temperature, after which a 4 mm high triangle was cut, and SERS measurements were taken.

2.4. Calculation of the Limit of Detection

The detection limit was obtained by the following formula:

$$I_m = I_{bl} + k\,\sigma_{bl} \tag{1}$$

where I_m is the minimum distinguishable intensity of the signal, I_{bl} is the Raman signal generated by a blank measurement of the SERS substrate in the absence of the analyte. k is the proportionality constant, and σ_{bl} is the standard deviation of blank measurements [35]. In addition, the amount of analyte providing 3 times the σ_{bl} value as a signal equal to or greater than the signal of the blank was considered (using k = 3 proposed by Kaiser [36]).

$$I = m\,C_m + I_{bl} \tag{2}$$

C_m was calculated by substituting I_m obtained by Equation (1) into I of the quantified linear function in Equation (2). m is the slope of the calibration curve at the concentration of interest, and C_m is the concentration at the limit of detection.

2.5. Instruments

Optical microscopy (Zeiss Primo star, ZEISS International, Jena, Germany) was used to obtain the color shift of the LbL model compared to the non-LbL model. Field emission scanning electron microscopy (FE-SEM, Hitachi SU8010, Hitachi, Tokyo, Japan) was used to image the surface and cross section of the substrate. The cross-sectional view was obtained using this cellulose membrane (thickness of around 20 µm) and by fracturing after immersing it in cryo liquid. The silver/chitosan nanocomposite layered samples were pre-treated with a Pt coating and then subjected to analysis. A universal testing machine (Instron 3400 series) was used for micro-tensile testing of the LbL fabricated paper samples. The Raman signals were measured using a C12710 Raman spectrometer from Hamamatsu. This device has a built-in laser with a wavelength of 785 mm. Here, the laser output was 50 mW (Raman mode) or 3 mW (SERS mode) and the acquisition time was 1500 ms. Raman intensity values were determined from 10 spots and averaged.

2.6. Statistics

Statistical analyses using Student's t-test and the standard deviation (of all error bars) were conducted using SPSS 18 (SPPS, Inc. Chicago, IL, USA) and Microsoft Excel (Microsoft, Inc. Redmond, WA, USA).

3. Results and Discussion

3.1. Characterization of Silver/Chitosan Nanocomposite Layered Paper

3.1.1. Physical Properties

To confirm the in situ formation of silver/chitosan nanocomposites on paper, the optical properties of the LbL model and the non-LbL model were compared. The first cycle performed on cellulose paper was identical in both models, i.e., chitosan immersion followed by the reduction of the silver nanoparticles (Ag NPs). The LbL model underwent repeated production steps sequentially, while in the non-LbL model, the reduction of Ag NPs was performed without submersion in chitosan. Comparing the optical micrographs of the two models in Figure 2a, a dramatic color change in the non-LbL model was observed. The distinct decrease in the brightness of the non-LbL sample is presumably due to the interference of the optical path, judging from the increase in the size or the aggregation of Ag NPs. The paper formulated by the non-LbL model turned darker during the cycling process because the spacing of the paper fibers became narrow. When the same molar concentration of silver ions was added at each cycle in the LbL model, fiber spaces were possibly preserved by the chitosan multilayer. Since chitosan can act as a spacer between Ag NPs, the aggregation of Ag NPs is prevented by chitosan in the LbL model, as illustrated in Figure 2b [37,38]. The optical intensities in both red and green maintained less than a 20% change in RG chromaticity (Figure S1). This observation indicated that the aggregation of Ag NPs was prevented by crosslinked chitosan in the LbL model, such that nanoparticles of similar sizes could be distributed without aggregation or unwanted growth.

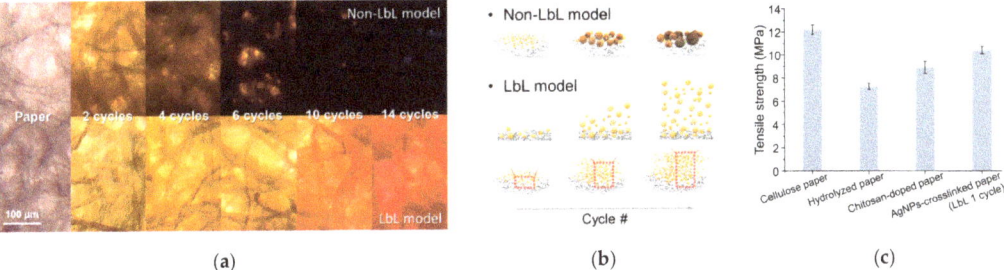

Figure 2. (a) Optical micrographs of LbL and non-LbL paper that underwent the fabrication process for 14 cycles, representing the effects of chitosan on colloidal stability; (b) Illustration showing how chitosan oligomer prevents the aggregation of particles during the LbL process; (c) Changes in the tensile strength of the substrate when proceeding with each step, implying mechanical enhancement by chitosan self-assembly and crosslinks with silver nanoparticles.

A micro-tensile test was conducted to evaluate the physical properties of the nanoscale material inside the nanocomposite layered paper. With the acid-catalyzed glycosidic hydrolysis, the tensile strength of the hydrolyzed paper was significantly reduced compared to that of the cellulose paper (Figure 2c). Meanwhile, the physical strength of the substrate was recovered through the doped chitosan crosslinked with Ag NPs.

3.1.2. Morphology of the Silver/Chitosan Nanocomposite

The distribution and conformation of the nanoparticles are two of the major sources of SERS enhancement. Accordingly, the morphologies of the silver/chitosan nanocomposites on cellulose paper were characterized by SEM. Chemically untreated chromatography paper was chosen as a control paper; however, it was easily torn by the electron beam of the SEM and was photographed at low magnification. Figure 3 shows the evenly spread Ag NPs over the surface of the cellulose fiber as a consequence of LbL cycling. The size of the Ag NPs did not increase by more than 50 nm, even when the cycling was repeated. The histogram distribution also confirmed that the Ag NP reduction rates were consistent throughout the cycles, exhibiting an average nanoparticle size of 26.99 ± 5.74 nm (Figure S2). We believe that the particle size is not affected by further solution immersion steps as the citrate works as capping agent, stabilizing and inhibiting the over-growth of Ag NPs while also preventing their aggregation and coagulation formed in the previous cycle. Sodium citrate can also chemically crosslink with chitosan between protonated amines and carboxylate ions through a heat treatment [39,40]. Since the paper after the dipping step in the citrate-containing reductant goes through an oven-drying process at about 60 degrees, the above reaction is likely to occur. Chitosan not only binds to silver nanoparticles but also binds to the citrate capping agent to form a stable three-dimensional layer. Therefore, it appears that the silver ions are prevented from diffusing and, consequently, have a constant reduction rate and maintain a uniform particle size over multiple cycles.

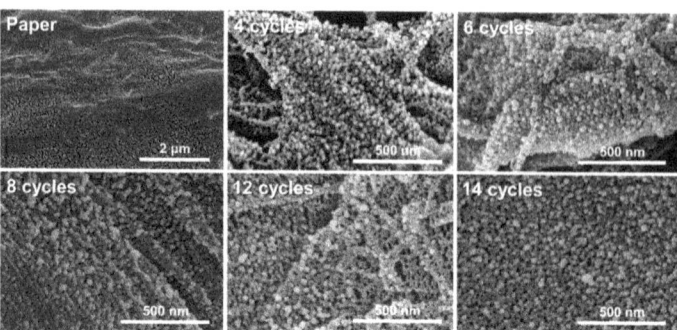

Figure 3. SEM micrographs of the resulting LbL papers after each cycle (from top right: original paper; 4, 6, 8, 12, and 14 cycles) where silver nanoparticles are evenly anchored to the surface of fibers without significant changes in particle size.

This corresponds to the overall Ag NP sizes in each cycle, 20 to 30 nm, as calculated from the SEM images, implying that the Ag NPs created by the LbL cycling did not aggregate but maintained a relatively constant size. It is well known that constant size and regularity of plasmonic nanoparticles are crucial factors related to SERS performance outcomes because these factors can affect the formation of local electromagnetic fields on the surfaces of the nanoparticles [41]. In the LbL model, Ag NPs between the chitosan multilayers not only prevented aggregation but also maintained a suitable size of the nanoparticles for the SERS signal.

Figure 4 presents an SEM image of a cross section of the nanocomposite layer on the cellulose surface (the specifications of the materials are shown in the methodology section). A cross-sectional view demonstrates the fabricated multilayer (thickness of approx. 575 nm at 14 cycles) and its nanoporous structure. Notably, the nanoporous structure was well refined and evenly formed over the layers with similar pore sizes of up to 30 nm in diameter (Figure S3). Chitosan oligomers associated with the surface shrank to themselves, while the high concentration of hydroxide induced self-assembly of these oligomers, and the structure was then fixed after being dried out. This nanoporous structure brings more functions to our substrate; it can promote the high acquisition of SERS signals as a 'spacer', but it can also selectively filtrate for target analytes by molecular size to allow for low matrix effects due to proteins in biological samples.

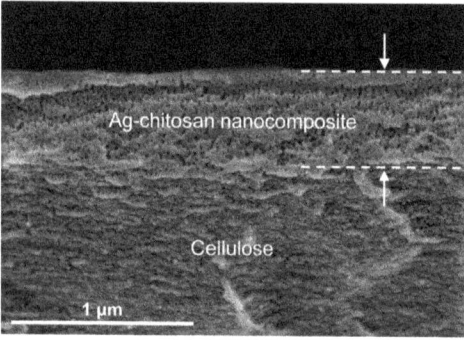

Figure 4. Cross-sectional view of Ag–chitosan nanocomposite on the cellulose substrate (thickness of Ag–chitosan nanocomposite, approx. 575 nm; diameter of nanopores, up to 30 nm).

3.1.3. Raman Spectroscopy

The chemical structures of each paper layer up to 14 cycles were analyzed by Raman spectroscopy using a 785 nm incident laser at 50 mW. Figure 5 shows the Raman spectra of the untreated cellulose paper, the chitosan-doped cellulose paper, the Ag NP-crosslinked paper, and the LbL 14-cycle paper. The high-intensity peak at 1090 cm^{-1} represents C-O ring stretching and/or glycosidic ring stretching [42,43]. Bands from ring stretches were detected in all samples. Chitosan and cellulose have similar molecular structures, with the difference being the existence of an amine group, NH_2 or $NHCOCH_3$, located at the C2 site in the case of chitosan. The Raman band of the amine group in chitosan was located at 1593 cm^{-1} [44], and the silver peak was measured in the LbL 1-cycle sample at 789 cm^{-1}. Comparing the Raman signals of the nanocomposite layered paper and the untreated cellulose paper, the position of the cellulose peak in the LbL 14-cycle paper was 1085 cm^{-1}, which shifted to a wavenumber lower than that of the control paper. Studies of deformation mechanisms have shown that a shift in the Raman band is indicative of stress in the fiber [45,46]. The Raman shift to a lower wavenumber means that the vibrational frequency of the molecule is decreased, which could be considered as evidence of the lengthening of the chemical bond due to tensile stress. As the silver/chitosan nanocomposites were repeatedly deposited, stress was applied to the C-O stretching motion of cellulose, which is almost parallel to the chain axis, and a shift of the Raman band was observed [47].

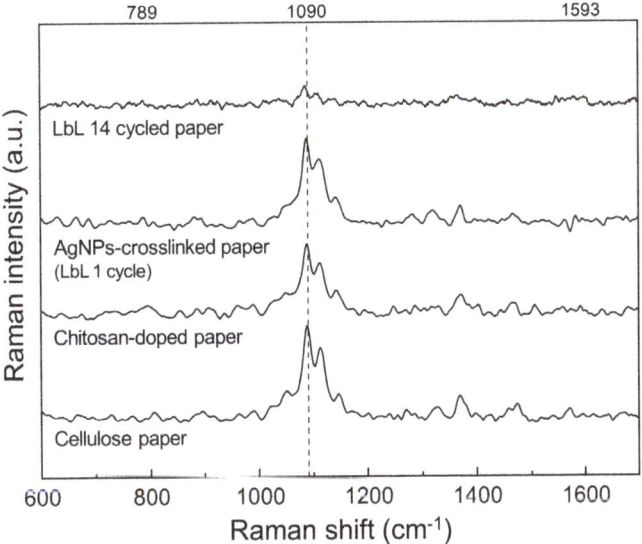

Figure 5. Raman spectra obtained from original cellulose, chitosan-doped, LbL 1-cycle, and LbL 14-cycle substrates, where the yellow bands represent the chemical motifs of the following: glycosidic ring stretching, 1090 cm^{-1}; amine group in chitosan, 1593 cm^{-1}; and silver, 789 cm^{-1}.

3.2. SERS Measurement

3.2.1. Detection of 4-Aminothiophenol

Figure 6 shows the SERS intensity with increasing number of synthesis cycles. The standard 4-aminothiophenol (4-ATP) was employed to study the SERS performance of the silver/chitosan nanocomposite layered paper. The characteristic peak of 4-ATP is at 1070 cm^{-1}, corresponding to C-S stretching vibration [48]. Each cycled LbL paper showed amplification of the Raman signal with increasing cycle number as compared to the untreated paper. It appears that the silver nanoparticles inside the nanocomposite were spaced by chitosan, effectively increasing the number of hot spots. A strong electromagnetic field occurred with the interparticle distance decreased to a few nanometers; the chitosan backbone structure prevented the silver nanoparticles from aggregating, while still keeping them quite close. In addition, the three-dimensional structure of cellulose paper and chitosan appears to have contributed to the increased hot spot density due to the porous structures of these components.

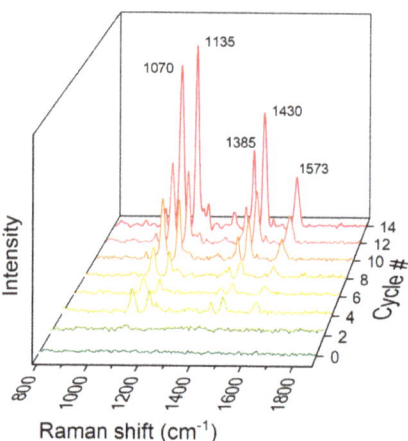

Figure 6. SERS spectra showing an increment in each peak of 4-ATP (12.5 ppm) with increasing number of LbL cycles.

For quantitative analysis, a series of solutions with different concentrations of 4-ATP were measured via SERS, as shown in Figure 7. The intensity of the Raman signal at 1070 cm^{-1} increased with a rise in the concentration of 4-ATP. The bands at 1135, 1385, and 1430 cm^{-1} indicate b$_2$ vibration modes that are selectively enhanced via the charge transfer mechanism, so their quantification is unstable [49,50]. Among several bands, 1070 cm^{-1}, representing C-S stretching vibration, was chosen as a specific peak for quantitative analysis. The coefficient of determination (R^2) was determined to be 0.936 according to a linear regression analysis. The detection limit was found to be 5.13 ppb, which is equivalent to approximately 41 nM. This is comparable sensitivity to that of other rapid-testing SERS substrates and very refined nanomaterials achieving nanomolar detection of environmental pollutants, while ours retains feasibility in terms of the fabrication and wettability of the paper material. We look forward to the use of this substrate as a superb candidate platform for on-site biosensors [25,51].

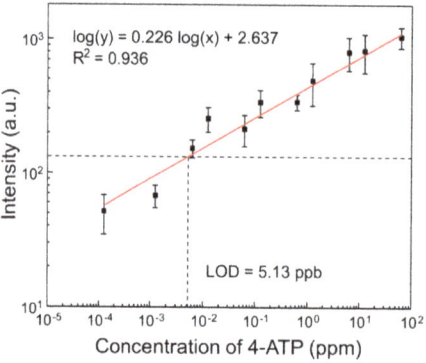

Figure 7. SERS intensity at 1070 cm^{-1} obtained from a series of different concentrations of 4-ATP dropped onto prepared SERS substrates (analyte concentration ranging from 0.00125 ppm to 12.5 ppm).

3.2.2. Application to Biosensing Approaches

While our SERS substrate has shown competent functionality, further potential was observed when recalling the traits of paper celluloses: large surface area, conformation of the scaffold structure, capillary flow, and free evaporation, to name but a few. This implies that this substrate can be used to implement novel biosensing applications, for instance, the real-time monitoring of bacterial metabolites during cultivation [52]. The nanoporous structure observed via SEM is thought to filter large matrix molecules like proteins, increase the surface area, and specifically target small molecules. Further, capillary flow and free evaporation have been considered a simple but effective strategy to concentrate analytes.

In paper, the cellulose fibers are irregularly interspersed, and it is expected that the spaces inside show microtubule-like behavior; thus, we tested the efficiency of analyte-containing fluid transport in the paper. After the chromatography process was carried out with ethanol as a solvent, an isosceles triangle with a height of 4 mm was cut out and used for 10 SERS measurements from different spots (Figure 8a). The Raman signals of the control and the experimental sample with 12.5 ppm of 4-ATP at 1070 cm^{-1} were 823.39 and 1455.02, respectively, showing an improvement by approximately 76% ($p = 0.0006$, $p < 0.001$; differences for which p was less than 0.01 were regarded as statistically significant), as shown in Figure 8b. It was noted that the solvent migrated together with the analyte, contributing to an increase in the molecular density of the analyte around the hot spots. Also, the relative standard deviation (%RSD) of the Raman signal was reduced from 32.1% to 17.7%. Consequently, the capillary phenomenon, enabled by the characteristics of the paper, enhanced the detection sensitivity of the paper sensor.

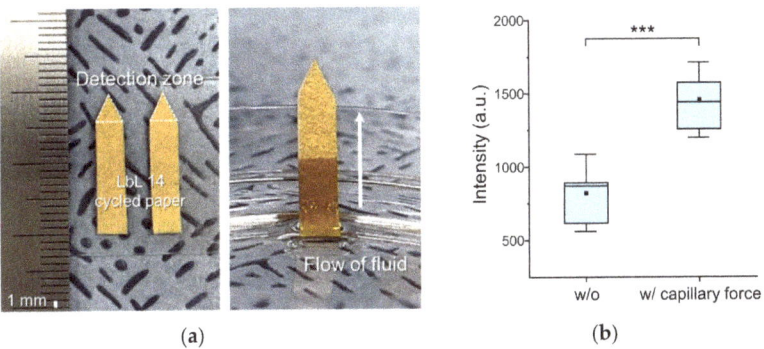

Figure 8. (a) Photograph of LbL paper substrate cut into an arrow shape with a lateral transportation and detection zone where the sample liquid moves and is vaporized, consequently focusing analyte molecules on the tip; (b) Signal enhancement by simply cutting the LbL paper substrate (black dot, mean; black solid line in box, median; box height, sample variability from 25% to 75%; error bar, standard deviation; *** $p < 0.001$).

4. Conclusions

A new approach to generating high-density hot spots in a paper matrix was introduced herein. The layer-by-layer process with a pH-based self-assembly step enabled feasible and robust fabrication that resulted in good traits regarding mechanical characterization and surface-enhance Raman spectrometry. The synthesized Ag nanoparticles maintained a certain size even after repeated cycles, at an average of 26.99 ± 5.74 nm, which is suitable for amplifying the electromagnetic field and contributing to enhanced SERS signals. These findings show that the cellulose, chitosan, and silver nanoparticles were strongly bonded by coordinate bonds, indicating that coating on fibrils was successfully achieved. In SERS signal analysis using 4-ATP, sufficiently enhanced signals were obtained to detect 5.13 ppb. Meanwhile, combining the general traits of paper celluloses and the functionality of this nanocomposite offers potential for novel biosensing applications, such as real-time monitoring during microbial cultivation and lateral flow sensing, as we mentioned. Our results obtained by employing a capillary-actuated fluid transport scheme showed how this substrate can be used for applications ranging from simple analyte concentration up to a more complicated sensing approach. We expect that this multilayered paper will serve in the detection and monitoring of various disease factors in human body fluids, including blood, tears, and sweat, as well as environmental samples.

Supplementary Materials: The following supporting information can be downloaded at: https://www.mdpi.com/article/10.3390/bios12050266/s1, Figure S1: RG chromaticity diagram of the LbL and non-LbL model paper samples up to 14 cycles. The number of cycles of both models increases along the direction of the arrow. Inset pictures are optical micrographs of the cellulose paper and 14 cycles in both models; Figure S2: Histogram of the diameters of the Ag NPs overall; Figure S3: Cross-sectional SEM image of an Ag–chitosan nanocomposite with pore size measurements; Figure S4: Tensile strength of silver/chitosan nanocomposite layered papers from cellulose paper (0 cycles) to 14 cycles [53].

Author Contributions: Conceptualization, H.J.K. and H.N.; methodology, H.J.K.; validation, Y.K., H.J.K. and H.N.; formal analysis, Y.K.; investigation, Y.K.; resources, H.N.; data curation, Y.K.; writing—original draft preparation, Y.K.; writing—review and editing, H.J.K., S.H.L. and H.N.; visualization, Y.K. and H.J.K.; supervision, H.N.; project administration, Y.K.; funding acquisition, H.N. All authors have read and agreed to the published version of the manuscript.

Funding: This research was funded by a National Research Foundation of Korea (NRF) grant funded by the Korean government (MEST) (No. 2019003588).

Institutional Review Board Statement: Not applicable.

Informed Consent Statement: Not applicable.

Data Availability Statement: The data presented in this study are available in https://figshare.com/search?q=10.6084%2Fm9.figshare.19635069, (accessed on 16 March 2022).

Conflicts of Interest: The authors declare no conflict of interest.

References

1. Su, S.; Zhang, C.; Yuwen, L.; Chao, J.; Zuo, X.; Liu, X.; Song, C.; Fan, C.; Wang, L. Creating SERS hot spots on MoS$_2$ nanosheets with in situ grown gold nanoparticles. *ACS Appl. Mater. Interfaces* **2014**, *6*, 18735–18741. [CrossRef] [PubMed]
2. Ogundare, S.A.; Van Zyl, W.E. A review of cellulose-based substrates for SERS: Fundamentals, design principles, applications. *Cellulose* **2019**, *26*, 6489–6528. [CrossRef]
3. Fierro-Mercado, P.M.; Hernández-Rivera, S.P. Highly sensitive filter paper substrate for SERS trace explosives detection. *Int. J. Spectrosc.* **2012**, *2012*, 716527. [CrossRef]
4. Chen, A.; Deprince, A.E.; Demortière, A.; Joshi-Imre, A.; Shevchenko, E.V.; Gray, S.K.; Welp, U.; Vlasko-Vlasov, V.K. Self-assembled large au nanoparticle arrays with regular hot spots for SERS. *Small* **2011**, *7*, 2365–2371. [CrossRef]
5. Restaino, S.M.; White, I.M. A critical review of flexible and porous SERS sensors for analytical chemistry at the point-of-sample. *Anal. Chim. Acta* **2019**, *1060*, 17–29. [CrossRef]
6. Bantz, K.C.; Meyer, A.F.; Wittenberg, N.J.; Im, H.; Kurtuluş, Ö.; Lee, S.H.; Lindquist, N.C.; Oh, S.-H.; Haynes, C.L. Recent progress in SERS biosensing. *Phys. Chem. Chem. Phys.* **2011**, *13*, 11551. [CrossRef]
7. Moore, T.; Moody, A.; Payne, T.; Sarabia, G.; Daniel, A.; Sharma, B. In vitro and in vivo SERS biosensing for disease diagnosis. *Biosensors* **2018**, *8*, 46. [CrossRef]
8. Guarrotxena, N.; Liu, B.; Fabris, L.; Bazan, G.C. Antitags: Nanostructured tools for developing SERS-based ELISA analogs. *Adv. Mater.* **2010**, *22*, 4954–4958. [CrossRef]
9. Park, J.-H.; Cho, Y.-W.; Kim, T.-H. Recent advances in surface plasmon resonance sensors for sensitive optical detection of pathogens. *Biosensors* **2022**, *12*, 180. [CrossRef]
10. Schmidheini, L.; Tiefenauer, R.F.; Gatterdam, V.; Frutiger, A.; Sannomiya, T.; Aramesh, M. Self-assembly of nanodiamonds and plasmonic nanoparticles for nanoscopy. *Biosensors* **2022**, *12*, 148. [CrossRef]
11. Altug, H.; Oh, S.-H.; Maier, S.A.; Homola, J. Advances and applications of nanophotonic biosensors. *Nat. Nanotechnol.* **2022**, *17*, 5–16. [CrossRef] [PubMed]
12. Zhao, X.; Luo, X.; Bazuin, C.G.; Masson, J.-F. In situ growth of AuNPs on glass nanofibers for SERS sensors. *ACS Appl. Mater. Interfaces* **2020**, *12*, 55349–55361. [CrossRef] [PubMed]
13. He, Y.; Su, S.; Xu, T.; Zhong, Y.; Zapien, J.A.; Li, J.; Fan, C.; Lee, S.T. Silicon nanowires-based highly-efficient SERS-active platform for ultrasensitive DNA detection. *Nano Today* **2011**, *6*, 122–130. [CrossRef]

14. Wu, S.; Duan, N.; Shen, M.; Wang, J.; Wang, Z. Surface-enhanced Raman spectroscopic single step detection of Vibrio parahaemolyticus using gold coated polydimethylsiloxane as the active substrate and aptamer modified gold nanoparticles. *Microchim. Acta* **2019**, *186*, 401. [CrossRef]
15. Yu, X.; Cai, H.; Zhang, W.; Li, X.; Pan, N.; Luo, Y.; Wang, X.; Hou, J.G. Tuning chemical enhancement of SERS by controlling the chemical reduction of graphene oxide nanosheets. *ACS Nano* **2011**, *5*, 952–958. [CrossRef]
16. Lee, W.W.Y.; Silverson, V.A.D.; Mccoy, C.P.; Donnelly, R.F.; Bell, S.E.J. Preaggregated Ag nanoparticles in dry swellable gel films for off-the-shelf surface-enhanced raman spectroscopy. *Anal. Chem.* **2014**, *86*, 8106–8113. [CrossRef]
17. Panarin, A.Y.; Terekhov, S.N.; Kholostov, K.I.; Bondarenko, V.P. SERS-active substrates based on n-type porous silicon. *Appl. Surf. Sci.* **2010**, *256*, 6969–6976. [CrossRef]
18. Bandarenka, H.; Girel, K.; Zavatski, S.; Panarin, A.; Terekhov, S. Progress in the development of SERS-active substrates based on metal-coated porous silicon. *Materials* **2018**, *11*, 852. [CrossRef]
19. Li, K.; Liu, G.; Zhang, S.; Dai, Y.; Ghafoor, S.; Huang, W.; Zu, Z.; Lu, Y. A porous Au–Ag hybrid nanoparticle array with broadband absorption and high-density hotspots for stable SERS analysis. *Nanoscale* **2019**, *11*, 9587–9592. [CrossRef]
20. Chen, N.; Xiao, T.-H.; Luo, Z.; Kitahama, Y.; Hiramatsu, K.; Kishimoto, N.; Itoh, T.; Cheng, Z.; Goda, K. Porous carbon nanowire array for surface-enhanced Raman spectroscopy. *Nat. Commun.* **2020**, *11*, 4772. [CrossRef]
21. Lu, G.; Wang, G.; Li, H. Effect of nanostructured silicon on surface enhanced Raman scattering. *RSC Adv.* **2018**, *8*, 6629–6633. [CrossRef]
22. Kim, S.; Ansah, I.B.; Park, J.S.; Dang, H.; Choi, N.; Lee, W.C.; Lee, S.H.; Jung, H.S.; Kim, D.H.; Yoo, S.M.; et al. Early and direct detection of bacterial signaling molecules through one-pot au electrodeposition onto paper-based 3D SERS substrates. *Sens. Actuators B Chem.* **2022**, *358*, 131504. [CrossRef]
23. Yeh, Y.-J.; Chiang, W.-H. Ag microplasma-engineered nanoassemblies on cellulose papers for surface-enhanced raman scattering and catalytic nitrophenol reduction. *ACS Appl. Nano Mater.* **2021**, *4*, 6364–6375. [CrossRef]
24. Tegegne, W.A.; Su, W.-N.; Beyene, A.B.; Huang, W.-H.; Tsai, M.-C.; Hwang, B.-J. Flexible hydrophobic filter paper-based SERS substrate using silver nanocubes for sensitive and rapid detection of adenine. *Microchem. J.* **2021**, *168*, 106349. [CrossRef]
25. Lee, M.; Oh, K.; Choi, H.-K.; Lee, S.G.; Youn, H.J.; Lee, H.L.; Jeong, D.H. Subnanomolar sensitivity of filter paper-based SERS sensor for pesticide detection by hydrophobicity change of paper surface. *ACS Sens.* **2018**, *3*, 151–159. [CrossRef]
26. Kim, H.; Hyung, J.; Noh, H. Rationalization of in-situ synthesized plasmonic paper for colorimetric detection of glucose in ocular fluids. *Chemosensors* **2020**, *8*, 81. [CrossRef]
27. Siebe, H.S.; Chen, Q.; Li, X.; Xu, Y.; Browne, W.R.; Bell, S.E.J. Filter paper based SERS substrate for the direct detection of analytes in complex matrices. *Analyst* **2021**, *146*, 1281–1288. [CrossRef]
28. Yu, W.W.; White, I.M. Inkjet printed surface enhanced raman spectroscopy array on cellulose paper. *Anal. Chem.* **2010**, *82*, 9626–9630. [CrossRef]
29. Torul, H.; Çiftçi, H.; Çetin, D.; Suludere, Z.; Boyacı, I.H.; Tamer, U. Paper membrane-based SERS platform for the determination of glucose in blood samples. *Anal. Bioanal. Chem.* **2015**, *407*, 8243–8251. [CrossRef]
30. Wu, L.; Zhang, W.; Liu, C.; Foda, M.F.; Zhu, Y. Strawberry-like SiO$_2$/Ag nanocomposites immersed filter paper as SERS substrate for acrylamide detection. *Food Chem.* **2020**, *328*, 127106. [CrossRef]
31. Yin, G.; Bai, S.; Tu, X.; Li, Z.; Zhang, Y.; Wang, W.; Lu, J.; He, D. Highly sensitive and stable SERS substrate fabricated by co-sputtering and atomic layer deposition. *Nanoscale Res. Lett.* **2019**, *14*, 1–7. [CrossRef] [PubMed]
32. Hirai, Y.; Yabu, H.; Matsuo, Y.; Ijiro, K.; Shimomura, M. Arrays of triangular shaped pincushions for SERS substrates prepared by using self-organization and vapor deposition. *Chem. Commun.* **2010**, *46*, 2298. [CrossRef] [PubMed]
33. Yan, K.; Xu, F.; Wei, W.; Yang, C.; Wang, D.; Shi, X. Electrochemical synthesis of chitosan/silver nanoparticles multilayer hydrogel coating with pH-dependent controlled release capability and antibacterial property. *Colloids Surf. B Biointerfaces* **2021**, *202*, 111711. [CrossRef] [PubMed]
34. Chook, S.W.; Chia, C.H.; Zakaria, S.; Neoh, H.M.; Jamal, R. Effective immobilization of silver nanoparticles on a regenerated cellulose–chitosan composite membrane and its antibacterial activity. *New J. Chem.* **2017**, *41*, 5061–5065. [CrossRef]
35. Xiong, Z.; Lin, M.; Lin, H.; Huang, M. Facile synthesis of cellulose nanofiber nanocomposite as a SERS substrate for detection of thiram in juice. *Carbohydr. Polym.* **2018**, *189*, 79–86. [CrossRef]
36. Carré, M.; Excoffier, S.; Mermet, J.M. A study of the relation between the limit of detection and the limit of quantitation in inductively coupled plasma spectrochemistry. *Spectrochim. Acta Part B At. Spectrosc.* **1997**, *52*, 2043–2049. [CrossRef]
37. Cinteza, L.; Scomoroscenco, C.; Voicu, S.; Nistor, C.; Nitu, S.; Trica, B.; Jecu, M.-L.; Petcu, C. Chitosan-stabilized Ag nanoparticles with superior biocompatibility and their synergistic antibacterial effect in mixtures with essential oils. *Nanomaterials* **2018**, *8*, 826. [CrossRef]
38. Kalaivani, R.; Maruthupandy, M.; Muneeswaran, T.; Hameedha Beevi, A.; Anand, M.; Ramakritinan, C.M.; Kumaraguru, A.K. Synthesis of chitosan mediated silver nanoparticles (Ag NPs) for potential antimicrobial applications. *Front. Lab. Med.* **2018**, *2*, 30–35. [CrossRef]
39. Thanh, N.T.K.; Maclean, N.; Mahidine, S. Mechanisms of nucleation and growth of nanoparticles in solution. *Chem. Rev.* **2014**, *114*, 7610–7630. [CrossRef]
40. Khouri, J.; Penlidis, A.; Moresoli, C. Viscoelastic properties of crosslinked chitosan films. *Processes* **2019**, *7*, 157. [CrossRef]

41. Wang, A.; Kong, X. Review of recent progress of plasmonic materials and Nano-structures for surface-enhanced Raman scattering. *Materials* **2015**, *8*, 3024–3052. [CrossRef] [PubMed]
42. Wiley, J.H.; Atalla, R.H. Band assignments in the Raman spectra of celluloses. *Carbohydr. Res.* **1987**, *160*, 113–129. [CrossRef]
43. Kong, K.; Eichhorn, S.J. Crystalline and amorphous deformation of process-controlled cellulose-II fibres. *Polymer* **2005**, *46*, 6380–6390. [CrossRef]
44. Zając, A.; Hanuza, J.; Wandas, M.; Dymińska, L. Determination of N-acetylation degree in chitosan using Raman spectroscopy. *Spectrochim. Acta Part A Mol. Biomol. Spectrosc.* **2015**, *134*, 114–120. [CrossRef]
45. Wanasekara, N.D.; Michud, A.; Zhu, C.; Rahatekar, S.; Sixta, H.; Eichhorn, S.J. Deformation mechanisms in ionic liquid spun cellulose fibers. *Polymer* **2016**, *99*, 222–230. [CrossRef]
46. Eichhorn, S.J.; Sirichaisit, J.; Young, R.J. Deformation mechanisms in cellulose fibres, paper and wood. *J. Mater. Sci.* **2001**, *36*, 3129–3135. [CrossRef]
47. Gierlinger, N.; Schwanninger, M.; Reinecke, A.; Burgert, I. Molecular Changes during Tensile Deformation of Single Wood Fibers Followed by Raman Microscopy. *Biomacromolecules* **2006**, *7*, 2077–2081. [CrossRef]
48. Quynh, L.M.; Nam, N.H.; Kong, K.; Nhung, N.T.; Notingher, I.; Henini, M.; Luong, N.H. Surface-enhanced Raman spectroscopy study of 4-ATP on gold nanoparticles for basal cell carcinoma fingerprint detection. *J. Electron. Mater.* **2016**, *45*, 2563–2568. [CrossRef]
49. Kumar, G.; Soni, R.K. Silver nanocube- and nanowire-based SERS substrates for ultra-low detection of PATP and thiram molecules. *Plasmonics* **2020**, *15*, 1577–1589. [CrossRef]
50. Wang, Y.; Zou, X.; Ren, W.; Wang, W.; Wang, E. Effect of silvernanoplates on Raman spectra of p-aminothiophenol assembled on smooth macroscopic gold and silver surface. *J. Phys. Chem. C* **2007**, *111*, 3259–3265. [CrossRef]
51. Li, L.; Chin, W.S. Rapid fabrication of a flexible and transparent Ag Nanocubes@PDMS film as a SERS substrate with high performance. *ACS Appl. Mater. Interfaces* **2020**, *12*, 37538–37548. [CrossRef] [PubMed]
52. Mosier-Boss, P. Review on SERS of bacteria. *Biosensors* **2017**, *7*, 51. [CrossRef] [PubMed]
53. Azevedo, E.P.; Retarekar, R.; Raghavan, M.L.; Kumar, V. Mechanical properties of cellulose: Chitosan blends for potential use as a coronary artery bypass graft. *J. Biomater. Sci. Polym. Ed.* **2013**, *24*, 239–252. [CrossRef]

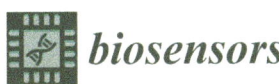

Article

Identifying the Posture of Young Adults in Walking Videos by Using a Fusion Artificial Intelligent Method

Posen Lee [1], Tai-Been Chen [2,3], Chin-Hsuan Liu [1,4,*], Chi-Yuan Wang [2], Guan-Hua Huang [3] and Nan-Han Lu [2,5,6]

1. Department of Occupation Therapy, I-Shou University, No. 8, Yida Road, Jiaosu Village, Yanchao District, Kaohsiung 82445, Taiwan; posenlee@isu.edu.tw
2. Department of Medical Imaging and Radiological Science, I-Shou University, No. 8, Yida Road, Jiaosu Village, Yanchao District, Kaohsiung 82445, Taiwan; ctb@isu.edu.tw (T.-B.C.); wang1b011@isu.edu.tw (C.-Y.W.); ed103911@edah.org.tw (N.-H.L.)
3. Institute of Statistics, National Yang Ming Chiao Tung University, No. 1001, University Road, Hsinchu 30010, Taiwan; ghuang@stat.nctu.edu.tw
4. Department of Occupational Therapy, Kaohsiung Municipal Kai-Syuan Psychiatric Hospital, No. 130, Kaisyuan 2nd Road, Lingya District, Kaohsiung City 80276, Taiwan
5. Department of Pharmacy, Tajen University, No. 20, Weixin Road, Yanpu Township, Pingtung County 90741, Taiwan
6. Department of Radiology, E-DA Hospital, I-Shou University, No. 1, Yida Road, Jiaosu Village, Yanchao District, Kaohsiung City 82445, Taiwan
* Correspondence: isu6a394@cloud.isu.edu.tw; Tel.: +886-7-6151100 (ext. 7516)

Abstract: Many neurological and musculoskeletal disorders are associated with problems related to postural movement. Noninvasive tracking devices are used to record, analyze, measure, and detect the postural control of the body, which may indicate health problems in real time. A total of 35 young adults without any health problems were recruited for this study to participate in a walking experiment. An iso-block postural identity method was used to quantitatively analyze posture control and walking behavior. The participants who exhibited straightforward walking and skewed walking were defined as the control and experimental groups, respectively. Fusion deep learning was applied to generate dynamic joint node plots by using OpenPose-based methods, and skewness was qualitatively analyzed using convolutional neural networks. The maximum specificity and sensitivity achieved using a combination of ResNet101 and the naïve Bayes classifier were 0.84 and 0.87, respectively. The proposed approach successfully combines cell phone camera recordings, cloud storage, and fusion deep learning for posture estimation and classification.

Keywords: iso-block postural identity; OpenPose; fusion deep learning

1. Introduction

The OpenPose algorithm is a deep learning method in which part affinity fields (PAFs) are used to detect the two-dimensional (2D) postures of humans in images [1]. The relationship between posture stability, motor function, and quality of life has been determined [2,3]. Moreover, the OpenPose algorithm has been used for checking the medication situations of patients and for their physical monitoring [4,5]. The evaluation of the cardinal symptoms of resting tremor and bradykinesia for Parkinson's disease has been conducted using an OpenPose-based deep learning method [6,7]. Furthermore, in [8], the OpenPose framework was used to create a human behavior recognition system for skeleton posture estimation. Quantitative gait (motor) variables can be estimated and recorded using pose tracking systems (e.g., OpenPose, AlphaPose, and Detectron) [9]. These factors are useful for measuring the quality of life of older adults [10–12]. Moreover, parkinsonian motion features have been created using deep-learning-based 2D OpenPose models [13,14]. For people with autism spectrum disorder, skeleton posture characteristics are correlated with long-term memory in the field of action recognition [15–17]. The physical function of a patient should be assessed according to their health data obtained using a skeleton pose tracking device and gait analysis [18–21]. Many neurological and musculoskeletal disorders are associated with problems related to postural movement, which can be estimated using a pose-capturing device [22]. Therefore, noninvasive tracking devices are used to record, analyze, measure, and detect the postural control of the body, which may indicate health problems in real time. In this study, fusion deep learning was used to generate dynamic joint node plots (DJNPs) by using OpenPose-based methods, and skewness in walking was qualitatively analyzed using convolutional neural networks (CNNs) [23]. An iso-block postural identity (IPI) method was used to perform the quantified analysis of postural control and walking behavior. This proposed approach combines cell phone camera recordings, cloud storage, and fusion deep learning for postural estimation and classification.

2. Materials and Methods

2.1. Research Ethics

All the experimental procedures were approved by the Institutional Review Board of E-DA Hospital [with approval number EMRP52110N (04/11/2021)]. Verbal and written information on all the experimental details was provided to all the participants before they provided informed consent. Written informed consent was obtained from the participants prior to experimental data collection.

2.2. Flow of Research

In this study, videos walking toward and away from a cell phone camera were recorded using the camera (Step 1 in Figure 1). The videos were recorded at 24-bit (RGB), 1080p resolution, and 30 frames per second. The videos were uploaded to Google Cloud through 5G mobile Internet or Wi-Fi (Step 2 in Figure 1). The workstation used in this study downloaded a video, extracted a single frame from the video, and then applied a fusion artificial intelligence (AI) method to this frame (Step 3 in Figure 1). In the aforementioned step, single frames were extracted from an input video (Step 3A), frames with static walking were identified using an OpenPose-based deep learning method (Step 3B), and the joint nodes of the input video were merged into a plot (Step 3C). The obtained DJNP was categorized as representing straight or skewed walking (Step 3D). CNNs were used to classify DJNPs into one of the aforementioned two groups. Two types of deep learning methods were used in the fusion AI method adopted in this study: an OpenPose-based deep learning method and CNN-based methods. The OpenPose-based method is useful for estimating the coordinates of joint nodes from an input image [1]. The adopted CNNs are suitable for the classification of images with high accuracy and robustness.

2.3. Participants

A total of 35 young adults without any health problems were recruited to participate in a walking experiment. The age range was 20.20 ± 1.08 years. The inclusion criteria were healthy adults who were willing to participate and could walk more than 5 m. People with musculoskeletal pain (such as muscle soreness), those who had drunk alcohol or taken sleeping pills within 24 h before the commencement of the experiment, and individuals with limited vision (such as nearsighted people without glasses) were excluded from this study.

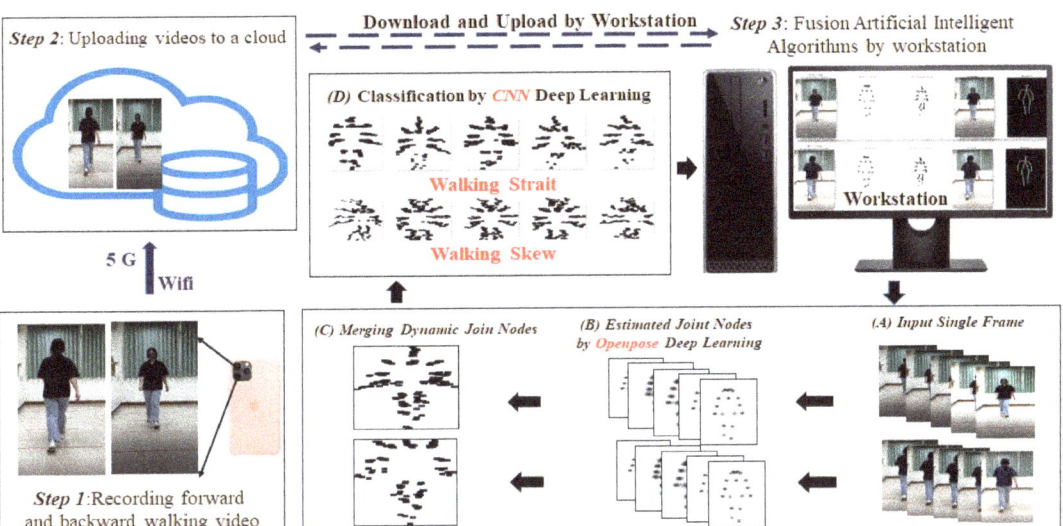

Figure 1. Flow of research.

2.4. Experimental Design

The experimental setup is depicted in Figure 2. The total length of the experimental space was greater than 7 m. The ground was level, free of debris, and smooth to ensure a straight and smooth walking path. The cell phone was placed 1 m above the ground (approximately equal to the height of a medium-sized adult holding a cell phone) and 2 m from the endpoint of the walking path. The entire body of a participant was recorded during the walk. The participants were required to wear walking shoes and not slippers while walking. Participants walked away from the cell phone and then turned back and walked toward the cell phone. The participants walked for 5 m toward and away from the camera three times each. One video was captured for each 5-m walk; thus, six videos were recorded for each participant. A series of single (static) frames was extracted from a video every 0.3 s. For example, for a 3-s input video, 10 frames were extracted to estimate the coordinates of joint nodes. A static frame of one DJNP was extracted per 0.3 s for one video. For example, a 10 s walking video with frame rate 30 (frames/second), the total static frame in one DJNP are 90 frames (i.e., 90 = 10 (second) × 30 (frames/second) × 0.3 (second)). Hence, the DJNP was a variety of frames according to the length of a walking video. The filmmakers are not medical experts but are trained in motion assessment. The video is analyzed by an expert in image analysis and an occupational therapist specializing in rehabilitation Table 1 lists the number of participants and the mean and standard deviation (STD) of velocity (m/s) and time (s) for each group.

Table 1. Information on the number of participants and the mean and standard deviation (STD) of velocity (m/s) and time (s) for each group.

Group	N	Mean Velocity (m/s)	STD Velocity (m/s)	Mean Time (s)	STD Time (s)
Skew	102	0.68	0.08	7.48	0.84
Straight	108	0.69	0.08	7.39	0.91

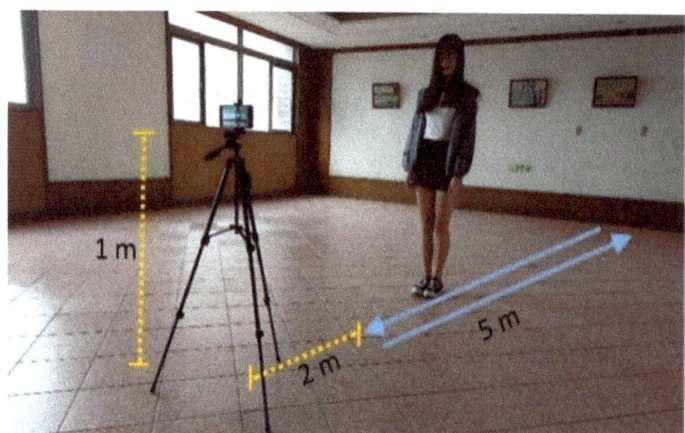

Figure 2. Experimental setup (the cell phone was placed 1 m above the floor and 2 m from the participant).

2.5. Measurement of Joint Nodes through Openpose-Based Deep Learning

OpenPose is a well-known system that uses a bottom-up approach for real-time multiperson body pose estimation. In the proposed OpenPose-based method, PAFs are used to obtain a nonparametric representation for associating body parts with individuals in an image [1]. This bottom-up method achieves high accuracy in real time, regardless of the number of people in the image. It can be used to detect the 2D poses of multiple people in an image and to perform single-person pose estimation for each detection. In this study, the OpenPose algorithm was mainly used to output a heat map of joint nodes (Figure 3). The center coordinates of joint nodes were estimated by using the geometric centroid formula.

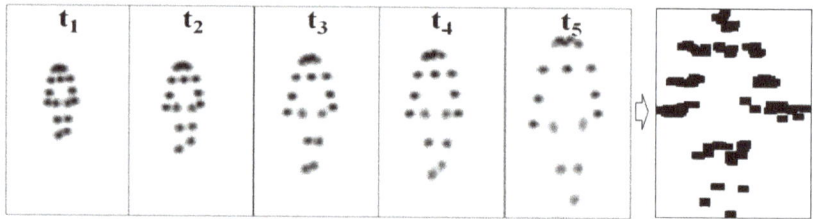

Figure 3. Dynamic joint node plot (DJNP) (right) obtained by merging the heat maps of joint nodes from t_1 to t_5 by using the OpenPose algorithm.

2.6. Definition of the Control and Experimental Groups

The data for the control group comprised DJNPs that indicated straightforward walking toward and away from the camera. The experimental group comprised DJNPs that indicated skewed walking. The data for the control and experimental groups comprised 102 and 108 DJNPs, respectively, which were classified using different CNNs.

2.7. Classification Using Pretrained CNNs and Machine Learning Classifiers

Pretrained CNNs were used to extract the features of DJNPs, and machine learning classifiers were used to construct classification models. The eight pre-trained CNNs used in this study were AlexNet, DenseNet201, GoogleNet, MobileNetV2, ResNet101, ResNet50, VGG16, and VGG19. Moreover, the three machine learning classifiers used in this study were logistic regression (LR), naïve Bayes (NB), and support vector machine (SVM).

CNNs have a high learning capacity, which makes them suitable for image classification. They extract features and learn data according to variations in the breadth and depth of features. Table 2 lists the features that were extracted by CNNs and served as the inputs for the LR, NB, and SVM. A deep CNN network comprises five types of primary layers: a convolutional layer, a pooling layer, a rectified linear unit layer, fully connected layers, and a softmax layer. Information on the pretrained CNNs used in this study is provided in Table 2. The fully connected layers of the CNNs extracted and stored the features of the input image. In the present study, eight CNNs and three classifiers with four batch sizes and 20 random splits were adopted. The four batch sizes selected in this study for the CNNs were 5, 8, 11, and 14. The total number of investigated models was 8 (CNNs) × 3 (machine learning techniques) × 4 (batch size settings) × 20 (instances of random splitting) = 1920. Therefore, the 1920 models represent the 1920 possible combinations of one CNN, classifier, batch size, and random data split. CNNs have demonstrated utility and efficiency in image feature extraction in the fields of biomedicine and biology [23–27].

Table 2. Information on the adopted convolutional neural networks.

CNN	Image Size	Layers	Parametric Size (MB)	Layer of Features
AlexNet	227 × 227	25	227	17th (4096 × 9216)
DenseNet201	224 × 224	709	77	706th (1000 × 1920)
GoogleNet	224 × 224	144	27	142nd (1000 × 1024)
MobileNetV2	224 × 224	154	13	152nd (1000 × 1280)
ResNet101	224 × 224	347	167	345th (1000 × 2048)
ResNet50	224 × 224	177	96	175th (1000 × 2048)
VGG16	224 × 224	41	27	33rd (4096 × 25,088)
VGG19	224 × 224	47	535	39th (4096 × 25,088)

LR is a process of modeling the probability of a discrete outcome when an input variable is given. This process is often used to analyze associations between two or more predictors or variables. LR does not require the existence of a linear relationship between inputs and output variables. This method is useful when the response variable is binary, but the explanatory variables are continuous. LR is also an effective analysis method for classification problems. The LR method is used for the development of classification models in the field of machine learning because of its capacity to provide hierarchical or tree-like structures. Many fields have adopted LR for prediction and classification. LR is suitable for classification problems related to health issues, such as whether a person has a specific ailment or disease when a set of symptoms are given.

NB classifiers are based on Bayes' theorem with a naïve independence hypothesis between the adopted predictors or features. These classifiers are the most suitable ones for solving classification problems in which no dependency exists between a particular feature and other features of a certain class. NB classifiers offer high flexibility for linear or nonlinear relations among variables (features or predictors) in classification problems and provide increased accuracy when combined with kernel density estimation. NB classifiers exhibit higher performance for categorical input data than for numerical input data. These classifiers are easy to implement and computationally inexpensive, perform well on large datasets with high dimensionality, and are extremely sensitive to feature selection.

SVM classifiers are highly powerful classifiers that can be used to solve two-class pattern recognition problems. They transform the original nonlinear data into a higher-dimensional space and then create a separating hyperplane defined by various support vectors in this space to maximize the margin between two datasets. Data can be linearly separated in the higher-dimensional space by using a kernel function. Many useful kernels are available to improve the classification performance and reduce the false rate. SVM is a supervised learning method for the classification of linear and nonlinear data and is generally used for the classification of high-dimensional or nonlinear data.

The computing time of using SVM is in linear time, rather than by expensive iterative approximation, which is performed by many other types of classifiers. The LR, NB, and SVM methods were applied as deep and machine learning methods to extract features of DJNPs and classify the postural control of the straight and skewed walking groups.

2.8. Validation of Classification Performance

The data for the control and experimental groups comprised 102 and 108 DJNPs, respectively. A random splitting schema was employed to separate the training (70%) and testing (30%) sets; 71 and 31 samples from the control group were used for training and testing, respectively, and 76 and 32 samples from the experimental group were used for training and testing, respectively. Testing sets and confusion matrices were used to evaluate the models with respect to the kappa value, accuracy, sensitivity, specificity, positive predictive value (PPV), and negative predictive value (NPV). These indices were sorted in the ascending order of the corresponding kappa value, and a radar plot was then generated to present the aforementioned indices of the adopted models.

3. Results

In this study, 70% of the samples of each group were randomly used to train the adopted classifiers, and the remaining 30% of samples were used to perform validation. Figure 4 shows a scatter plot for the specificity and sensitivity of the 1920 models for the validation dataset. The maximum specificity and sensitivity of 0.84 and 0.87, respectively, were achieved by the ResNet101 and NB classifiers, respectively.

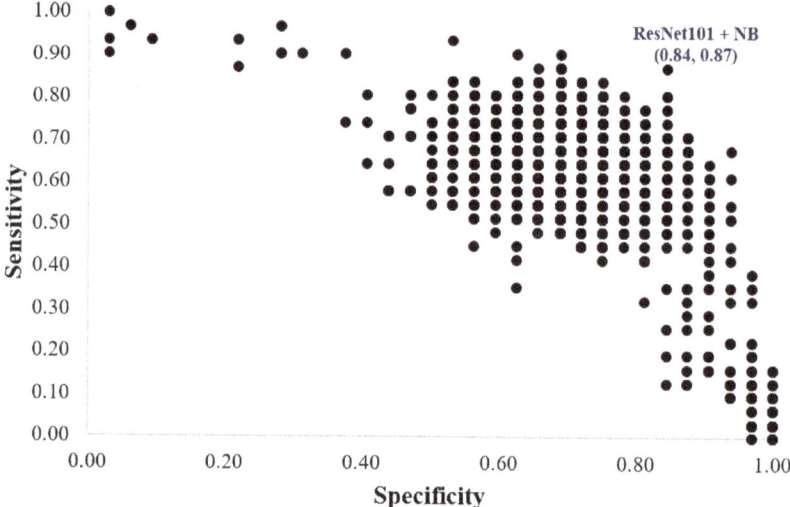

Figure 4. Scatter plot for the specificity and sensitivity of the 1920 models for the validation dataset.

In Figure 5, a radar plot was constructed for six performance indices with the results sorted by the maximum kappa value for 96 models (the abbreviations of the investigated models are written in Appendix A). The best performing model was M53, which is a combination of ResNet101 and naïve Bayes. The kappa, accuracy, sensitivity (Sen), specificity (Spe), PPV, and NPV values were 0.71, 0.86, 0.87, 0.84, 0.84, and 0.87, respectively. All of the performance indices are over 0.7. The optimized model, ResNet101 with naïve Bayes, had acceptable agreement results and the highest accuracy.

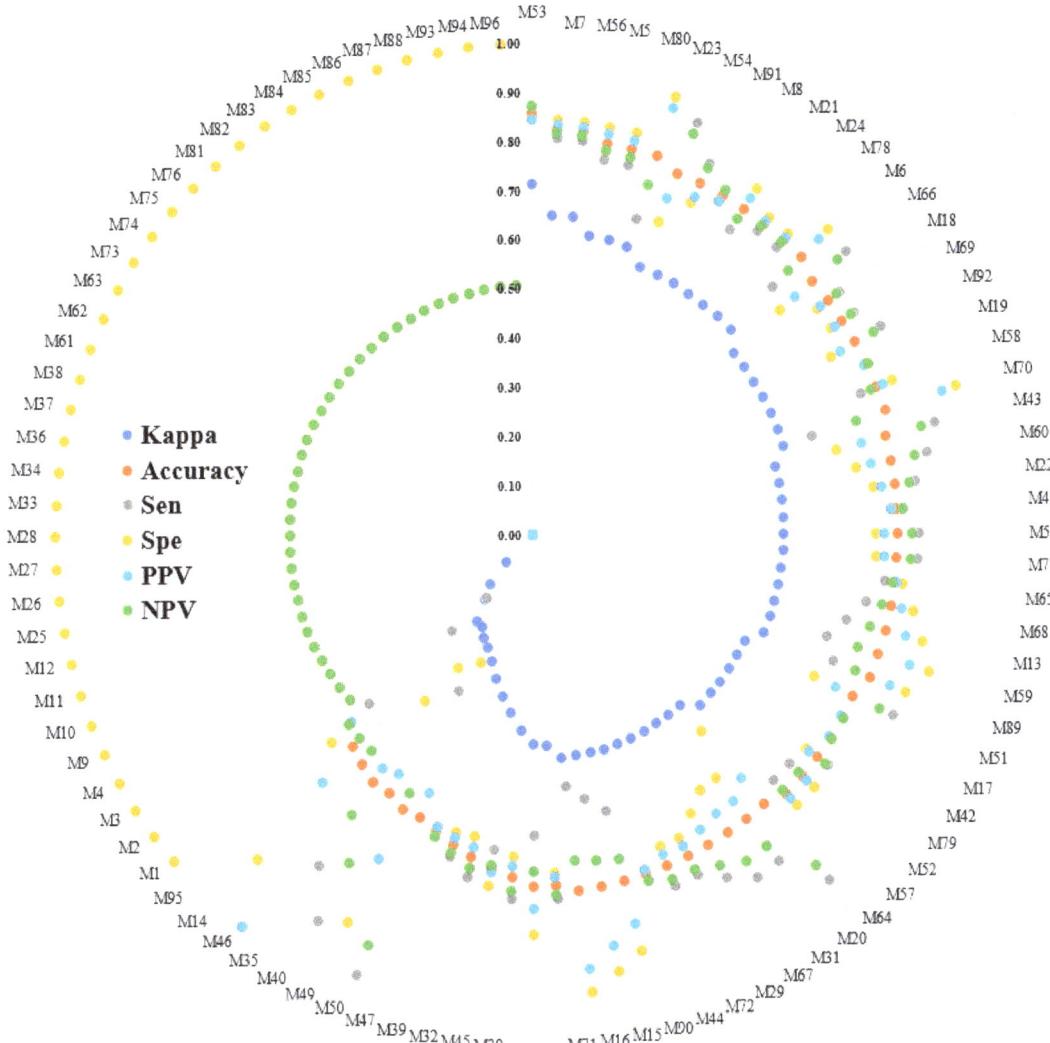

Figure 5. Radar plot of the six performance indices sorted in the ascending order of the kappa value for 96 models (the abbreviations are explained in the Appendix A). Sen represents the sensitivity, and Spe represents the specificity.

Table 3 lists the 13 models with kappa values greater than 0.59. These models comprised four (30.8%) AlexNet models, three DenseNet201 models (23.1%), three ResNet101 models (23.1%), two VGG16 models (15.4%), and one VGG19 model (7.7%). AlexNet, DenseNet201, and ResNet101 accounted for 10 of the aforementioned 13 models (76.9%). SVM and NB were the main machine learning classifiers that performed well in this study. The numbers of the aforementioned 13 models with SVM and NB classifiers were 3 and 10, respectively. Thus, NB performed well. Finally, the batch sizes of the 13 models were 5, 8, 11, and 14 useable in this work.

Table 3. Models with kappa values greater than 0.59.

CNN	Classifier	Batch Size	Model	Kappa	Accuracy	Sen	Spe	PPV	NPV
ResNet101	NB	5	M53	0.71	0.86	0.87	0.84	0.84	0.87
AlexNet	NB	11	M7	0.65	0.83	0.81	0.84	0.83	0.82
ResNet101	NB	14	M56	0.65	0.83	0.81	0.84	0.83	0.82
AlexNet	NB	5	M5	0.62	0.81	0.77	0.84	0.83	0.79
VGG16	NB	14	M80	0.62	0.81	0.77	0.84	0.83	0.79
DenseNet201	SVM	11	M23	0.62	0.81	0.68	0.94	0.91	0.75
ResNet101	NB	8	M54	0.59	0.79	0.90	0.69	0.74	0.88
VGG19	NB	11	M91	0.59	0.79	0.84	0.75	0.77	0.83
AlexNet	NB	14	M8	0.59	0.79	0.81	0.78	0.78	0.81
DenseNet201	SVM	5	M21	0.59	0.79	0.74	0.84	0.82	0.77
DenseNet201	SVM	14	M24	0.59	0.79	0.77	0.81	0.80	0.79
VGG16	NB	8	M78	0.59	0.79	0.77	0.81	0.80	0.79
AlexNet	NB	8	M6	0.59	0.79	0.71	0.88	0.85	0.76

4. Discussion

4.1. Measurement of Postural Control

IPIs were used to measure the skewness or displacement. Figure 6 illustrates the fusion of a DJNP with the IPI generated for a series of time points. In this study, an IPI was created every 0.3 s, and all the IPIs were fused with DJNPs.

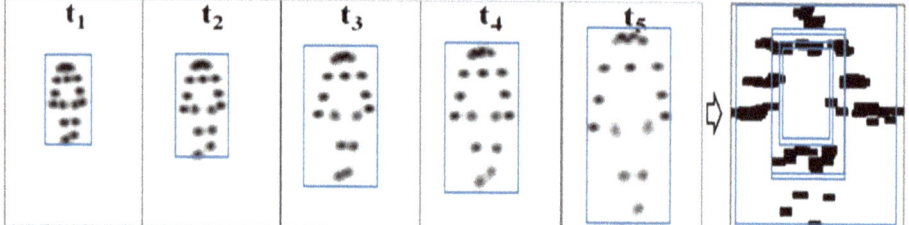

Figure 6. Iso-block postural identity (IPI) generated for a series of times and fusion of the IPI with a DJNP (right).

Figure 7 presents the skewness or displacement for a walking video at three time points (i.e., t_0, t_1, and t_2). Figure 7A,C,D,F depict DJNPs and IPIs for skewed walking. Figure 7B,E depict DJNPs and IPIs for straight walking. These DJNPs can be used to measure skewness and horizontal postural movement.

The parameters Θ_r and Θ_l represent the angles of the right and left sides of the body during captured images, respectively (Figure 7E). The ratio of two angles (i.e., $SR = \Theta_l/\Theta_r$) was used to measure the skewness tendency. When this ratio is >1, the body tends to skew to the right. When $SR = 1$, the body is almost straight. When SR is <1, the body tends to skew to the left. The displacement of the body between two time points was quantified by estimating the distance covered between these time points. For example, in Figure 7B,E, $D_{r,0,1}$ and $D_{l,0,1}$ represent the displacements of the right and left sides of the body, respectively, between t_0 and t_1. Similarly, $D_{r,1,2}$ and $D_{l,1,2}$ represent the displacements of the right and left sides of the body, respectively, between t_1 and t_2. Therefore, the ratio of $D_{r,i-1,i}$ to $D_{l,i-1,i}$ (i.e., $MD = D_{r,i-1,i}/D_{l,i-1,i}$, $i = 0, 1, 2$) could be used to determine the dominant side of body displacement. When MD was >1, the right side was the dominant side of displacement. When MD was 1, the walking posture was almost straight. Moreover, when MD was <1, the left side was the dominant displacement side.

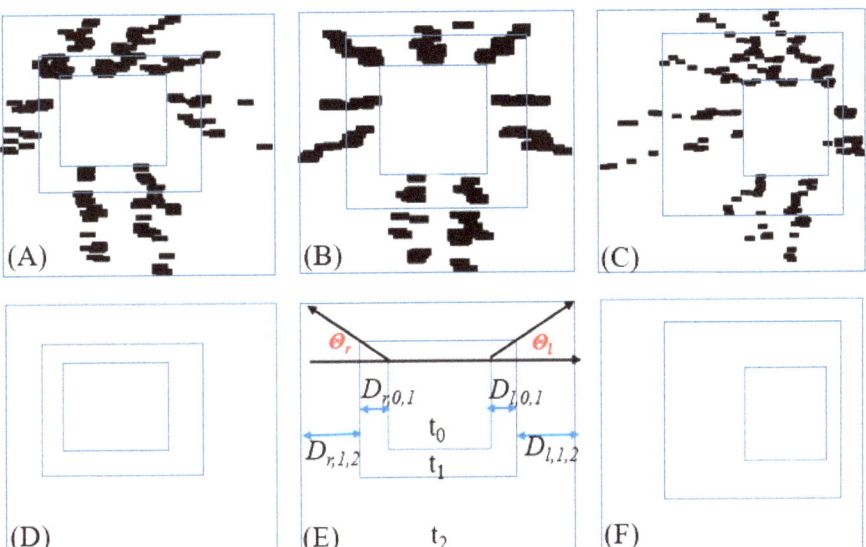

Figure 7. Graphical representation of the skewness or displacement for a walking video at three time points (i.e., t_0, t_1, t_2). (**A,D**), (**B,E**), and (**C,F**), respectively, present postural skew to the left, postural balance, and postural skew to the right with participants walking toward the camera.

4.2. Literature for Health Issues and Postural Control during Walking

Poor postural control during walking may indicate health problems. An individual's postural control considerably influences their quality of life [2,3]. Equipping participants with wearable devices that assess their posture can be challenging [4]. Nevertheless, this problem can be overcome by incorporating deep learning into Internet of things monitoring systems to effectively detect motion and posture [5]. Resting tremors and finger tapping have been detected using OpenPose-based deep learning methods [6,7]. Moreover, skeleton normality has been determined through the measurement of angles and velocities by using the aforementioned methods [8–10]. Such methods are useful for not only generating three-dimensional poses [11,12] but also for identifying the relationship between postural behavior and functional diseases, such as Parkinson's disease [6,13,14], autism spectrum disorder [15], and metatarsophalangeal joint flexions [16]. OpenPose-based deep learning methods can be used for skeleton, ankle, and foot motion [8,17] detection; physical function assessment [18,19]; and poststroke study [20].

Thus, noninvasive tracking devices play crucial roles in the recording [21], analysis, measurement, and detection of body posture, which may indicate health issues in real time.

5. Conclusions

In this study, fusion deep learning was applied to generate DJNPs by using an OpenPose-based method and quantify skewness by using CNNs. The adopted approach successfully incorporates cell phone camera recording, cloud storage, and fusion deep learning for posture estimation and classification. Moreover, the adopted IPI method can be used to perform a quantified analysis of postural control and walking behavior.

The research conducted in the present study can be considered preliminary. We developed the IPI method and attempted a quantified analysis of postural control and walking behavior to identify factors indicative of possible clinical gait disorders. However, at the time of writing, the research is in the preliminary phase and will remain as such until the automated analysis is completed through the IPI method. The highlights of our proposed method include its suitability for use with computer vision for identifying signs of gait problems for clinical application, as well as its replacement of a dynamic joint node plot. In addition, the IPI method is straightforward and allows for real-time monitoring. A video of walking behavior can be conveniently recorded in real-time by using a mobile device. A user can easily remove the background from the video and generate dynamic joint node coordinates through fusion AI methods. The developed IPI method allows for use with computer vision to identify postural characteristics for clinical applications.

Future studies can apply the proposed approach to individuals with health problems to validate this approach.

Author Contributions: Conceptualization, P.L., T.-B.C. and C.-H.L.; Data curation, T.-B.C., G.-H.H. and N.-H.L.; Formal analysis, P.L., T.-B.C. and C.-H.L.; Investigation, C.-Y.W.; Methodology, P.L., T.-B.C. and C.-H.L.; Project administration, P.L.; Software, T.-B.C.; Supervision, P.L. and C.-H.L.; Writing—original draft, T.-B.C. and C.-H.L.; Writing—review and editing, P.L. and C.-H.L. All authors have read and agreed to the published version of the manuscript.

Funding: Ministry of Science and Technology of Taiwan funded this research under the grant numbers MOST 110-2118-M-214-001.

Institutional Review Board Statement: The study was conducted in accordance with the guidelines of the Declaration of Helsinki. All experimental procedures were approved by the Institutional Review Board of the E-DA Hospital, Kaohsiung, Taiwan (approval number EMRP52110N).

Informed Consent Statement: Informed consent was obtained from all subjects involved in the study.

Data Availability Statement: Not applicable.

Conflicts of Interest: The authors declare no conflict of interest.

Appendix A

Table A1. The 96 combinations of investigated models with abbreviation are listed below.

CNN	Classifier	Batch Size	Model	CNN	Classifier	Batch Size	Model	CNN	Classifier	Batch Size	Model
AlexNet	LR	5	M1	GoogleNet	SVM	5	M33	ResNet50	NB	5	M65
AlexNet	LR	8	M2	GoogleNet	SVM	8	M34	ResNet50	NB	8	M66
AlexNet	LR	11	M3	GoogleNet	SVM	11	M35	ResNet50	NB	11	M67
AlexNet	LR	14	M4	GoogleNet	SVM	14	M36	ResNet50	NB	14	M68
AlexNet	NB	5	M5	MobileNetV2	LR	5	M37	ResNet50	SVM	5	M69
AlexNet	NB	8	M6	MobileNetV2	LR	8	M38	ResNet50	SVM	8	M70
AlexNet	NB	11	M7	MobileNetV2	LR	11	M39	ResNet50	SVM	11	M71
AlexNet	NB	14	M8	MobileNetV2	LR	14	M40	ResNet50	SVM	14	M72
AlexNet	SVM	5	M9	MobileNetV2	NB	5	M41	VGG16	LR	5	M73
AlexNet	SVM	8	M10	MobileNetV2	NB	8	M42	VGG16	LR	8	M74
AlexNet	SVM	11	M11	MobileNetV2	NB	11	M43	VGG16	LR	11	M75
AlexNet	SVM	14	M12	MobileNetV2	NB	14	M44	VGG16	LR	14	M76
DenseNet201	LR	5	M13	MobileNetV2	SVM	5	M45	VGG16	NB	5	M77
DenseNet201	LR	8	M14	MobileNetV2	SVM	8	M46	VGG16	NB	8	M78
DenseNet201	LR	11	M15	MobileNetV2	SVM	11	M47	VGG16	NB	11	M79
DenseNet201	LR	14	M16	MobileNetV2	SVM	14	M48	VGG16	NB	14	M80
DenseNet201	NB	5	M17	ResNet101	LR	5	M49	VGG16	SVM	5	M81
DenseNet201	NB	8	M18	ResNet101	LR	8	M50	VGG16	SVM	8	M82
DenseNet201	NB	11	M19	ResNet101	LR	11	M51	VGG16	SVM	11	M83
DenseNet201	NB	14	M20	ResNet101	LR	14	M52	VGG16	SVM	14	M84
DenseNet201	SVM	5	M21	**ResNet101**	**NB**	**5**	**M53**	VGG19	LR	5	M85
DenseNet201	SVM	8	M22	ResNet101	NB	8	M54	VGG19	LR	8	M86
DenseNet201	SVM	11	M23	ResNet101	NB	11	M55	VGG19	LR	11	M87
DenseNet201	SVM	14	M24	ResNet101	NB	14	M56	VGG19	LR	14	M88
GoogleNet	LR	5	M25	ResNet101	SVM	5	M57	VGG19	NB	5	M89
GoogleNet	LR	8	M26	ResNet101	SVM	8	M58	VGG19	NB	8	M90
GoogleNet	LR	11	M27	ResNet101	SVM	11	M59	VGG19	NB	11	M91
GoogleNet	LR	14	M28	ResNet101	SVM	14	M60	VGG19	NB	14	M92
GoogleNet	NB	5	M29	ResNet50	LR	5	M61	VGG19	SVM	5	M93
GoogleNet	NB	8	M30	ResNet50	LR	8	M62	VGG19	SVM	8	M94
GoogleNet	NB	11	M31	ResNet50	LR	11	M63	VGG19	SVM	11	M95
GoogleNet	NB	14	M32	ResNet50	LR	14	M64	VGG19	SVM	14	M96

References

1. Cao, Z.; Hidalgo, G.; Simon, T.; Wei, S.E.; Sheikh, Y. OpenPose: Realtime Multi-Person 2D Pose Estimation Using Part Affinity Fields. *IEEE Trans. Pattern Anal. Mach. Intell.* **2019**, *43*, 172–186. [CrossRef]
2. Ali, M.S. Does spasticity affect the postural stability and quality of life of children with cerebral palsy? *J. Taibah Univ. Med Sci.* **2021**, *16*, 761–766. [CrossRef]
3. Park, E.-Y. Path analysis of strength, spasticity, gross motor function, and health-related quality of life in children with spastic cerebral palsy. *Health Qual. Life Outcomes* **2018**, *16*, 70. [CrossRef] [PubMed]
4. Roh, H.; Shin, S.; Han, J.; Lim, S. A deep learning-based medication behavior monitoring system. *Math. Biosci. Eng.* **2021**, *18*, 1513–1528. [CrossRef]
5. Manogaran, G.; Shakeel, P.M.; Fouad, H.; Nam, Y.; Baskar, S.; Chilamkurti, N.; Sundarasekar, R. Wearable IoT Smart-Log Patch: An Edge Computing-Based Bayesian Deep Learning Network System for Multi Access Physical Monitoring System. *Sensors* **2019**, *19*, 3030. [CrossRef] [PubMed]
6. Park, K.W.; Lee, E.-J.; Lee, J.S.; Jeong, J.; Choi, N.; Jo, S.; Jung, M.; Do, J.Y.; Kang, D.-W.; Lee, J.-G.; et al. Machine Learning–Based Automatic Rating for Cardinal Symptoms of Parkinson Disease. *Neurology* **2021**, *96*, e1761–e1769. [CrossRef] [PubMed]
7. Heldman, D.A.; Espay, A.; LeWitt, P.A.; Giuffrida, J.P. Clinician versus machine: Reliability and responsiveness of motor endpoints in Parkinson's disease. *Park. Relat. Disord.* **2014**, *20*, 590–595. [CrossRef]
8. Lin, F.-C.; Ngo, H.-H.; Dow, C.-R.; Lam, K.-H.; Le, H. Student Behavior Recognition System for the Classroom Environment Based on Skeleton Pose Estimation and Person Detection. *Sensors* **2021**, *21*, 5314. [CrossRef]
9. Mehdizadeh, S.; Nabavi, H.; Sabo, A.; Arora, T.; Iaboni, A.; Taati, B. Concurrent validity of human pose tracking in video for measuring gait parameters in older adults: A preliminary analysis with multiple trackers, viewing angles, and walking directions. *J. Neuroeng. Rehabilitation* **2021**, *18*, 1–16. [CrossRef]
10. Ota, M.; Tateuchi, H.; Hashiguchi, T.; Ichihashi, N. Verification of validity of gait analysis systems during treadmill walking and running using human pose tracking algorithm. *Gait Posture* **2021**, *85*, 290–297. [CrossRef]
11. Rapczyński, M.; Werner, P.; Handrich, S.; Al-Hamadi, A. A Baseline for Cross-Database 3D Human Pose Estimation. *Sensors* **2021**, *21*, 3769. [CrossRef] [PubMed]
12. Pagnon, D.; Domalain, M.; Reveret, L. Pose2Sim: An End-to-End Workflow for 3D Markerless Sports Kinematics—Part 1: Robustness. *Sensors* **2021**, *21*, 6530. [CrossRef] [PubMed]
13. Sato, K.; Nagashima, Y.; Mano, T.; Iwata, A.; Toda, T. Quantifying normal and parkinsonian gait features from home movies: Practical application of a deep learning–based 2D pose estimator. *PLoS ONE* **2019**, *14*, e0223549. [CrossRef] [PubMed]
14. Rupprechter, S.; Morinan, G.; Peng, Y.; Foltynie, T.; Sibley, K.; Weil, R.S.; Leyland, L.-A.; Baig, F.; Morgante, F.; Gilron, R.; et al. A Clinically Interpretable Computer-Vision Based Method for Quantifying Gait in Parkinson's Disease. *Sensors* **2021**, *21*, 5437. [CrossRef]
15. Zhang, Y.; Tian, Y.; Wu, P.; Chen, D. Application of Skeleton Data and Long Short-Term Memory in Action Recognition of Children with Autism Spectrum Disorder. *Sensors* **2021**, *21*, 411. [CrossRef] [PubMed]
16. Takeda, I.; Yamada, A.; Onodera, H. Artificial Intelligence-Assisted motion capture for medical applications: A comparative study between markerless and passive marker motion capture. *Comput. Methods Biomech. Biomed. Eng.* **2020**, *24*, 864–873. [CrossRef]
17. Kobayashi, T.; Orendurff, M.S.; Hunt, G.; Gao, F.; LeCursi, N.; Lincoln, L.S.; Foreman, K.B. The effects of an articulated ankle-foot orthosis with resistance-adjustable joints on lower limb joint kinematics and kinetics during gait in individuals post-stroke. *Clin. Biomech.* **2018**, *59*, 47–55. [CrossRef] [PubMed]
18. Clark, R.A.; Mentiplay, B.F.; Hough, E.; Pua, Y.H. Three-dimensional cameras and skeleton pose tracking for physical function assessment: A review of uses, validity, current developments and Kinect alternatives. *Gait Posture* **2019**, *68*, 193–200. [CrossRef]
19. Albert, J.A.; Owolabi, V.; Gebel, A.; Brahms, C.M.; Granacher, U.; Arnrich, B. Evaluation of the Pose Tracking Performance of the Azure Kinect and Kinect v2 for Gait Analysis in Comparison with a Gold Standard: A Pilot Study. *Sensors* **2020**, *20*, 5104. [CrossRef]
20. Ferraris, C.; Cimolin, V.; Vismara, L.; Votta, V.; Amprimo, G.; Cremascoli, R.; Galli, M.; Nerino, R.; Mauro, A.; Priano, L. Monitoring of Gait Parameters in Post-Stroke Individuals: A Feasibility Study Using RGB-D Sensors. *Sensors* **2021**, *21*, 5945. [CrossRef]
21. Han, K.; Yang, Q.; Huang, Z. A Two-Stage Fall Recognition Algorithm Based on Human Posture Features. *Sensors* **2020**, *20*, 6966. [CrossRef] [PubMed]
22. Kidziński, Ł.; Yang, B.; Hicks, J.L.; Rajagopal, A.; Delp, S.L.; Schwartz, M.H. Deep neural networks enable quantitative movement analysis using single-camera videos. *Nat. Commun.* **2020**, *11*, 1–10. [CrossRef]
23. Lee, P.; Chen, T.-B.; Wang, C.-Y.; Hsu, S.-Y.; Liu, C.-H. Detection of Postural Control in Young and Elderly Adults Using Deep and Machine Learning Methods with Joint–Node Plots. *Sensors* **2021**, *21*, 3212. [CrossRef] [PubMed]
24. Bakator, M.; Radosav, D. Deep Learning and Medical Diagnosis: A Review of Literature. *Multimodal Technol. Interact.* **2018**, *2*, 47. [CrossRef]
25. Lee, J.-G.; Jun, S.; Cho, Y.-W.; Lee, H.; Kim, G.B.; Seo, J.B.; Kim, N. Deep Learning in Medical Imaging: General Overview. *Korean J. Radiol.* **2017**, *18*, 570–584. [CrossRef] [PubMed]
26. Suzuki, K. Overview of deep learning in medical imaging. *Radiol. Phys. Technol.* **2017**, *10*, 257–273. [CrossRef] [PubMed]
27. Ravi, D.; Wong, C.; Deligianni, F.; Berthelot, M.; Andreu-Perez, J.; Lo, B.; Yang, G.-Z. Deep Learning for Health Informatics. *IEEE J. Biomed. Health Informatics* **2016**, *21*, 4–21. [CrossRef]

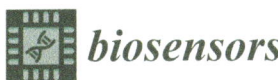

Communication

Masticatory Myoelectric Side Modular Ratio Asymmetry during Maximal Biting in Women with and without Temporomandibular Disorders

Felipe Acácio de Paiva [1], Kariny Realino Ferreira [2], Michelle Almeida Barbosa [2] and Alexandre Carvalho Barbosa [1,2,3,*]

1 MSc Program in Health Sciences, Federal University of Juiz de Fora, Juiz de Fora 35020-360, Brazil
2 Institute of Health Sciences, Federal University of Juiz de Fora, Juiz de Fora 35020-360, Brazil
3 PhD and MSc Program in Physical Education, Federal University of Juiz de Fora, Juiz de Fora 35020-360, Brazil
* Correspondence: alexandre.barbosa@ufjf.br

Abstract: There is no consensus on the role of electromyographic analysis in detecting and characterizing the asymmetries of jaw muscle excitation in patients with temporomandibular disorders (TMD). To analyze the TMD patients (n = 72) in comparison with the healthy controls (n = 30), the surface electromyography (sEMG) of the temporalis anterior muscle (TA) and masseter muscle (M) was recorded while a maximal biting task was performed. The differences in the asymmetry of the relationship between the masseter muscles were assessed in a module to determine the sensitivity (Sn) of binomial logistic models, based on the dominance of the TA or the M muscle, in accurately predicting the presence of TMD. All assumptions were met, and comparisons between the groups showed significant differences for the TA muscle ratio (p = 0.007), but not for the M muscle ratio (p = 0.13). The left side was predominant over the right side in the TMD group for both the TA (p = 0.02) and M muscles (p = 0.001), while the non-TMD group had a higher frequency of the right side. Binary logistic regression showed a significant model (χ^2 = 9.53; p = 0.002) for the TA muscle with Sn = 0.843. The model for the M muscle also showed significance (χ^2 = 8.03; p = 0.005) with Sn = 0.837. The TMD patients showed an increased TA muscle ratio and asymmetry of left dominance, compared to the healthy subjects. Both of the binomial logistic models, based on muscle dominance TA or M, were moderately sensitive for predicting the presence of TMD.

Keywords: electromyography; facial pain; temporomandibular joint disorders; jaw muscles; diagnosis

1. Introduction

The prevalence of temporomandibular disorders (TMD) is 27–38% in the adult population [1]. Chronic TMD affects the patient's ability to work and interact in the social environment, and results in an impaired quality of life [2,3]. An accurate diagnosis of TMD is critical for treatment planning and increases the chances of successful outcomes. Evidence suggests that individuals with TMD have a lower rate of motor unit discharge in painful muscles [4–6] and early fatigue, compared with individuals without TMD [7,8]. Surface electromyography (sEMG) provides a direct and objective assessment of muscle excitation [4,5] and can aid in the diagnosis of TMD, particularly the assessment of masticatory muscle activity in patients with impaired function and altered jaw movement patterns [9,10].

Some studies suggest that the use of sEMG to assess masticatory muscle excitation can discriminate against women with and without TMD [5,11–13]. In this sense, some features of muscle functionality in TMD patients have been reported, but the results of specific thresholds for raw electromyography of the masticatory muscles showed poor responsiveness and accuracy in discriminating between healthy and TMD patients [14,15].

One possible solution to this is to compare the excitation asymmetries between the sides and muscles to prioritize intervention [10]. However, no consensus has been reached on the usefulness of sEMG and the presence of muscle excitation asymmetries in TMD patients [14].

Aside from the above-mentioned issues, understanding the musculoskeletal impairments associated with TMD diagnoses is critical to providing effective treatments. Therefore, clarifying the relationship between the excitation of the major jaw muscles between sides during biting could provide insights into managing patients with this complex disorder. In this sense, the primary objective of the present study was to evaluate the difference in the modular relationship between the excitation of the side-to-side muscles by electromyography of the TA and M in TMD patients and healthy subjects, bilaterally. A secondary objective was to evaluate the possible differences, considering a nominal side-to-side predominance in both groups, and to establish possible predictive models with combined sensitivity and specificity analysis. The first hypothesis was that the TMD patients would have an increased asymmetry of ratio and dominance, compared with the healthy subjects. The second hypothesis was that a binomial logistic model, based on the dominance of the TA or M muscle, would be able to accurately predict the presence of TMD.

2. Materials and Methods

2.1. Participants

Participants (Table 1) were recruited through public invitations, via recruitment posters and personal contacts. A sample of 112 women were interested in participating. The inclusion criterion for the TMD group was a diagnosis of TMD arthralgia that was associated with myofascial pain, according to the Diagnostic Criteria for Temporomandibular Disorders (RDC/TMD), for at least 6 months' duration. The RDC/TMD is internationally recognized as the gold standard for TMD diagnosis [16]. The assessment included external palpation, using a calibrated pressure algometer (MED.DOR pressure algometry, Governador Valadares, Brazil) [17]. Internal to the mouth, the index finger was calibrated using the pressure algometer to palpate the medial pterygoideus muscles. The inclusion criteria for both groups were having a minimum of 28 permanent teeth and an age between 18 and 45 years. All patients were evaluated by a dentist for periodontal problems. The exclusion criteria for both groups were as follows: a history of trauma to the face and temporomandibular joints; systemic diseases such as arthritis; fibromyalgia; pain due to confirmed migraine; headache or neck pain unrelated to TMD; ongoing use of analgesics, anti-inflammatory drugs, muscle relaxants or psychotropic medications; acute infections or other serious dental, ear, eye, nose, or throat conditions; and neurologic or cognitive deficits. After the initial screening, 10 participants were excluded. The 102 included participants were divided into 2 groups, according to RDC/TMD axis I: 1. The non-TMD group ($n = 30$ individuals without TMD), 2. The TMD group ($n = 72$ individuals with TMD). This cross-sectional study was approved by the Ethics Committee of the Federal College of Juiz de Fora (number 68457617.6.0000.5147). Participants were informed of the benefits and potential risks before signing a written informed consent form, before participating in the study. An a priori sample size was calculated based on a previous study. An effect size of 0.88 was considered (variable: side-to-side electrical excitation %), with $\alpha = 0.05$ and a power (1-β) of 0.95. The analysis yielded an actual sample power of 0.949, with a total sample size of 60 participants. Considering a drop-out of 20%, the recommended sample included at least 72 participants. G-Power software (version 3.1.5, Franz Faul, College of Kiel, Düsseldorf, Germany) was used to calculate the sample size.

Table 1. Participants' Characteristics.

Characteristic		TMD	Non-TMD	p
N		72	30	-
Age (years)		29 (6)	29 (4)	0.44
Weight (Kg)		64 (13)	68 (16)	0.18
Height (cm)		163 (6)	164 (5)	0.41
Bite Force (kgf)		13.2 (4.3)	15.1 (2.6)	0.09
Severity (Sample %)	None	0	100	-
	Low	62.5	0	-
	Moderate	37.5	0	-
	Severe	0	0	-
Pain Side Predominance	Left	57%	-	-
	Right	20%	-	-
	Both	23%	-	-

2.2. Electromyography

All the sEMG procedures and the device's specifications were in accordance with the recommendations of the International Society of Electrophysiology and Kinesiology (https://isek.org/, accessed on 25 June 2021). The conversion of analog to digital signals was performed by an A/D board with an input range of 16-bit resolution, a sampling frequency of 2 kHz, a joint-rejection module of more than 100 dB, a signal-to-noise ratio of less than 03 µV root mean square, and an impedance of 109 Ω. The sEMG signals were recorded as root mean square in µV, using surface Meditrace™ (Ludlow Technical Products, Gananoque, ON, Canada) Ag/AgCl electrodes with a diameter of 2 cm and a center-to-center spacing of 2 cm, placed in transverse alignment, parallel to the underlying fibers at a muscle site. Differential bipolar sensors were attached to the electrodes to reduce the constant noise. A reference electrode was placed on the left lateral humeral epicondyle. The sEMG signals were amplified and filtered (Butterworth 4th order, 20–450 Hz bandpass filter, 60 Hz notch filter). All information was recorded and processed using Miotec Suite® software (Miotec Biomedical Equipments, Porto Alegre, RS, Brazil) [7,8,18]. Before placement of the sEMG electrodes, the skin was cleaned with 70% alcohol to remove fatty residues, followed by exfoliation with a special sandpaper for the skin and a second cleaning with alcohol. As the TM and M electrodes' locations were not described in the Surface Electromyography for the Non-Invasive Assessment of Muscles (SENIAM) site (http://seniam.org/, accessed on 25 June 2021), the electrodes were placed on both the left and right sides, according to previous studies' descriptions [7,8,18].

2.3. Maximal Voluntary Isometric Contraction

The excitation of M and TA muscles was assessed during a maximal bite force test. Each participant performed a 10 s maximal isometric contraction (MVIC), while biting on a load cell (maximum tension–compression = 200 Kgf, precision of 0.1 Kgf, maximum measurement error = 0.33%; Miotec™ Biomedical Equipment, Porto Alegre, RS, Brazil). Subjects were asked to sit comfortably while the adapted arms of the load cell were positioned on the incisors (Figure 1). A disposable material was used to cover the adapted arms for each subject. Forward head posture was controlled during all procedures by positioning the load cell closer to the participant so that participants could bite in their natural head posture. Standardized verbal commands ("begin", "continue biting", and "stop") were used by the same experimenter for all recordings. A 5 s familiarization period was followed by a 3 min pause before the task. The load cell was coupled and synchronized with the electromyograph.

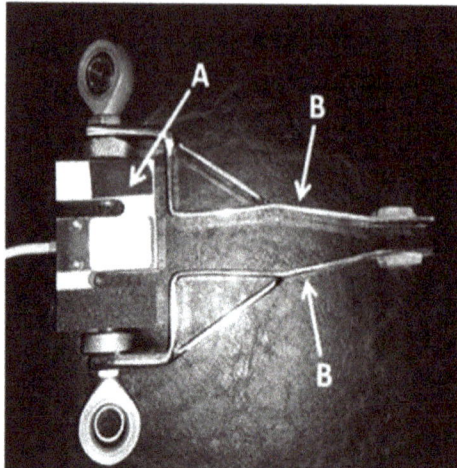 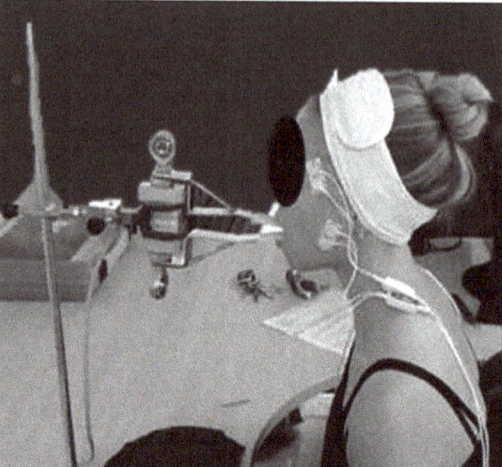

Figure 1. The adapted load cell. (**A**) laboratory-grade load cell; (**B**) adapted arms.

2.4. Data Extraction

All data were extracted offline using Miotec Suite™ software (Miotec™, Biomedical Equipments). Because the load cell was synchronized with the electromyography channels, the trained rater determined the interval based on the increase in force. After three 1 s windows of rest were collected, onset was defined by three times the standard deviation from the average rest intervals, plus the mean itself (Figure 2). The interval began when the signal exceeded the onset threshold. Conversely, the end of the interval was defined by the same threshold. For statistical analysis, the mean values of the force intervals were used [7]. The sEMG ratio was calculated using the maximum value (in µV), divided by the minimum value (in µV), so that the difference could always be modular (with positive values). Thus, the difference values were displayed regardless of the side. To determine the sEMG side predominance, a nominal classification was used. If the voltage on the right side had the highest value, the participant's result was classified as "1". Conversely, if the left side was higher than the right side, the result was classified as "2".

2.5. Statistical Analysis

The between-group differences were assessed using the independent samples t-tests. The 95% confidence interval was also used to set the lower and the upper limits of significance. The effect size (ES) was set using Cohen's d coefficient. The magnitude of the ES was qualitatively interpreted using the following thresholds: <0.2, trivial; 0.2–0.6, small; 0.6–1.2, moderate; 1.2–2.0, large; 2.0–4.0, very large; and >4.0, huge [19]. The Chi-square test, with continuity correction, was used to verify the frequency differences for nominal side predominance. To provide a predictive model, binary logistic regressions were performed for M and TA analysis. The assumptions of the absence of multicollinearity (Variance Inflation Factor [VIF] less than 5) and outliers were evaluated. The best fit model was judged based on the values of the Chi-square test, Nagelkerk's R^2 and odds ratio (OR), considering its confidence intervals (OR [95% CI]). In addition, the likelihood ratio test, Akaike Information Criteria (AIC), and Bayesian Information Criteria (BIC) values were inspected to assess the model fit (i.e., the lower the better). The sensitivity (Sn) and the specificity (Sp) were also investigated for each model. The correlation between the pain side and the outcome variables were assessed using Pearson's coefficient (r), accompanied by the adjusted coefficient of determination (r^2), which is used to measure how well a statistical model predicts an outcome. They were qualitatively interpreted using the following thresholds: <0.1, trivial; 0.11–0.3, small; 0.31–0.5, moderate; 0.51–0.7, large; 0.71–0.9, very large; and >0.9, nearly perfect [19]. All data analysis was performed using the JAMOVI software (v. 1.6.15.0, The JAMOVI Project, 2022), with significance level set at 5%.

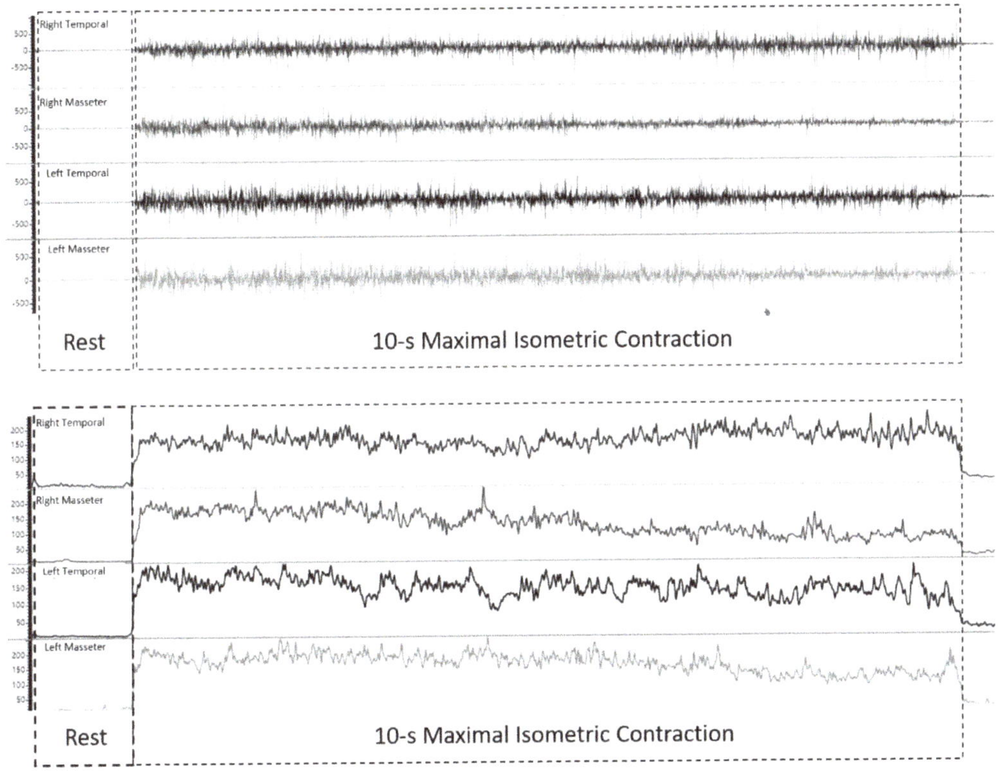

Figure 2. Example of the raw (image above–in μV) and processed RMS signal (image below–in μV).

3. Results

The between-group comparisons showed significant differences for the TA muscle ratio (TMD: 2.17 [1.74] μV vs. non-TMD: 1.50 [1.28] μV; $p = 0.007$; 95% CI: −0.43 to −0.04; ES = 0.35 [small]), but not for the M muscle ratio (TMD: 1.80 [1.46] μV vs. non-TMD: 1.29 [0.23] μV; $p = 0.13$; 95% CI: −0.23 to 0.02; ES = 0.19 [trivial]). In terms of frequency, the left side was predominant over the right side on the TMD group for both the TA muscle (46.6% vs. 31.4%; $\chi^2 = 5.41$; $p = 0.02$) and the M muscle (46% vs. 30.9%; $\chi^2 = 11$; $p = 0.001$), while the non-TMD group showed a higher frequency of the right side (TA: 13.5% vs. 8.4% and M: 17% vs. 6.4%). The side of pain was only significantly and positively correlated to the temporal ratio index ($r = 0.30$; $p = 0.007$).

The binary logistic regression showed a significant model (likelihood $\chi^2 = 9.53$; $p = 0.002$; Nagelkerk's $R^2 = 0.119$) for the TA muscle, with a 1.07 μV cutoff point. The VIF values confirmed the absence of collinearity (VIF = 1), and the low AIC (=136) and BIC (=141) confirmed the model fit. The model's Sn was 0.843, with an Sp of 0.431 for an OR of 4.08 (95% CI = 1.599 to 10.400). The M muscle regression model also showed significance, with a cutoff point of 1.11 μV (likelihood $\chi^2 = 8.03$; $p = 0.005$; Nagelkerk's $R^2 = 0.056$). The VIF (=1), AIC (=137), and BIC (=142) values confirmed the absence of collinearity and the model fit. The analysis highlighted an OR of 3.64 (95% CI = 1.429 to 9.255), with an Sn of 0.837 and an Sp of 0.415.

4. Discussion

The results showed that the TA muscle percentage was two times significantly higher in the TMD group, compared with the non-TMD group. Moreover, the left side was electromyographically predominant in the TMD patients. Conversely, the right side was predominant in the non-TMD participants. The results also showed a predictive value in distinguishing the TMD and non-TMD patients, when considering the TA (OR = 4.08) or the M's (OR = 3.64) frequency of asymmetry, with a high Sn to detect those with TMD. The primary hypothesis was partially confirmed because differences were observed only in the TA muscle.

Other studies examined the responsiveness of individual variables to distinguish the subjects with TMD from those without TMD. One study examined the pressure–pain threshold (PPT) in 200 subjects of both sexes, aged 19–27 years [20]. Each subject described the result of pressure algometry for the superficial and deep parts of the masseter muscle, the anterior and posterior parts of the temporalis muscle, and the tissues adjacent to the lateral and dorsal parts of the temporomandibular joint capsule, by selecting the pain intensity on a visual analog scale (VAS) each time. A receiver operating characteristic curve analysis showed a specificity of 95.3% in identifying healthy subjects and a sensitivity of 58.4% in identifying patients with TMD symptoms, at a cut-off point of 7.4 VAS and an accuracy of 68.1%. Another study examined a sample of 49 women who were divided into the following three groups: TMJ osteoarthritis, asymptomatic disk displacement, and control group [21]. The authors aimed to determine a cut-off point for PPT and determined the sensitivity and specificity. The specificity determined was 89.6% and the sensitivity was 70%, for a cutoff point of 1.36 kgf/cm^2 (area under the curve = 0.90). In a previous study, PPT, sensitivity, and specificity were found to be 0.67 and 0.85 for the masseter muscle, and 0.77 and 0.87 for the temporal muscle, respectively, with a cutoff point one standard deviation below the mean PPT of subjects who did not have TMD [20]. Given these results, pressure algometry has severe limitations when used as a single diagnostic tool because of its limited ability to detect true positives (Sn).

The sEMG technique has also been studied, but methodological problems tend to compromise its ability to predict and distinguish the TMD patients from the healthy controls. A previous study showed altered coactivation and coordination strategies of the jaw muscles during mastication, resulting in higher relative energy expenditure and impaired differential recruitment [22]. Another study showed that women with TMD myalgia had greater jaw muscle work than healthy control subjects [9]. However, the same study showed that the activity of the temporalis anterior muscle (TA) and the masseter muscle (M) were similar when comparing the right and left sides in both the TMD and healthy groups, but the TMD group had greater M activity, compared to TA activity. Other studies examined the electromyographic muscle asymmetry between the sides when comparing TMD and healthy subjects [10,13], but the authors reported no differences at rest or during isometric contractions. One study showed the moderate accuracy (0.74–0.84) of raw sEMG in the TA, M, and the suprahyoid muscles in diagnosing TMD at rest, and in the suprahyoid muscles during maximal contraction on parafilm [11]. In addition, the sensitivity ranged from 71.3% to 80% and the specificity ranged from 60.5% to 76.6%. Such conflicting results are often due to different methods of analyzing the electromyographic signal; differences in how TMD patients have been previously diagnosed; and the inclusion of small samples, combined with the lack of sample size calculation. In the present study, the gold standard method for TMD diagnosis was used in conjunction with a large sample size and an a priori calculated power of 0.95. These procedures were performed to ensure further inference on the assessment of asymmetry, instead of the usual raw values for sEMG analysis. Despite the moderate Sp in the current analysis, the main objective was to identify the women with TMD, instead of their healthy counterparts. The analysis yielded values of over 80% sensitivity for the detection of TMD, using nominal side-predominance, with well-established cutoff points. The ideal Sn value is 100%, meaning that all individuals with TMD are detected [23]. However, this value is rarely achieved in clinical or even research studies. Given the possible effect-size bias associated with an inappropriate sample size (type I error), a post-hoc power calculation would demonstrate the value of the results. In the present work, the two-sided post hoc power calculation returned that the power was 0.96 or 96%, with a maximum possible power of 1 or 100% considering the input ES of 0.35, with the sample of 102 participants.

An important issue that must be addressed is the predominance of pain to the left side (57%) over the right side (20%), and over the combination of both sides (23%) for the occurrence of pain (see Table 1). That predominance could be a possible confounding factor that may lead to an interpretation bias of the current results. In fact, the single significant correlation occurred between the pain location and the temporal ratio. However, it was classified as small ($r = 0.30$; $p = 0.007$), with a trivial coefficient of determination ($r^2 = 0.09$). This result means that only 9% of the data fits the predicted model. As a positive correlation, the pain would increase following the increase in the temporal ratio in the TMD patients, but not in an exact linear trend. This means that muscle excitation would also weakly increase proportionally to the pain predominance. The impact of such a left predominance of pain in TMD patients should be further studied, but in the present work its relevance is questionable.

The current study did not aim to establish which side is predominant for all people with TMD, as this may vary according to the location, population age, and other factors to be set in further studies. Instead, the present results reinforce the sEMG as an important factor to account for TMD evaluation, using an alternative index and a nominal classification. As noticed, the imbalance is not restricted to TMD patients, but it is also present (in a different direction) for healthy people. However, the modular ratio showed the intensification of the index for TMD. A limitation of the present study was the cross-sectional design, which did not allow cause–effect inferences. The present study also focused on women in a limited age range. Those with other levels of functional limitations might show a different pattern than their male counterparts of the same age. Not all intrinsic factors were addressed (such as the predominant side for chewing), and the results could be biased by those issues. However, as it also constitutes a memory recall, it was not possible to be sure of such factors for the analysis. Instead, they were pondered by the most usual factors set in previous studies.

5. Conclusions

TMD patients exhibit increased TA muscle ratio and an asymmetry of left dominance, compared with healthy subjects. Both binomial logistic models, based on TA or M muscle predominance, were moderately sensitive to predicting the presence of TMD.

Author Contributions: Conceptualization, A.C.B. and M.A.B.; methodology, A.C.B.; software, K.R.F. and A.C.B.; validation, K.R.F., M.A.B. and F.A.d.P.; formal analysis, F.A.d.P. and A.C.B.; investigation, F.A.d.P., M.A.B. and K.R.F.; resources, A.C.B.; data curation, F.A.d.P.; writing—original draft preparation, A.C.B. and M.A.B.; writing—review and editing, A.C.B.; visualization, F.A.d.P.; supervision, A.C.B. and M.A.B.; project administration, M.A.B. and A.C.B.; funding acquisition, A.C.B. All authors have read and agreed to the published version of the manuscript.

Funding: This research was funded by Fundação de Amparo à Pesquisa de Minas Gerais–FAPEMIG, grant number APQ 02040/18. This study was also supported, in part, by the Coordenação de Aperfeiçoamento de Pessoal de Nível Superior—Brazil (CAPES)—Finance Code 001. This research was funded by the Federal University of Juiz de Fora, supporting the APC.

Institutional Review Board Statement: The study was conducted in accordance with the Declaration of Helsinki and approved by the Ethics Committee of the Federal University of Juiz de Fora (protocol code 68457617.6.0000.5147), for studies involving humans.

Informed Consent Statement: Informed consent was obtained from all subjects involved in the study.

Data Availability Statement: Data are available only upon a request to the authors.

Acknowledgments: Special thanks to the UFJF-GV Department of Physical Therapy, MSc in Health Sciences–UFJF/GV and PhD/MSc in Physical Education Programs–UFJF/UFV.

Conflicts of Interest: The authors declare no conflict of interest.

References

1. Gözler, S. Myofascial Pain Dysfunction Syndrome: Etiology, Diagnosis, and Treatment. In *Temporomandibular Joint Pathology-Current Approaches and Understanding*; InTech: London, UK, 2018; pp. 17–45.
2. Harper, D.E.; Schrepf, A.; Clauw, D.J. Pain Mechanisms and Centralized Pain in Temporomandibular Disorders. *J. Dent. Res.* **2016**, *95*, 1102–1108. [CrossRef] [PubMed]
3. La Touche, R.; Paris-Alemany, A.; Hidalgo-Pérez, A.; López-de-Uralde-Villanueva, I.; Angulo-Diaz-Parreño, S.; Muñoz-García, D. Evidence for Central Sensitization in Patients with Temporomandibular Disorders: A Systematic Review and Meta-analysis of Observational Studies. *Pain Pract.* **2018**, *18*, 388–409. [CrossRef]
4. Xu, L.; Fan, S.; Cai, B.; Fang, Z.; Jiang, X. Influence of sustained submaximal clenching fatigue test on electromyographic activity and maximum voluntary bite forces in healthy subjects and patients with temporomandibular disorders. *J. Oral Rehabil.* **2017**, *44*, 340–346. [CrossRef] [PubMed]
5. Machado, M.B.; Nitsch, G.S.; Pitta, N.C.; de Oliveira, A.S.; Machado, M.B.; Nitsch, G.S.; Pitta, N.C.; de Oliveira, A.S. Tempo de ativação muscular em portadoras de disfunção temporomandibular durante a mastigação. *Audiol.-Commun. Res.* **2014**, *19*, 202–207. [CrossRef]
6. Woźniak, K.; Lipski, M.; Lichota, D.; Szyszka-Sommerfeld, L. Muscle Fatigue in the Temporal and Masseter Muscles in Patients with Temporomandibular Dysfunction. *Biomed Res. Int.* **2015**, *2015*, 1–6. [CrossRef]
7. Barbosa, M.A.; Tahara, A.K.; Ferreira, I.C.; Intelangelo, L.; Barbosa, A.C. Effects of 8 weeks of masticatory muscles focused endurance exercises on women with oro-facial pain and temporomandibular disorders: A placebo randomised controlled trial. *J. Oral Rehabil.* **2019**, *46*, 885–894. [CrossRef]
8. Leite, W.B.; Oliveira, M.L.; Ferreira, I.C.; Anjos, C.F.; Barbosa, M.A.; Barbosa, A.C. Effects of 4-Week Diacutaneous Fibrolysis on Myalgia, Mouth Opening, and Level of Functional Severity in Women With Temporomandibular Disorders: A Randomized Controlled Trial. *J. Manip. Physiol. Ther.* **2020**, *43*, 806–815. [CrossRef]
9. Valentino, R.; Cioffi, I.; Vollaro, S.; Cimino, R.; Baiano, R.; Michelotti, A. Jaw muscle activity patterns in women with chronic TMD myalgia during standardized clenching and chewing tasks. *CRANIO®* **2021**, *39*, 157–163. [CrossRef]
10. Hotta, G.H.; de Oliveira, A.I.S.; de Oliveira, A.S.; Pedroni, C.R. Electromyography and asymmetry index of masticatory muscles in undergraduate students with temporomandibular disorders. *Braz. J. Oral Sci.* **2015**, *14*, 176–181. [CrossRef]
11. dos Santos Berni, K.C.; Dibai-Filho, A.V.; Pires, P.F.; Rodrigues-Bigaton, D. Accuracy of the surface electromyography RMS processing for the diagnosis of myogenous temporomandibular disorder. *J. Electromyogr. Kinesiol.* **2015**, *25*, 596–602. [CrossRef]
12. Santana-Mora, U.; López-Ratón, M.; Mora, M.J.; Cadarso-Suárez, C.; López-Cedrún, J.; Santana-Penín, U. Surface raw electromyography has a moderate discriminatory capacity for differentiating between healthy individuals and those with TMD: A diagnostic study. *J. Electromyogr. Kinesiol.* **2014**, *24*, 332–340. [CrossRef]
13. Rodrigues-Bigaton, D.; Berni, K.C.S.; Almeida, A.F.N.; Silva, M.T. Activity and asymmetry index of masticatory muscles in women with and without dysfunction temporomandibular. *Electromyogr. Clin. Neurophysiol.* **2010**, *50*, 333–338. [PubMed]
14. Piekartz, H.; Schwiddessen, J.; Reineke, L.; Armijo-Olivio, S.; Bevilaqua-Grossi, D.; Biasotto Gonzalez, D.A.; Carvalho, G.; Chaput, E.; Cox, E.; Fernández-de-las-Peñas, C.; et al. International consensus on the most useful assessments used by physical therapists to evaluate patients with temporomandibular disorders: A Delphi study. *J. Oral Rehabil.* **2020**, *47*, 685–702. [CrossRef]
15. Szyszka-Sommerfeld, L.; Sycińska-Dziarnowska, M.; Budzyńska, A.; Woźniak, K. Accuracy of Surface Electromyography in the Diagnosis of Pain-Related Temporomandibular Disorders in Children with Awake Bruxism. *J. Clin. Med.* **2022**, *11*, 1323. [CrossRef] [PubMed]
16. Manfredini, D.; Guarda-Nardini, L.; Winocur, E.; Piccotti, F.; Ahlberg, J.; Lobbezoo, F. Research diagnostic criteria for temporomandibular disorders: A systematic review of axis i epidemiologic findings. *Oral Surg. Oral Med. Oral Pathol. Oral Radiol. Endodontology* **2011**, *112*, 453–462. [CrossRef] [PubMed]
17. Jerez-Mayorga, D.; dos Anjos, C.F.; de Cássia Macedo, M.; Fernandes, I.G.; Aedo-Muñoz, E.; Intelangelo, L.; Barbosa, A.C. Instrumental validity and intra/inter-rater reliability of a novel low-cost digital pressure algometer. *PeerJ* **2020**, *8*, e10162. [CrossRef] [PubMed]
18. Fassicollo, C.E.; Graciosa, M.D.; Graefling, B.F.; Ries, L.G.K. Temporomandibular dysfunction, myofascial, craniomandibular and cervical pain: Effect on masticatory activity during rest and mandibular isometry. *Rev. Dor* **2017**, *18*, 103–112. [CrossRef]
19. Hopkins, W.G.; Marshall, S.W.; Batterham, A.M.; Hanin, J. Progressive statistics for studies in sports medicine and exercise science. *Med. Sci. Sports Exerc.* **2009**, *41*, 3–13. [CrossRef]
20. Więckiewicz, W.; Woźniak, K.; Piątkowska, D.; Szyszka-Sommerfeld, L.; Lipski, M. The Diagnostic Value of Pressure Algometry for Temporomandibular Disorders. *Biomed Res. Int.* **2015**, *2015*, 1–8. [CrossRef]
21. Cunha, C.O.; Pinto-Fiamengui, L.M.S.; Castro, A.C.P.C.; Lauris, J.R.P.; Conti, P.C.R. Determination of a pressure pain threshold cut-off value for the diagnosis of temporomandibular joint arthralgia. *J. Oral Rehabil.* **2014**, *41*, 323–329. [CrossRef]

22. Fassicollo, C.E.; Garcia, D.M.; Machado, B.C.Z.; de Felício, C.M. Changes in jaw and neck muscle coactivation and coordination in patients with chronic painful TMD disk displacement with reduction during chewing. *Physiol. Behav.* **2021**, *230*, 113267. [CrossRef] [PubMed]
23. Gadotti, I.; Vieira, E.; Dj, M. Importance and clarification of measurement properties in rehabilitation. *Rev. Bras. Fisioter.* **2006**, *10*, 137–146. [CrossRef]

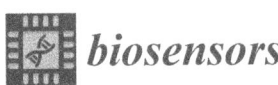

Review

Salivary Diagnostics in Pediatrics and the Status of Saliva-Based Biosensors

Hayeon Min [1,†], Sophie Zhu [1,†], Lydia Safi [1], Munzer Alkourdi [1], Bich Hong Nguyen [2], Akshaya Upadhyay [1] and Simon D. Tran [1,*]

[1] McGill Craniofacial Tissue Engineering and Stem Cells Laboratory, Faculty of Dental Medicine and Oral Health Science, McGill University, 3640 University Street, Montreal, QC H3A 0C7, Canada
[2] CHU Sainte Justine Hospital, Montreal, QC H3T 1C5, Canada
* Correspondence: simon.tran@mcgill.ca
† These authors contributed equally to this work.

Abstract: Salivary biomarkers are increasingly being used as an alternative to diagnose and monitor the progression of various diseases due to their ease of use, on site application, non-invasiveness, and most likely improved patient compliance. Here, we highlight the role of salivary biosensors in the general population, followed by the application of saliva as a diagnostic tool in the pediatric population. We searched the literature for pediatric applications of salivary biomarkers, more specifically, in children from 0 to 18 years old. The use of those biomarkers spans autoimmune, developmental disorders, oncology, neuropsychiatry, respiratory illnesses, gastrointestinal disorders, and oral diseases. Four major applications of salivary proteins as biomarkers are: (1) dental health (caries, stress from orthodontic appliances, and gingivitis); (2) gastrointestinal conditions (eosinophilic esophagitis, acid reflux, appendicitis); (3) metabolic conditions (obesity, diabetes); and (4) respiratory conditions (asthma, allergic rhinitis, small airway inflammation, pneumonia). Genomics, metabolomics, microbiomics, proteomics, and transcriptomics, are various other classifications for biosensing based on the type of biomarkers used and reviewed here. Lastly, we describe the recent advances in pediatric biosensing applications using saliva. This work guides scientists in fabricating saliva-based biosensors by comprehensively overviewing the potential markers and techniques that can be employed.

Keywords: biosensors; biomaterials; oral diagnostics; pediatric population; salivary diagnostics; salivary biomarkers

1. Introduction

Currently, blood and urine tests are commonly carried out to assess one's immune status, neuropsychiatric state, and development status. However, invasive screening, diagnostic, and prognostic tests induce a high-stress level in the pediatric population and their parents. Recent research has shown that salivary biomarkers can be an alternative non-invasive test, particularly useful in reducing stress in children between 0 and 18. This study aims to screen the current research on the use of salivary biomarkers in diagnosing autoimmune diseases, developmental disorders, and cancer, as well as neuropsychiatric, pulmonary, gastrointestinal, and oral diseases. It is an effort to highlight the role of saliva as a sample for its utilization in biosensing applications (Figure 1).

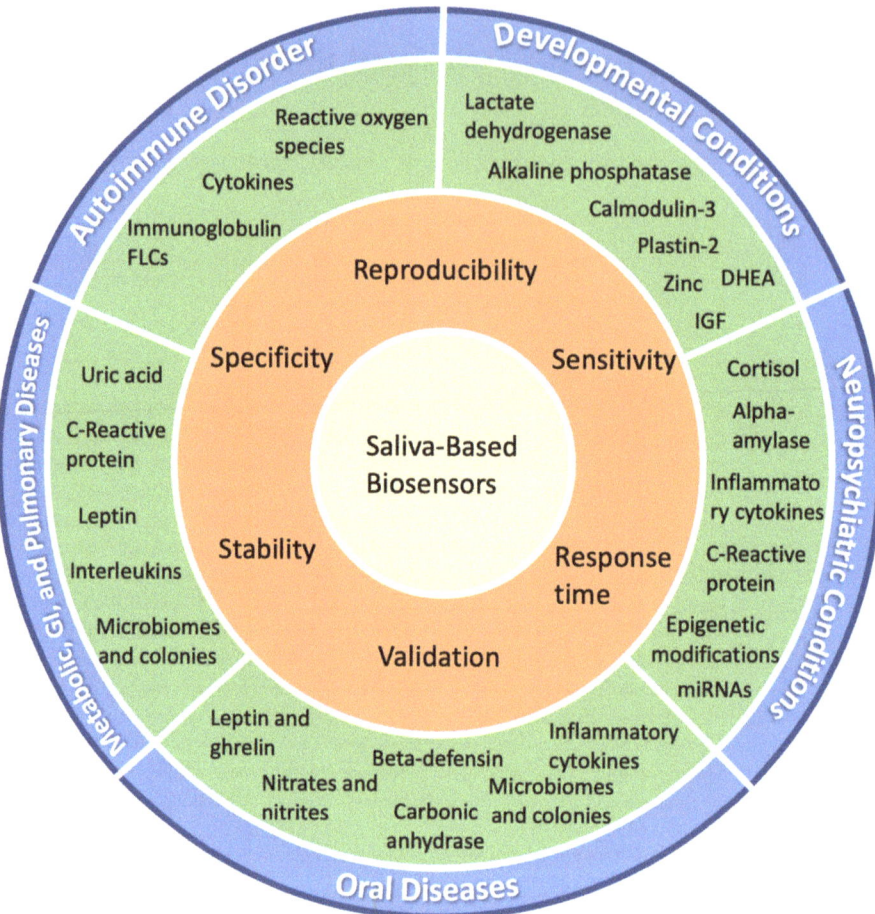

Figure 1. Prospects for saliva-based biosensors: various biomarkers have been identified in systemic conditions; discussed here are autoimmune disorders, developmental conditions, neuropsychiatric conditions, metabolic disorders, gastrointestinal disorders, pulmonary diseases, and oral diseases. For biosensing applications, they should be assessed for: their reproducibility at different time points, locations, and populations; specificity towards the marker and disease; sensitivity, meaning they should be able to detect as low a concentration of the markers as possible, ideally lower than a clinically available test; the response time of the assay, preferably shorter for quicker results; and validation in clinical conditions in larger population sizes.

2. Materials and Methods

2.1. Study Design

This study involved an Ovid database search with the following search strategy: (1) saliva.mp. (69,706 articles); (2) salivary diagnostics.mp. (172 articles); (3) saliva*.mp. (131,830 articles); (4) oral.mp. (767,765 articles); (5) 1 or 2 or 3 or 4 (876,003 articles); (6) biomarkers.mp. or Biomarkers, Tumor/or Biomarkers/or Biomarkers, Pharmacological/(639,768 articles); (7) 5 and 6 (24,223 articles); (8) pediatrics.mp. or Pediatrics/or Child/(1,892,565 articles); (9) 7 and 8 (1285 articles).

2.2. Study Participants

The publication year was limited to "2015 to current", resulting in a total of 698 articles that fit the criteria above at the time of preparing this manuscript in August 2022. We established inclusion and exclusion criteria for this study to filter those articles further. Inclusion criteria: the research paper must focus on using salivary biomarkers to diagnose a specific disease or disorder in the pediatric population, between 0 years old and 18 years old. Exclusion criteria: review articles and case reports were excluded.

2.3. Data Collection

We selected 161 articles and divided them into 7 sections: pulmonary and gastrointestinal diseases; developmental disorders; infectious diseases; neuropsychiatric diseases; oral diseases; oncology; and autoimmune diseases. There were: 9 articles related to autoimmune diseases; 27 articles for developmental disorders; 7 articles for infectious diseases; 57 articles for neuropsychiatric diseases; 27 articles for oral diseases; 3 articles for oncology; and 31 for pulmonary and gastrointestinal diseases. Each section is further divided into 5 specific applications of salivary biomarkers: metabolomics, proteomics, genomics, transcriptomics, and microbiomics.

3. Salivary Biomarkers as Diagnostic Tools in Autoimmune Disorders

3.1. Metabolomics

A study by Aral et al. investigated the salivary oxidative status of children with Type I Diabetes Mellitus (T1DM) and its implications regarding the risk of periodontal disease (PD) development. The authors observed that, when compared to their healthy counterparts, children with T1DM have a greater Oxidative Stress Index (OSI) ($p < 0.05$) [1]. To explain this finding, the authors observe that chronic hyperglycemia impairs reactive oxygen species (ROS) elimination. The elevated ROS produces tissue damage, thus contributing to the development of PD. This finding highlights the potential of salivary OSI as a prognostic tool for PD in children with T1DM, which would enable physicians to intervene earlier to improve the course of the patient's periodontal disease and, by extension, the duration of their diabetes.

3.2. Proteomics

A study by Collin et al. compared the salivary levels of several cytokines in children with Juvenile Idiopathic Arthritis (JIA) to those in healthy children. While IL-8 levels initially seemed to be higher in children with JIA, the authors ultimately concluded that there was no significant difference in the level of any investigated cytokines across the two group [2]. To explain this finding, the authors highlight that the children with JIA were taking immunosuppressive therapy throughout the study, which could hold their immune activity, and thus salivary cytokine levels, in check. Despite this, it could be possible to create a prognostic tool for children with JIA based on salivary cytokine levels. Such a tool would help monitor the children's response to therapy and the prognosis of their symptoms.

Immunoglobulin-free light chains (FLCs) were identified as a strong predictor in the prognosis of Pediatric-Onset Multiple Sclerosis (POMS), and its relapse [3]. Detecting the higher levels of free light chains early can potentially enable physicians to initiate stronger therapy to reduce the severity of the children's symptoms. Additionally, compared to current prognostic modalities, saliva collection is significantly less invasive than a lumbar puncture; it avoids gadolinium's potentially harmful deposition in the brain from repeated MRIs.

In a similar fashion to the studies above, Gomez Hernandez et al. investigated the saliva of children with Sjogren's Syndrome (SS) for cytokines, chemokines, and biomarkers (CCBM) that can serve as a diagnostic instrument for the condition [4]. The authors found 43 CCBM levels significantly elevated in children with SS, compared to healthy controls. Judging that number is too high for practical use; the authors recommend a test based on

IL-27 and CCL-4 alone, or a quintuple test of IL-27, MIA, CCL-4, TNFRSF18 and TNFA, to aid in diagnosing SS. The authors encourage the pursuit of further studies to link these CCBM to Sjogren's, as identifying such salivary biomarkers, which would appear early before the onset of symptoms, would enable physicians to intervene early and avert the course of the disease. A common limitation of the studies reviewed here is the small sample size. Indeed, the authors of the above papers invite further research to consolidate their findings. Further, other markers pertaining to transcriptomics and genomics can be explored for such conditions (Table 1).

Table 1. Investigated autoimmune disorders and their respective biomarkers.

	Disease	Observed Biomarker	Methodology	Ref.
1.	Type I Diabetes Mellitus	Oxidative Stress Index (OSI), assessed by examining: - Total Antioxidant Status (TAS) - Total Oxidant Status (TOS)	Commercially available assay kits (Rel Assay, Mega Tıp, Gaziantep, Turkey)	[1]
2.	Juvenile Idiopathic Arthritis	TNF-alpha, TNFRSF1B, MMP-1, MMP-2, MMP-3, MMP-13, IL-1alpha, IL-1beta, IL-1 RII, IL-2, IL-6, IL-6Ralpha, IL-8, IL-10, IL-12, CCL2, CCL3, CCL11, CCL22, CXCL9, S100A8	Customized R&D-bead based immunoassay (R&D SYSTEMS/Bio-Techne; Minneapolis, MN, USA)	[2]
3.	Pediatric-Onset Multiple Sclerosis	FLC as Monomers & Dimers (kapapaM, lambdaM, kappaD, lambdaD)	Gel Analysis & Blotting using rabbit antibodies to human Ig kappa and lambda light chains	[3]
4.	Sjogren's Syndrome	IL27, MIA, CCL4, TNFRSF18 and TNF-alpha (Among others)	Multiplex fluorescent microparticle-based immunoassays	[4]

4. Salivary Biomarkers as Diagnostic Tools in Developmental Conditions
4.1. Metabolomics

Bone-specific alkaline phosphatase (B-ALP) is a bone formation marker whose levels fluctuate with puberty. Al-Khatieeb et al. hypothesized that the level of ALP and LDH could affect the compliance of patients to monoblock therapy for orthoskeletal treatment. A high level of these enzymes was observed but was not significant after performing statistical analysis [5]. In another study, ALP, protein concentration, and chronological age with cervical vertebral maturation stages (CVMS) were used as non-invasive biomarkers to determine skeletal maturity. Salivary levels of ALP in conjunction with chronological age were accurate predictors for CVMS in 53.2% of cases [6]. ALP levels were co-related with variable stages of skeletal maturity ($p = 0.0003$) [7].

The early diagnosis and intervention of those with Autism Spectrum Disorder (ASD) have been linked with enhanced functional outcomes. The diagnosis, intervention, and prognosis would be facilitated by biomarker sampling, particularly salivary zinc concentrations. Low salivary zinc in those with ASD may contribute to the pathogenesis of autism [8]. Salivary metabolites were found to be higher in children experiencing pain when compared to those not experiencing pain. Collecting these non-invasive biomarkers may contribute to future pain management interventions in children with ASD [9].

4.2. Proteomics

It was found that insulin-like growth factor (IGF-1) and insulin-like growth factor binding protein-3 (IGFBP-3) may be used to estimate skeletal maturity. It was found that low salivary IGF-1 levels were present during puberty and lowered as pubertal growth ended. As a result, these salivary levels may be used to predict the completion of skeletal growth and may help predict when children would be most amenable to orthodontic treatments [10,11].

Increased levels of salivary proinflammatory markers, such as interleukin-6 (IL-6) and c-reactive protein (CRP), have been associated with child maltreatment. IL-6 secretions have been found to follow a clear circadian rhythm, suggesting that a disrupted rhythm is indicative of a dysfunctional inflammatory system. These findings suggest that a disrupted IL-6 rhythm, and, as a result, a disrupted inflammatory system, may be linked with childhood traumas (p = 0.031) [12]. Mucosal secretory immunoglobulin A (s-IgA) plays a critical role in the immune system. It has been found that acute psychosocial stress stimulates s-IgA secretion in adults and children who have undergone maltreatment. This is suggestive of child maltreatment prematurely aging their immune system [13]. Familial social and economic instability in early childhood has been linked to immune system dysregulation, as is evidenced by DNA shedding of the Epstein-Barr virus (EBV) salivary biomarkers. Traumatic early childhood events resulted in a 100% increase in EBV DNA shedding among previously infected adolescents. This indicates that the salivary biomarkers of EBV may be indicative of childhood trauma [14].

The protein composition of saliva has been studied from early on to find associated markers for the diagnosis and prognosis of ASD [15,16]. The mass spectrometric analysis of a patient cohort of 132 proteins were increased in ASD-positive patients, 25 of which were associated with a severe to moderate group of the elevated proteins, suggested as biomarkers for ASD calmodulin-3, plastin-2, and protein s100-a7 [17].

4.3. Genomics

Those with Cleft Lip Palate (CLP), one of the most common congenital malformations of the head and neck, are found to be more likely to present with accompanying anomalies including Defects of Enamel (DDE). Matrix Metallopeptidase 2 (MMP2), a membrane-bound protein containing collagen-degrading capabilities, plays a crucial role in tooth formation and mineralization. The findings suggest that MMP2 may play a role in a genomic approach to establish any potential risks for those with CLP [18]. Supernumerary teeth are one of the most common dental anomalies seen in the pediatric population. An immunohistochemistry panel showed that those with supernumerary teeth presented with an enhanced expression of Wingless (Wnt) and Sonic Hedgehog (SHH) proteins, both of which are pro-tumorigenic proteins [19].

It has been shown that psychological stress elicits telomere shortening. Through salivary samples via PCR testing, it was found that families with an ASD child endure exceeding levels of psychological stress [20]. Using these biomarkers may contribute to the early diagnosis of any psychological stress and respective intervention, which would optimize mental well-being and the quality of life. Maternal stress affects an infant's neurocognitive development before, during, and post-pregnancy. Certain CpGs were found to be linked genetically, including YAP1, TOMM20, and CSMD1.

Additionally, two differentiated methylation groups (DMR), DAXX and ARL4D, were found to be related to maternal stress measures. An early assessment of maternal stress may contribute to preventative health measures for the infant, further optimizing their health and the quality of life [21]. Upon examining polymorphisms of the STS and SULT2A1 genes, dehydroepiandrosterone (DHEA) and its sulfated form, DHEA-A, and their relationship to Attention Deficit Hyperactivity Disorder (ADHD), it was found that the levels of DHEA were positive correlated with attention. This may highlight the potential role of ADHD and its pathogenesis with regard to STS polymorphisms and neurosteroid levels [22] (Table 2).

Table 2. Most commonly recurring developmental conditions and their respective biomarkers.

	Disease	Observed Biomarker	Methodology	Ref.
1.	Autism Spectrum Disorder	Salivary zinc	Plasma emission spectroscopy	[8]
		16s rRNA	16s RNA gene amplicon sequencing	[23,24]
		Calmodulin-3 Plastin-2 S100-a7	Bio-Rad protein assay	[17]
2.	Skeletal Maturity	LDH	Spectrophotometry	[5]
		ALP	ALP and protein assay	[6]
		Salivary B-ALP	ELISA	[7]
		IGF-1 IGFBP-3	Spectrophotometry	[10,11]
3.	Attention Deficit Hyperactivity Disorder	DHEA CpG methylation	TaqMan assay	[22]

4.4. Transcriptomics

Circulating microRNA (miRNA) was compared to cerebrospinal fluid miRNA levels when assessing miRNA as a biomarker for pediatric concussions. Six miRNAs had similar changes in both CSF and salivary levels, including miR-182-5p, miR-221-3p, mir-26b-5p, miR-320c, miR-29c-3p, and miR-30e-5p. More specifically, concentrations of miR-320c were found to be directly correlated with attention deficit. This suggests that salivary miRNA may be an accurate potential biomarker for traumatic brain injuries [25].

Several miRNAs have been found to potentially be used as biomarkers in diagnosing and treating those with ASD. The most accurate miRNAs to differentiate between typically developing children and those with ASD were miR-23a-3p, miR-32-5p, and miR-628-5p [24].

4.5. Microbiomics

ASD has been linked with many comorbidities, including gastrointestinal abnormalities, dental disease, and allergies. Oral and gut microbiomes are suggested to play important roles in inflammation and immune dysfunction pathogenesis. More specifically, 16S rRNA gene amplicon sequencing helps distinguish the oral and gut macrobiotics of patients with ASD. Altering the oral and gut microbiome may potentially address and ameliorate co-morbidities associated with those with ASD [23].

5. Salivary Biomarkers as Diagnostic Tools in Neuropsychiatry

5.1. Metabolomics

A plethora of evidence supports that measuring salivary cortisol and alpha-amylase levels serves as stress biomarkers. The application of salivary stress biomarkers spans from pediatric dental anxiety to internalizing or externalizing disorders. The partial hypofunction of hypothalamus-pituitary-adrenal (HPA) was found to be associated with pediatric patients suffering from ADHD by assessing the cortisol levels to induced stress, which was found to be reduced in positive patients (p = 0.034) [26]. In addition, salivary immune biomarker secretory immunoglobin A (s-IgA) is often measured alongside HPA biomarkers to explore the interactions between stress, the HPA axis, and the immune system [27]. Obtaining samples through saliva is a great alternative to blood collection in the pediatric population, especially for children with cerebral palsy. In patients with cerebral palsy, the sympathetic nervous system predominates, causing vasoconstriction and making peripheral venous blood more difficult to access. A study demonstrated, with non-invasive salivary diagnostics, that higher levels of inflammatory markers in patients with cerebral palsy are associated with excessive constipation and a reduced quality of life [28].

While using salivary stress biomarkers, such as cortisol and alpha-amylase, as a diagnostic tool is largely favorable, they are far from perfect. For instance, they cannot distinguish between acute fear and chronic anxiety [29]. Additionally, salivary cortisol concentrations reflect free serum cortisol concentrations, which is the unbound and biologically active 5% of total cortisol under basal conditions. On the other hand, measuring plasma cortisol concentration yields total cortisol. In other words, salivary cortisol can only be a surrogate for free serum cortisol concentrations [30]. Another study demonstrated that the validity of assessing manganese exposure through saliva samples needs further study. The correlation between manganese exposure in water and salivary levels is the weakest of the candidate biomarkers, including saliva, hair, and toenails [31].

5.2. Proteomics

Soluble salivary immune mediators such as C-reactive protein (CRP), interleukin-6 (IL-6), IL-1beta, IL-8, tumor necrosis factor-alpha (TNF-alpha), and secretory immunoglobin A (s-IgA), can be measured in salivary samples and serve as markers for systemic inflammation, including gingival inflammation [32]. In the case of children and youth with Obsessive-Compulsive Disorder (OCD), the elevated salivary levels of lysozyme, alpha-amylase, secretory s-IgA, CRP, IL-6, IL-1beta, and TNF-alpha are found to be associated with OCD diagnosis and symptom severity [32,33]. Melatonin secretion can also be detected and collected in saliva to evaluate one's sleep [34], with the possibility of an at-home collection [35].

5.3. Genomics

Salivary extracellular vesicles (EVs) are reliable diagnostic biomarkers for detecting mild traumatic brain injury (TBI). Genetic profiling with the real-time PCR of salivary EVs showed that more than 50 genes, and more significantly three of them (CDC2, CSNK1A1, and CTSD), are upregulated in emergency department patients and in concussion clinic patients, compared to control groups ($p < 0.05$) [36]. Salivary DNA samples can also help researchers determine epigenetic changes in maltreated school-aged low-income children. The increase or the decrease in methylation varies depending on the sex of the child and the timing of maltreatment. In general, the mean difference in methylation between maltreated children and the control group was 6.2%. Epigenetic modifications are also seen in the glucocorticoid receptor gene (nuclear receptor subfamily 3, group C, member 1 genes), dopaminergic gene (ankyrin repeat and kinase domain containing 1) and alcohol-metabolizing gene (aldehyde dehydrogenase 2), which are particularly important for the development of psychopathology in maltreated children [37].

5.4. Transcriptomics

MicroRNA (miRNA) expression in the saliva is shown to be an accurate biomarker for traumatic brain injury (TBI) in Hicks' study. The 2018 article published in the Journal of Neurotrauma compared changes in miRNA concentration after childhood TBI in CSF and in saliva. A total of 214 miRNAs were detected in CSF, where 63% of them were also present in saliva, and 10% had parallel changes in both saliva and CSF. Six miRNAs had similar changes in both CSF and saliva: miR-182-5p, miR-221-3p, mir-26b-5p, miR-320c, miR-29c-3p, and miR-30e-5p; three of them were related to neuronal development. Attention difficulty reported by the child and parent was directly correlated with the concentration of miR-320c [25].

Another study explored the relationship between miRNA expression in saliva and detecting prolonged concussion symptoms [38]. Researchers could accurately identify patients with prolonged symptoms using levels of 5 miRNAs (miR-320c-1, miR-133a-5p, miR-769-5p, let-7a-3p, and miR-1307-3p) and logistic regression (area under the curve, 0.856; 95% CI, 0.822–0.890). One month after injury, the expression of three miRNAs was associated with specific symptoms: miR-320c-1 was associated with memory difficulty; miR-629 with headaches; and let-7b-5p with fatigue. Similarly, a study compared salivary miRNA expression in two groups of children: those with persistent post-concussive symptoms (PPCS); and those without PPCS, at three different time points (within one week of injury, one to two weeks post-injury and four weeks post-injury) [39]. The study analyzed a total of 827 miRNAs, 91 of which had higher expression levels than the calculated background threshold and were included in the differential gene expression analysis. Among these 91 miRNAs, 13 had significantly different expression levels in children with PPCS at all the time points (Table 3).

Table 3. Neuropsychiatric conditions and their respective biomarkers.

	Condition	Observed Biomarker	Methodology	Ref.
1.	Stress	s-IgA	s-IgA ELISA kit (EUROIMMUN AG; Luebeck, Germany)	[27]
		Cortisol	Commercial ELISA kit (Salimetrics, USA)	[27]
		Alpha-amylase	Commercially available chemoimmunoluminiscence assay kits (Cobas integra400 plus, Roche Diagnostics, Risch-Rotkreuz, Switzerland) and analyzer (Cobas e411, Roche Diagnostics, Risch-Rotkreuz, Switzerland)	[29]
2.	Cerebral Palsy	IL-1β IL-6 IL-8 IL-10 TNF-α	CBA Cytokine Inflammatory Kit (Becton Dickinson, CA, USA)	[28]
3.	Systemic Inflammation	C-reactive proteins	Commercially available enzyme-linked immunoassay kit from Salimetrics, Suffolk, UK	[32]
		Cytokine concentrations (IL-1β, IL-6, IL-8, and TNF-α)	MILLIPLEX MAP HCYTOMAG-60K-04 kit (Millipore, Billerica, MA, USA)	[31]
		s-IgA	Colorimetric immunoenzymatic assay (ELISA) using an s-IgA saliva kit (DiaMetra, Milano, Italy)	[31]
4.	Mild TBI	CDC2, CSNK1A1 and CTSD	NanoSight NS500 instrument (Nanosight, Malvern, UK), transmission electron microscopy, Western blot analysis, Taqman	[36]
		miR-182-5p, miR-221-3p, mir-26b-5p, miR-320c, miR-29c-3p, miR-30e-5p	Oragene RE-100 saliva collection kit (DNA Genotek; Ottawa, Canada)	[25]
5.	Child Maltreatment	ALDH2, ANKK1 and NR3C1	Oragene DNA Self-Collection kits	[37]
6.	Prolonged Concussion Syndrome	miR-320c-1, miR-133a-5p, miR-769-5p, let-7a-3p, and miR-1307-3p	Plasma/Serum Circulating and Exosomal RNA Purification Kits (Norgen Biotek)	[38,40]
		hsa-miR-95-3p, hsa-miR-301a-5p, hsa-miR-626, hsa-miR-548y, hsa-miR-203a-5p, hsa-miR-548e-5p, hsa-miR-585-3p, hsa-miR-378h, hsa-miR-1323, hsa-miR-183-5p, hsa-miR-200a-3p, hsa-miR-888-5p, hsa-miR-199a-3p + hsa-miR-199b-3p	nCounter® human V3 miRNA assay kit (NanoString Technologies Inc., Seattle, WA, USA)	[39]
7.	Depression	EBV	QiaAmp blood kit (Qiagen, Valencia, CA, USA)	[40]

5.5. Microbiomics

A study measured the number of EBV copies shed in saliva and assessed depressive symptoms using the Center for Epidemiologic Studies-Depression scale in female and male adolescents aged 11–17 years. Their study showed that the presence of salivary shedding of reactivated EBV is linked to depressive symptoms in female adolescents only. In fact, the interaction between sex and depressive symptoms with EBV reactivation was statistically significant ($p < 0.01$) [40].

6. Salivary Biomarkers as Diagnostic Tools in Metabolic, Gastrointestinal, and Pulmonary Diseases

6.1. Metabolomics

A pilot cohort study revealed that hepatic steatosis, or non-alcoholic fatty liver disease (NAFLD)—an important feature linked to metabolic syndrome—can be detected by elevated salivary uric acid levels in children with obesity. Saliva was sampled using a non-invasive swab collection device and analyzed using gas chromatography-mass spectrometry. Moreover, salivary uric acid increased was associated with elevated homeostatic model assessment-insulin resistance values. Despite the small sample, its findings revealed the hopeful use of salivary markers as a screening and preventive tool for hepato-metabolic comorbidities, including hepatic steatosis, with high sensitivity, specificity, and accuracy among children with obesity [41].

6.2. Proteomics

Studies have confirmed a significant increase in CRP and insulin concentrations in the saliva of children with obesity. An observational study in Spain followed a cohort of children from ages 8 to 12 and measured the levels of circulating inflammatory cytokines to detect the signs of obesity-related inflammation and glucose intolerance, a predisposing factor responsible for the progression of diabetes and metabolic syndrome. Increased salivary CRP, leptin, and insulin levels in assays detected differences in the body-mass index, dietary characteristics, and physical activity levels in a sex-dependent manner [42]. A large cohort study constructed and evaluated a continuous approach to a scoring system for metabolic syndrome risk factors adapted to children. The diagnostic tool proposed by Shi et al. incorporates a combination of clinical parameters, such as waist circumference and systolic blood pressure. It uses salivary measures of fasting glucose and high-density lipoprotein cholesterol as surrogates of plasma measures. In addition to finding correlations between obesity and the salivary measures of insulin, CRP, and adiponectin, the progressive nature of their suggested scoring system, as opposed to the binary definition of the disease in adults, revealed a higher level of sensitivity for pediatric populations [43].

Evaluating systemic changes in saliva can also be a potential tool for diagnosing, predicting, and monitoring pulmonary diseases in pediatrics. Like obesity, salivary CRP is suggested to be a predictor of pediatric acute respiratory illness, more importantly in pediatric pneumonia. The clinical utility of salivary CRP can be seen in an acute pediatric setting and helps predict serum CRP above 100 mg/L with high specificity. This can replace the invasive use of venipuncture in young outpatients [44]. Finally, salivary biosensors can detect early childhood asthma and predict asthma exacerbations. In their analytical cross-sectional study of children aged 6 to 12, Zamora-Mendoza et al. proposed a non-invasive method based on immunoassay and surface-enhanced Raman spectroscopy. The study identified the proteomic profile of bronchial inflammation, including elevated levels of IL-8, IL-10, and sCD163 [45]. Another small cohort study conducted by Okazaki et al. revealed that salivary surfactant protein D (SP-D) in children with asthma using ELISA was much higher than in healthy controls. This reflected the degree of bronchial inflammation in response to allergen exposure causing airway resistance and correlated with the increased indices measured by the forced oscillation technique. Increased salivary SP-D levels were associated with a higher degree of asthma exacerbation [46].

In the field of liver diseases, proteomic methodologies were also applied to look for a non-invasive method of monitoring. With the salivary cytokine profile using ELISA quantification, Davidovich et al. were able to reflect a similar pattern of serum inflammatory parameters describing the immunosuppressive status in liver-transplanted children undergoing tacrolimus therapy. The potential markers of inflammation in saliva using proteomics were identified, such as the reduced levels of IL-6 and IL-10 and the elevated levels of IL-1b [47].

6.3. Microbiomics

Two studies examined oral microbiota dysbiosis using bacterial 16S rRNA gene sequence analysis in children with various liver diseases. Iwasawa et al. showed that subjects with Pediatric-Onset Primary Sclerosing Cholangitis (PSC) presented significantly decreased Haemophilus and increased Oribacterium colonies in their saliva, compared to healthy participants to patients with Ulcerative Colitis (UC). By observing significant differences between PSC and UC salivary bacterial profiles, microbiome markers in the saliva can help distinguish these two diseases and provide accurate diagnosis in a non-invasive manner [48]. Another cohort study performed microbial profiling from oral swabs in children diagnosed with non-alcoholic fatty liver disease. Systemic inflammation, cirrhosis, and advanced liver disease progression were associated with increased levels of oral *Veillonella* and *Prevotella* [49]; however, further microbial profiling is needed with larger heterogeneous sample sizes, as mentioned previously (Table 4).

Table 4. Common metabolic, gastrointestinal, and pulmonary conditions and their respective biomarkers.

	Condition	Observed Biomarker	Methodology	Ref.
1.	**Non-Alcoholic Fatty Liver Disease**	Uric acid	Gas chromatography-mass spectrometry	[41]
		Veillonella colonies *Prevotella* colonies	Bacterial 16S rRNA gene sequencing	[49]
2.	**Liver Graft versus Host Rejection**	IL-6 IL-10 IL-1b	ELISA	[47]
3.	**Primary Sclerosing Cholangitis**	*Haemophilus* colonies *Oribacterium* colonies	Bacterial 16S rRNA gene sequencing	[48]
4.	**Obesity**	Insulin CRP Leptin Adiponectin	Multiplex magnetic bead assays	[42] [43]
5.	**Pediatric Pneumonia**	CRP CP-D	ELISA ELISA	[44] [46]
6.	**Asthma**	IL-8 IL-10 sCD163	Immunoassay and surface-enhanced Raman spectroscopy	[45]

7. Salivary Biomarkers as Diagnostic Tools in Oral Diseases

In clinical practice, caries, gingivitis, and periodontitis diagnosis is mostly based on clinical, visual, and radiological findings. The following section overviews research where various proteins, microbes, and metabolites, were associated with childhood caries or periodontal disease. This research can be a basis for biochemical diagnostic tools in dental settings. Adopting such a biochemical diagnosis can improve treatment outcomes by enabling dentists to tailor therapeutic interventions to a patient's specific biochemical needs (Table 5).

Table 5. Oral diseases and their respective studied biomarkers.

	Disease	Observed Biomarker	Methodology	Ref.
1.	Dental Caries	Leptin and Ghrelin	Multiplex Magnetic Bead Panels on a Luminex 200 Platform	[50]
		NO (measured as total nitrates and nitrites)	Griess reaction method	[51]
		Carbonic Anhydrase-VI	Zymography method	[52]
		Beta-defensin-2 Histatin-5	ELISA	[53]
		IL6 IL8 TNF-alpha	ELISA	[54,55]
		Streptococcus mutans spp. *C. albicans* *Paludibacter* *Neisseria* (Among others)	16S rRNA	[56,57]
2.	Periodontal Disease	Phosphate	Multiplex Magnetic Bead Panels	[58]
		Alkaline Phosphatase (In T1DM patients only)	DEA-AMP Method	[59]

7.1. Metabolomics

In the case of dental caries, one study by Alqaderi et al. associated a later bedtime in Kuwaiti children with an increased incidence of caries [50]. To explain this association, the authors highlight that a later bedtime leads to changes in hormonal levels, notably a lower leptin level and a higher ghrelin level. This hormonal change leads to more frequent, carbohydrate-rich snacking in children, thus predisposing them to caries. This observation opens the door for cost-efficient, easy-to-implement sleep interventions in susceptible children to reduce their caries risk. Additionally, these hormonal changes can be detected relatively simply and non-invasively in saliva. Another study by Syed et al. associated a lower level of salivary nitric oxide (NO) and its metabolites with an increased risk of caries in children. This association can be explained by the antimicrobial role of NO in protection against caries [51]. Thus, screening children for salivary NO levels enables dentists to identify those at high-risk for caries, and tailor a dietary intervention with relatively easier compliance to raise their NO levels, and thus protect them from caries.

As for gingivitis and periodontal disease, Goodson et al. found an association between dietary phosphate intake and gingivitis in children. Indeed, phosphate acts as a local pro-inflammatory in the gingiva by reducing IL-4 production and raising that of IL-1b [58]. Thus, by screening children for salivary phosphate levels, we can identify those at high-risk for gingivitis and intervene by reducing their dietary intake to protect them from caries. Lastly, a study by Sridharan et al., focusing on periodontal disease in children with Type I Diabetes Mellitus (T1DM), observed that children with a higher alkaline phosphatase level had a greater gingival index and pocket pocking depth [59]. Thus, evaluating the salivary level of alkaline phosphatase in children with T1DM enables dentists to intervene early to avert the course of the disease and improve the children's outcomes.

7.2. Proteomics

This sub-section will also focus only on caries lesions. A study by de-Sousa et al. [52] found an association between the activity of carbonic anhydrase-VI (CA-VI) and caries incidence in children. Indeed, a lower activity level of salivary CA-VI predisposes children to caries and can thus be used as a prognostic factor for caries development. Another work by Jurczak et al. associated higher levels of salivary b-defensin-2 and histatin 5, two proteins with antimicrobial properties, with more advanced carious lesions [53]. Higher levels of 1β, IL-6, IL-8, IL-10, and TNF-a are seen to be increased in gingivitis and caries-prone children [54,55]. Lastly, while this does not constitute a salivary biomarker, Hertel et al. observed a higher level of Mucin 5b, Mucin 7, and IgA, in the pellicle of caries-active children compared to their caries-free counterparts [60].

While the authors of the studies above recognize a limitation in their work, namely their small sample sizes, they encourage the pursuit of larger-scale trials to confirm their observed associations. Much like we would test gene panels to identify a defective gene in an individual, to diagnose and prognose a suspected genetic disorder, one could do a "salivary biomarker screen", which would include the various metabolites, microbes, and proteins associated with oral disease. Such a screening tool would enable dentists to pinpoint a patient's biochemical risk factors for oral disease and develop individualized treatment plans for their patients.

7.3. Microbiomics

This sub-section focuses exclusively on childhood caries. One study by Kim et al. observed that caries-free Korean children had greater diversity in their oral microbiota than their caries-active counterparts [61]. Additionally, children with caries had greater proportions of bacteria that exhibit pro-caries behavior, such as *Streptococcus* and *Granulicatella*, which invade epithelial cells, as well as *Staphylococcus* and *Veillonella*, which are involved in D-alanine metabolism. In contrast, caries-free children had greater proportions of bacteria that antagonize caries formation, notably *Neisseria* and *Lautropia*, which are involved in linoleic acid metabolism, and *Capnocytophaga*, which is involved in flavonoid biosynthesis. Another study by Hemadi et al. observed higher salivary levels of *Streptococcus mutans spp., C. albicans,* and *Prevotella* spp. in children with caries, compared to their caries-free counterparts [56]. Lastly, Manzoor et al. observed higher levels of sugar fermenters, such as *Paludibacter* and *Labrenzia*, in children with caries [57].

8. Current Status and Advances in Saliva-Based Biosensors

The importance of saliva as a diagnostic tool came into light during the advent of the COVID-19 pandemic. Its non-invasiveness and the ease of collection ensured the safety of healthcare workers; nonetheless, nasopharyngeal swabs remained the gold standard. It evidenced how saliva can become an essential part of diagnostic procedures. Antibody antigen-based reactions can be efficiently utilized and detected by colorimetric or spectrophotometric changes. A prototype for a saliva-based MMP8 detector using specific antibodies and surface acoustic wave (SAW) technology was developed for periodontal disease and was seen to have comparable sensitivity and specificity to the standard ELISA-based methods [62] (Figure 2).

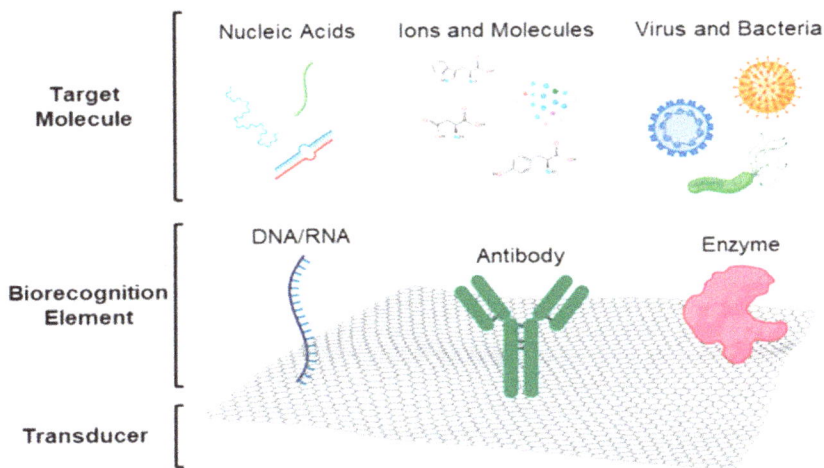

Figure 2. A typical saliva-based biosensor. Briefly, it consists principally of three components, a surface (carbon-based or metal) to accommodate the biorecognition element (probes, antibodies, or enzymes), which captures the target (genomic material, antibodies, proteins, etc.). The molecular interactions induce colorimetric or spectrometric changes, which can be observed with their corresponding detection technologies. Image used with permission from Goldoni et al., 2021 [63].

Stefan-van Staden et al. proposed a new method of assay of estradiol (E2), testosterone (T2), and dihydrotestosterone (DHT) based on stochastic microsensors that allow the earlier detection and prevention of hormonal, metabolic, and developmental problems in children. This could replace the classical measurement of electrochemical markers using ELISA or liquid chromatography-tandem mass spectrometry. The biosensor is designed using diamond paste as the matrix and three different electroactive materials: maltodextrin, a-cyclodextrin, and 5,10,15,20-tetraphenyl-21H,23H porphyrin [64]. The response to stochastic microsensors is based on channel conductivity, which is the degree of alteration of a current traversing a channel under a controlled potential of 125 mV when a steroidal hormone binds onto the channel wall. By manipulating the channel conductivity of analytes, stochastic sensors are described as having high reliability and selectivity, which could overcome the limitations of the standard method, such as its insufficient sensitivity for children's saliva. The results demonstrated that, compared to the standard method using ELISA, the stochastic biosensor could perform reliable pattern recognition, identification, and the quantification of the three hormones at very low concentrations in saliva samples [64].

Lukose et al. also highlighted optical technologies using photonics to rapidly screen abnormal health conditions and viral infections rapidly and universally through saliva. The article explored optical spectroscopy techniques that more precisely involve the UV-visible-infrared region, including surface plasmon resonance, Raman, IR spectroscopy, and laser-induced fluorescence [65]. For instance, a previous section of our paper discussed the potential use of surface-enhanced Raman spectroscopy to detect the proteomic characteristics of asthma in children. Non-invasive, photonic-based biosensors constitute a hopeful field of new diagnostic tools due to their capacity to provide the remote, contactless evaluation and identification of conditions, including communicable diseases such as COVID-19. In addition to detecting viral, bacterial, and parasitical infections, photonics can be applied in a wide range of health conditions, such as various cancers, oral diseases, metabolic and systemic diseases, as well as the detection of drug-related biomarkers in saliva [65]. Finally, Lukose and al. suggested the possibility of a multi-modal approach in which a combination of photonics tools, accompanied by artificial intelligence, could further optimize the specificity and sensitivity of these promising biosensors.

9. Conclusions

We have reviewed several methodologies that performed with good sensitivity and specificity, as well as additional advantages covering some of the important limitations of standard diagnostic tests performed today in the pediatric population. Acknowledging its non-invasiveness and ubiquitous applications, saliva as a probing biofluid sample remains highly attractive. It requires further investigations with larger samples and better analytical and comparative evidence. The pursuit of further studies on these biomarkers can be highly impactful. Indeed, salivary diagnostic/prognostic tools are less invasive and less harmful than current tools and enable physicians to intervene early, altering the course of the disease and significantly reducing suffering and disability in patients.

While sensitivity and specificity to the target molecules are satisfactory in the studies explored, the specificity to a particular condition remains a challenge. For example, pro-inflammatory markers can be commonly identified in autoimmune disorders, stress, poor oral health, and pulmonary conditions. Identifying a marker highly specific to each condition is imperative. Nonetheless, diagnosing infectious diseases like COVID-19, and periodontal diseases, using microbiome-specific screens, specific proteins in ASD, and miRNAs in various systemic conditions, are promising as salivary biosensor applications.

Author Contributions: Conceptualization, A.U., S.Z., H.M., L.S., M.A., B.H.N. and S.D.T.; writing—original draft preparation, S.Z., H.M., L.S., M.A. and A.U.; writing—review and editing, A.U., H.M., S.Z., B.H.N. and S.D.T.; supervision, S.D.T.; project administration, A.U., S.D.T. and B.H.N. All authors have read and agreed to the published version of the manuscript.

Funding: This research received no external funding.

Institutional Review Board Statement: Not applicable.

Informed Consent Statement: Not applicable.

Data Availability Statement: Not applicable.

Conflicts of Interest: The authors declare no conflict of interest.

References

1. Aral, C.A.; Nalbantoglu, O.; Nur, B.G.; Altunsoy, M.; Aral, K. Metabolic control and periodontal treatment decreases elevated oxidative stress in the early phases of type 1 diabetes onset. *Arch. Oral Biol.* **2017**, *82*, 115–120. [CrossRef] [PubMed]
2. Collin, M.; Ernberg, M.; Christidis, N.; Hedenberg-Magnusson, B. Salivary biomarkers in children with juvenile idiopathic arthritis and healthy age-matched controls: A prospective observational study. *Sci. Rep.* **2022**, *12*, 3240. [CrossRef] [PubMed]
3. Ganelin-Cohen, E.; Tartakovsky, E.; Klepfish, E.; Golderman, S.; Rozenberg, A.; Kaplan, B. Personalized Disease Monitoring in Pediatric Onset Multiple Sclerosis Using the Saliva Free Light Chain Test. *Front. Immunol.* **2022**, *13*, 821499. [CrossRef] [PubMed]
4. Gomez Hernandez, M.P.; Starman, E.E.; Davis, A.B.; Withanage, M.H.H.; Zeng, E.; Lieberman, S.M.; Brogden, K.A.; Lanzel, E.A. A distinguishing profile of chemokines, cytokines and biomarkers in the saliva of children with Sjogren's syndrome. *Rheumatology* **2021**, *60*, 4765–4777. [CrossRef]
5. Al-Khatieeb, M.M.; Rafeeq, R.A.; Saleem, A.I. Relationship between Orthodontic Force Applied by Monoblock and Salivary Levels of Alkaline Phosphatase and Lactate Dehydrogenase Enzymes. *J. Contemp. Dent. Pract.* **2018**, *19*, 1346–1351. [CrossRef]
6. Alhazmi, N.; Trotman, C.A.; Finkelman, M.; Hawley, D.; Zoukhri, D.; Papathanasiou, E. Salivary alkaline phosphatase activity and chronological age as indicators for skeletal maturity. *Angle Orthod.* **2019**, *89*, 637–642. [CrossRef]
7. Hegde, S.S.; Revankar, A.V.; Patil, A.K. Identification of bone-specific alkaline phosphatase in saliva and its correlation with skeletal age. *Indian J. Dent. Res. Off. Publ. Indian Soc. Dent. Res.* **2018**, *29*, 721–725. [CrossRef]
8. Deshpande, R.R.; Dungarwal, P.P.; Bagde, K.K.; Thakur, P.S.; Gajjar, P.M.; Kamath, A.P. Comparative evaluation of salivary zinc concentration in autistic and healthy children in mixed dentition age group-pilot study. *Indian J. Dent. Res. Off. Publ. Indian Soc. Dent. Res.* **2019**, *30*, 43–46. [CrossRef]
9. Symons, F.J.; ElGhazi, I.; Reilly, B.G.; Barney, C.C.; Hanson, L.; Panoskaltsis-Mortari, A.; Armitage, I.M.; Wilcox, G.L. Can biomarkers differentiate pain and no pain subgroups of nonverbal children with cerebral palsy? A preliminary investigation based on noninvasive saliva sampling. *Pain Med.* **2015**, *16*, 249–256. [CrossRef]

10. Almalki, A. Association of Salivary IGF and IGF/IGFBP-3 Molar Ratio with Cervical Vertebral Maturation Stages from Pre-Adolescent to Post-Adolescent Transition Period-A Cross-Sectional Exploratory Study. *Int. J. Environ. Res. Public Health* **2022**, *19*, 5172. [CrossRef]
11. Almalki, A.; Thomas, J.T.; Khan, A.R.A.; Almulhim, B.; Alassaf, A.; Alghamdi, S.A.; Joseph, B.; Alqerban, A.; Alotaibi, S. Correlation between Salivary Levels of IGF-1, IGFBP-3, IGF-1/IGFBP3 Ratio with Skeletal Maturity Using Hand-Wrist Radiographs. *Int. J. Environ. Res. Public Health* **2022**, *19*, 3723. [CrossRef]
12. Hori, H.; Izawa, S.; Yoshida, F.; Kunugi, H.; Kim, Y.; Mizukami, S.; Inoue, Y.; Tagaya, H.; Hakamata, Y. Association of childhood maltreatment history with salivary interleukin-6 diurnal patterns and C-reactive protein in healthy adults. *Brain Behav. Immun.* **2022**, *101*, 377–382. [CrossRef]
13. Marques-Feixa, L.; Castro-Quintas, A.; Palma-Gudiel, H.; Romero, S.; Morer, A.; Rapado-Castro, M.; Martin, M.; Zorrilla, I.; Blasco-Fontecilla, H.; Ramirez, M.; et al. Secretory immunoglobulin A (s-IgA) reactivity to acute psychosocial stress in children and adolescents: The influence of pubertal development and history of maltreatment. *Brain Behav. Immun.* **2022**, *103*, 122–129. [CrossRef]
14. Schmeer, K.K.; Ford, J.L.; Browning, C.R. Early childhood family instability and immune system dysregulation in adolescence. *Psychoneuroendocrinology* **2019**, *102*, 189–195. [CrossRef]
15. Ngounou Wetie, A.G.; Wormwood, K.L.; Russell, S.; Ryan, J.P.; Darie, C.C.; Woods, A.G. A Pilot Proteomic Analysis of Salivary Biomarkers in Autism Spectrum Disorder. *Autism Res.* **2015**, *8*, 338–350. [CrossRef]
16. Ngounou Wetie, A.G.; Wormwood, K.L.; Charette, L.; Ryan, J.P.; Woods, A.G.; Darie, C.C. Comparative two-dimensional polyacrylamide gel electrophoresis of the salivary proteome of children with autism spectrum disorder. *J. Cell. Mol. Med.* **2015**, *19*, 2664–2678. [CrossRef]
17. Mota, F.S.B.; Nascimento, K.S.; Oliveira, M.V.; Osterne, V.J.S.; Clemente, J.C.M.; Correia-Neto, C.; Lima-Neto, A.B.; van Tilburg, M.F.; Leal-Cardoso, J.H.; Guedes, M.I.F.; et al. Potential protein markers in children with Autistic Spectrum Disorder (ASD) revealed by salivary proteomics. *Int. J. Biol. Macromol.* **2022**, *199*, 243–251. [CrossRef]
18. Lavor, J.R.; Lacerda, R.H.W.; Modesto, A.; Vieira, A.R. Maxillary incisor enamel defects in individuals born with cleft lip/palate. *PLoS ONE* **2020**, *15*, e0244506. [CrossRef]
19. Talaat, D.M.; Hachim, I.Y.; Afifi, M.M.; Talaat, I.M.; ElKateb, M.A. Assessment of risk factors and molecular biomarkers in children with supernumerary teeth: A single-center study. *BMC Oral Health* **2022**, *22*, 117. [CrossRef]
20. Nelson, C.A.; Varcin, K.J.; Coman, N.K.; De Vivo, I.; Tager-Flusberg, H. Shortened Telomeres in Families with a Propensity to Autism. *J. Am. Acad. Child Adolesc. Psychiatry* **2015**, *54*, 588–594. [CrossRef]
21. Sharma, R.; Frasch, M.G.; Zelgert, C.; Zimmermann, P.; Fabre, B.; Wilson, R.; Waldenberger, M.; MacDonald, J.W.; Bammler, T.K.; Lobmaier, S.M.; et al. Maternal-fetal stress and DNA methylation signatures in neonatal saliva: An epigenome-wide association study. *Clin. Epigenet.* **2022**, *14*, 87. [CrossRef] [PubMed]
22. Wang, L.-J.; Chan, W.-C.; Chou, M.-C.; Chou, W.-J.; Lee, M.-J.; Lee, S.-Y.; Lin, P.-Y.; Yang, Y.-H.; Yen, C.-F. Polymorphisms of STS gene and SULT2A1 gene and neurosteroid levels in Han Chinese boys with attention-deficit/hyperactivity disorder: An exploratory investigation. *Sci. Rep.* **2017**, *7*, 45595. [CrossRef] [PubMed]
23. Kong, X.; Liu, J.; Cetinbas, M.; Sadreyev, R.; Koh, M.; Huang, H.; Adeseye, A.; He, P.; Zhu, J.; Russell, H.; et al. New and Preliminary Evidence on Altered Oral and Gut Microbiota in Individuals with Autism Spectrum Disorder (ASD): Implications for ASD Diagnosis and Subtyping Based on Microbial Biomarkers. *Nutrients* **2019**, *11*, 2128. [CrossRef] [PubMed]
24. Sehovic, E.; Spahic, L.; Smajlovic-Skenderagic, L.; Pistoljevic, N.; Dzanko, E.; Hajdarpasic, A. Identification of developmental disorders including autism spectrum disorder using salivary miRNAs in children from Bosnia and Herzegovina. *PLoS ONE* **2020**, *15*, e0232351. [CrossRef]
25. Hicks, S.D.; Johnson, J.; Carney, M.C.; Bramley, H.; Olympia, R.P.; Loeffert, A.C.; Thomas, N.J. Overlapping MicroRNA Expression in Saliva and Cerebrospinal Fluid Accurately Identifies Pediatric Traumatic Brain Injury. *J. Neurotrauma* **2018**, *35*, 64–72. [CrossRef]
26. Angeli, E.; Korpa, T.; Johnson, E.O.; Apostolakou, F.; Papassotiriou, I.; Chrousos, G.P.; Pervanidou, P. Salivary cortisol and alpha-amylase diurnal profiles and stress reactivity in children with Attention Deficit Hyperactivity Disorder. *Psychoneuroendocrinology* **2018**, *90*, 174–181. [CrossRef]
27. Yirmiya, K.; Djalovski, A.; Motsan, S.; Zagoory-Sharon, O.; Feldman, R. Stress and immune biomarkers interact with parenting behavior to shape anxiety symptoms in trauma-exposed youth. *Psychoneuroendocrinology* **2018**, *98*, 153–160. [CrossRef]
28. Ferreira, A.C.F.M.; Eveloff, R.J.; Freire, M.; Santos, M.T.B.R. The Impact of Oral-Gut Inflammation in Cerebral Palsy. *Front. Immunol.* **2021**, *12*, 619262. [CrossRef]
29. AlMaummar, M.; AlThabit, H.O.; Pani, S. The impact of dental treatment and age on salivary cortisol and alpha-amylase levels of patients with varying degrees of dental anxiety. *BMC Oral Health* **2019**, *19*, 211. [CrossRef]
30. Llorens, M.; Barba, M.; Torralbas, J.; Nadal, R.; Armario, A.; Gagliano, H.; Betriu, M.; Urraca, L.; Pujol, S.; Montalvo, I.; et al. Stress-related biomarkers and cognitive functioning in adolescents with ADHD: Effect of childhood maltreatment. *J. Psychiatr. Res.* **2022**, *149*, 217–225. [CrossRef]
31. Ntihabose, R.; Surette, C.; Foucher, D.; Clarisse, O.; Bouchard, M.F. Assessment of saliva, hair and toenails as biomarkers of low level exposure to manganese from drinking water in children. *Neurotoxicology* **2018**, *64*, 126–133. [CrossRef]

32. Cullen, A.E.; Tappin, B.M.; Zunszain, P.A.; Dickson, H.; Roberts, R.E.; Nikkheslat, N.; Khondoker, M.; Pariante, C.M.; Fisher, H.L.; Laurens, K.R. The relationship between salivary C-reactive protein and cognitive function in children aged 11–14years: Does psychopathology have a moderating effect? *Brain Behav. Immun.* **2017**, *66*, 221–229. [CrossRef]
33. Santos, M.T.B.R.; Diniz, M.B.; Guare, R.O.; Ferreira, M.C.D.; Gutierrez, G.M.; Gorjao, R. Inflammatory markers in saliva as indicators of gingival inflammation in cerebral palsy children with and without cervical motor control. *Int. J. Paediatr. Dent.* **2017**, *27*, 364–371. [CrossRef]
34. Ghaziuddin, N.; Shamseddeen, W.; Bertram, H.; McInnis, M.; Wilcox, H.C.; Mitchell, P.B.; Fullerton, J.M.; Roberts, G.M.P.; Glowinski, A.L.; Kamali, M.; et al. Salivary melatonin onset in youth at familial risk for bipolar disorder. *Psychiatry Res.* **2019**, *274*, 49–57. [CrossRef]
35. Mandrell, B.N.; Avent, Y.; Walker, B.; Loew, M.; Tynes, B.L.; Crabtree, V.M. In-home salivary melatonin collection: Methodology for children and adolescents. *Dev. Psychobiol.* **2018**, *60*, 118–122. [CrossRef]
36. Cheng, Y.; Pereira, M.; Raukar, N.; Reagan, J.L.; Queseneberry, M.; Goldberg, L.; Borgovan, T.; LaFrance, W.C., Jr.; Dooner, M.; Deregibus, M.; et al. Potential biomarkers to detect traumatic brain injury by the profiling of salivary extracellular vesicles. *J. Cell. Physiol.* **2019**, *234*, 14377–14388. [CrossRef]
37. Cicchetti, D.; Hetzel, S.; Rogosch, F.A.; Handley, E.D.; Toth, S.L. An investigation of child maltreatment and epigenetic mechanisms of mental and physical health risk. *Dev. Psychopathol.* **2016**, *28*, 1305–1317. [CrossRef]
38. Johnson, J.J.; Loeffert, A.C.; Stokes, J.; Olympia, R.P.; Bramley, H.; Hicks, S.D. Association of Salivary MicroRNA Changes with Prolonged Concussion Symptoms. *JAMA Pediatr.* **2018**, *172*, 65–73. [CrossRef]
39. Miller, K.E.; MacDonald, J.P.; Sullivan, L.; Venkata, L.P.R.; Shi, J.; Yeates, K.O.; Chen, S.; Alshaikh, E.; Taylor, H.G.; Hautmann, A.; et al. Salivary miRNA Expression in Children with Persistent Post-concussive Symptoms. *Front. Public Health* **2022**, *10*, 890420. [CrossRef]
40. Ford, J.L.; Stowe, R.P. Depressive symptoms are associated with salivary shedding of Epstein-Barr virus in female adolescents: The role of sex differences. *Psychoneuroendocrinology* **2017**, *86*, 128–133. [CrossRef]
41. Troisi, J.; Belmonte, F.; Bisogno, A.; Lausi, O.; Marciano, F.; Cavallo, P.; Guercio Nuzio, S.; Landolfi, A.; Pierri, L.; Vajro, P. Salivary markers of hepato-metabolic comorbidities in pediatric obesity. *Dig. Liver Dis.* **2019**, *51*, 516–523. [CrossRef] [PubMed]
42. Alqaderi, H.; Hegazi, F.; Al-Mulla, F.; Chiu, C.-J.; Kantarci, A.; Al-Ozairi, E.; Abu-Farha, M.; Bin-Hasan, S.; Alsumait, A.; Abubaker, J.; et al. Salivary Biomarkers as Predictors of Obesity and Intermediate Hyperglycemia in Adolescents. *Front. Public Health* **2022**, *10*, 800373. [CrossRef] [PubMed]
43. Shi, P.; Goodson, J.M.; Hartman, M.-L.; Hasturk, H.; Yaskell, T.; Vargas, J.; Cugini, M.; Barake, R.; Alsmadi, O.; Al-Mutawa, S.; et al. Continuous Metabolic Syndrome Scores for Children Using Salivary Biomarkers. *PLoS ONE* **2015**, *10*, e0138979. [CrossRef] [PubMed]
44. Gofin, Y.; Fanous, E.; Pasternak, Y.; Prokocimer, Z.; Zagoory-Sharon, O.; Feldman, R.; Codick, G.; Waisbourd-Zinman, O.; Fried, S.; Livni, G.; Schachter-Davidov, A. Salivary C-reactive protein-a possible predictor of serum levels in pediatric acute respiratory illness. *Eur. J. Pediatr.* **2021**, *180*, 2465–2472. [CrossRef]
45. Zamora-Mendoza, B.N.; Espinosa-Tanguma, R.; Ramirez-Elias, M.G.; Cabrera-Alonso, R.; Montero-Moran, G.; Portales-Perez, D.; Rosales-Romo, J.A.; Gonzalez, J.F.; Gonzalez, C. Surface-enhanced raman spectroscopy: A non invasive alternative procedure for early detection in childhood asthma biomarkers in saliva. *Photodiagn. Photodyn. Ther.* **2019**, *27*, 85–91. [CrossRef]
46. Okazaki, S.; Murai, H.; Kidoguchi, S.; Nomura, E.; Itoh, N.; Hashimoto, N.; Hamada, T.; Kawakita, A.; Yasutomi, M.; Ohshima, Y. The Biomarker Salivary SP-D May Indicate Small Airway Inflammation and Asthma Exacerbation. *J. Investig. Allergol. Clin. Immunol.* **2017**, *27*, 305–312. [CrossRef]
47. Davidovich, E.; Mozer, Y.; Polak, D. Salivary inflammatory cytokines echo the low inflammatory burden in liver-transplanted children. *Clin. Oral Investig.* **2021**, *25*, 2993–2998. [CrossRef]
48. Iwasawa, K.; Suda, W.; Tsunoda, T.; Oikawa-Kawamoto, M.; Umetsu, S.; Takayasu, L.; Inui, A.; Fujisawa, T.; Morita, H.; Sogo, T.; et al. Dysbiosis of the salivary microbiota in pediatric-onset primary sclerosing cholangitis and its potential as a biomarker. *Sci. Rep.* **2018**, *8*, 5480. [CrossRef]
49. Kordy, K.; Li, F.; Lee, D.J.; Kinchen, J.M.; Jew, M.H.; La Rocque, M.E.; Zabih, S.; Saavedra, M.; Woodward, C.; Cunningham, N.J.; et al. Metabolomic Predictors of Non-alcoholic Steatohepatitis and Advanced Fibrosis in Children. *Front. Microbiol.* **2021**, *12*, 713234. [CrossRef]
50. Alqaderi, H.; Tavares, M.; Al-Mulla, F.; Al-Ozairi, E.; Goodson, J.M. Late bedtime and dental caries incidence in Kuwaiti children: A longitudinal multilevel analysis. *Community Dent. Oral Epidemiol.* **2020**, *48*, 181–187. [CrossRef]
51. Syed, M.; Sachdev, V.; Chopra, R. Intercomparison of salivary nitric oxide as a biomarker of dental caries risk between caries-active and caries-free children. *Eur. Arch. Paediatr. Dent.* **2016**, *17*, 239–243. [CrossRef]
52. De-Sousa, E.T.; Lima-Holanda, A.T.; Nobre-Dos-Santos, M. Carbonic anhydrase VI activity in saliva and biofilm can predict early childhood caries: A preliminary study. *Int. J. Paediatr. Dent.* **2021**, *31*, 361–371. [CrossRef]
53. Jurczak, A.; Koscielniak, D.; Papiez, M.; Vyhouskaya, P.; Krzysciak, W. A study on beta-defensin-2 and histatin-5 as a diagnostic marker of early childhood caries progression. *Biol. Res.* **2015**, *48*, 61. [CrossRef]
54. Rinderknecht, C.; Filippi, C.; Ritz, N.; Fritschi, N.; Simmen, U.; Filippi, A.; Diesch-Furlanetto, T. Associations between salivary cytokines and oral health, age, and sex in healthy children. *Sci. Rep.* **2022**, *12*, 15991. [CrossRef]

55. Sharma, V.; Gupta, N.; Srivastava, N.; Rana, V.; Chandna, P.; Yadav, S.; Sharma, A. Diagnostic potential of inflammatory biomarkers in early childhood caries—A case control study. *Clin. Chim. Acta Int. J. Clin. Chem.* **2017**, *471*, 158–163. [CrossRef]
56. Hemadi, A.S.; Huang, R.; Zhou, Y.; Zou, J. Salivary proteins and microbiota as biomarkers for early childhood caries risk assessment. *Int. J. Oral Sci.* **2017**, *9*, e1. [CrossRef]
57. Manzoor, M.; Lommi, S.; Furuholm, J.; Sarkkola, C.; Engberg, E.; Raju, S.; Viljakainen, H. High abundance of sugar metabolisers in saliva of children with caries. *Sci. Rep.* **2021**, *11*, 4424. [CrossRef]
58. Goodson, J.M.; Shi, P.; Razzaque, M.S. Dietary phosphorus enhances inflammatory response: A study of human gingivitis. *J. Steroid Biochem. Mol. Biol.* **2019**, *188*, 166–171. [CrossRef]
59. Sridharan, S.; Sravani, P.; Satyanarayan, A.; Kiran, K.; Shetty, V. Salivary Alkaline Phosphatase as a Noninvasive Marker for Periodontal Disease in Children with Uncontrolled Type 1 Diabetes Mellitus. *J. Clin. Pediatr. Dent.* **2017**, *41*, 70–74. [CrossRef]
60. Hertel, S.; Hannig, M.; Hannig, C.; Sterzenbach, T. Mucins 5b and 7 and secretory IgA in the oral acquired pellicle of children with caries and caries-free children. *Arch. Oral Biol.* **2022**, *134*, 105314. [CrossRef]
61. Kim, B.-S.; Han, D.-H.; Lee, H.; Oh, B. Association of Salivary Microbiota with Dental Caries Incidence with Dentine Involvement after 4 Years. *J. Microbiol. Biotechnol.* **2018**, *28*, 454–464. [CrossRef] [PubMed]
62. Taylor, J.J.; Jaedicke, K.M.; van de Merwe, R.C.; Bissett, S.M.; Landsdowne, N.; Whall, K.M.; Pickering, K.; Thornton, V.; Lawson, V.; Yatsuda, H.; et al. A Prototype Antibody-based Biosensor for Measurement of Salivary MMP-8 in Periodontitis using Surface Acoustic Wave Technology. *Sci. Rep.* **2019**, *9*, 11034. [CrossRef] [PubMed]
63. Goldoni, R.; Farronato, M.; Connelly, S.T.; Tartaglia, G.M.; Yeo, W.-H. Recent advances in graphene-based nanobiosensors for salivary biomarker detection. *Biosens. Bioelectron.* **2021**, *171*, 112723. [CrossRef] [PubMed]
64. Van Staden, R.I.S.; Gugoasa, L.A.; Calenic, B.; Legler, J. Pattern recognition of estradiol, testosterone and dihydrotestosterone in children's saliva samples using stochastic microsensors. *Sci. Rep.* **2014**, *4*, 5. [CrossRef]
65. Lukose, J.; Barik, A.K.; Pai, K.M.; Unnikrishnan, V.K.; George, S.D.; Kartha, V.B.; Chidangil, S. Photonics of human saliva: Potential optical methods for the screening of abnormal health conditions and infections. *Biophys. Rev.* **2021**, *13*, 359–385. [CrossRef]

Disclaimer/Publisher's Note: The statements, opinions and data contained in all publications are solely those of the individual author(s) and contributor(s) and not of MDPI and/or the editor(s). MDPI and/or the editor(s) disclaim responsibility for any injury to people or property resulting from any ideas, methods, instructions or products referred to in the content.

MDPI
St. Alban-Anlage 66
4052 Basel
Switzerland
Tel. +41 61 683 77 34
Fax +41 61 302 89 18
www.mdpi.com

Biosensors Editorial Office
E-mail: biosensors@mdpi.com
www.mdpi.com/journal/biosensors

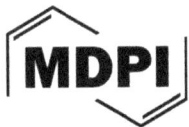

www.ingramcontent.com/pod-product-compliance
Lightning Source LLC
LaVergne TN
LVHW070730100526
838202LV00013B/1206